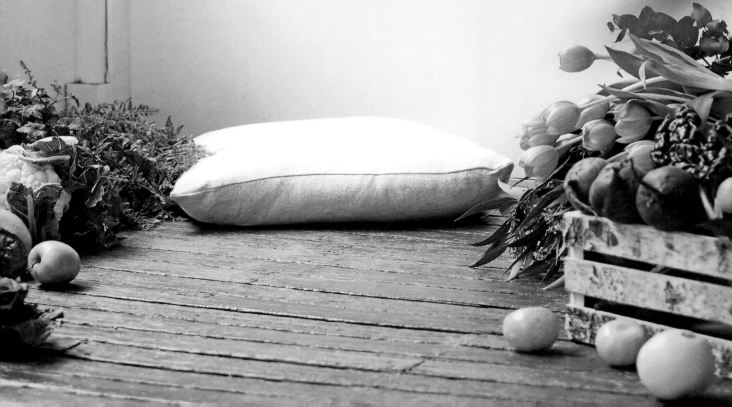
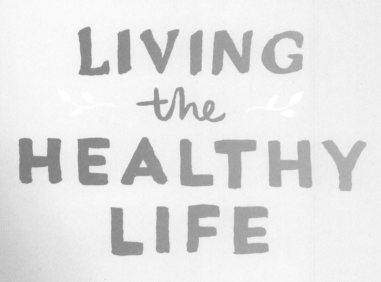

# LIVING
*the*
# HEALTHY
# LIFE

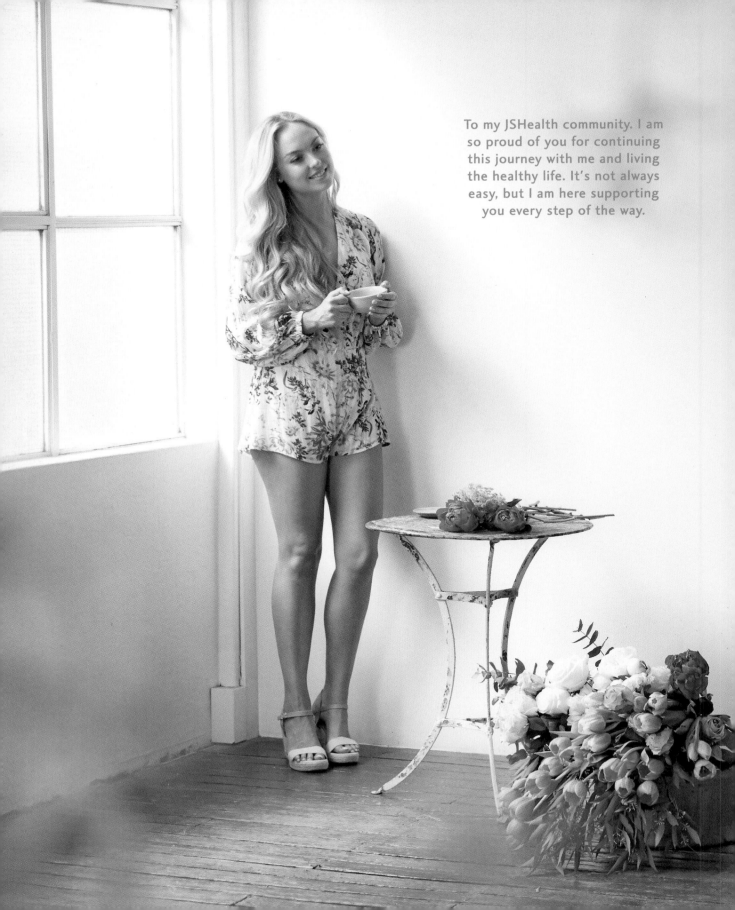

To my JSHealth community. I am so proud of you for continuing this journey with me and living the healthy life. It's not always easy, but I am here supporting you every step of the way.

# LIVING
*the*
# HEALTHY
# LIFE

## JESSICA SEPEL

bluebird
books for life

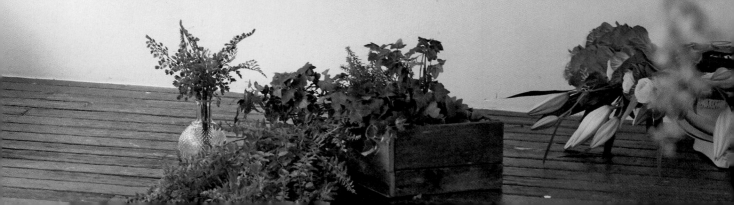

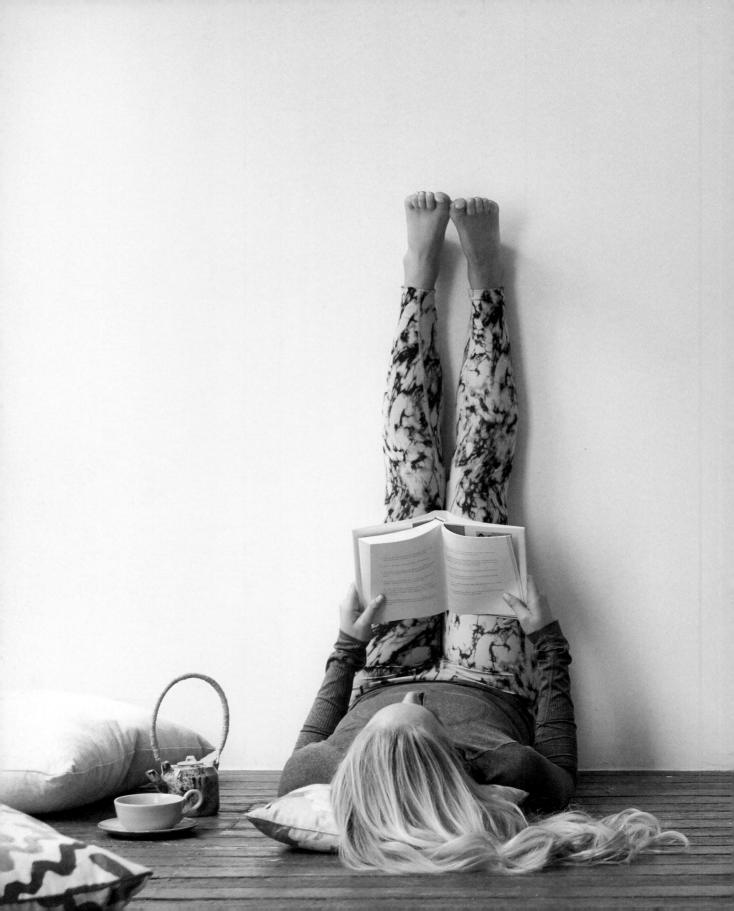

# CONTENTS

Introduction                                    6

**LIVING A HEALTHY LIFE**                       9
HEAL YOUR . . .
   Relationship with Food      10
   Relationship with Yourself  24
   Stress                      30
   Thyroid                     36
   Energy                      46
   Cleansing Functions         52
   Sleep                       60
   Weight Battles              64
   Lifestyle                   76
   Anxiety                     84
   Relationship with Others    90
   Nutrition                   96

**THE 8-WEEK ACTION PLAN**                    121

**HEALING RECIPES**                           132

Index                                         310

# HI THERE!

I'm Jessica Sepel – a nutritionist, health blogger and author.

While I've been officially studying health for over five years, it's always been my world. I grew up in South Africa, with an incredibly healthy family as my role models. My mum and dad were active, dedicated to wellbeing, and only served wholesome, nourishing food at home.

My grandmother was another huge healthy influence. I have vivid memories of her starting each day with lemon water and papaya (before that was a trend), taking supplements, walking and meditating. She took me to a health retreat at a young age, and I remember listening to the nutritionist's presentation and thinking, 'This is what I want to do'.

While processed foods weren't part of my upbringing, neither was deprivation. My family was all about balance. We were allowed treats in moderation. We were taught that food should be enjoyed. Living a healthy lifestyle was just the way it was, and I will be forever grateful for that. But somewhere along the way, that healthy life, and healthy relationship with food, was broken.

When I was 14, my family moved to Australia. I was going through puberty and insecure about my changing body. Then I **discovered dieting**. Food started ruling my life in an unhealthy way. I had low self-esteem and a negative body image, and this triggered me to severely restrict my food intake. I lost a lot of weight in a short period of time, and I was on the verge of an eating disorder. I thought being thin meant I would be more loveable. How wrong I was. It didn't make me feel any happier or any more loved – but that didn't stop me.

This was the beginning of years and years of dieting, weight obsession and food control. It was stressful and exhausting. I felt sad and alone and like I was never good enough. I lost sight of the blessings in my life, and I totally forgot about what my family had taught me about living with balance.

So, what changed? After school, I decided to study health and nutrition to better understand how the body works. I realised I had the knowledge (and power!) to heal my mind, heal my body, and, ultimately, change my life. I began experimenting in the kitchen and, slowly but surely, I started healing my broken relationship with food.

It wasn't long before I needed an outlet for my learning. I needed to share my experiences and journey with others, and that's when I launched my blog. I wrote honestly and candidly about fighting diets and finding balance, and people responded in a BIG way.

Fast forward to now, and the JSHealth community is one I feel so close to and so incredibly proud of. They motivate and inspire me to be the best version of myself.

We all struggle sometimes, myself included. I believe in journeys, not just outcomes. And I wear my heart on my sleeve. I'm not afraid to be vulnerable and speak my truth, and I encourage others to do the same. There's no reason why we should be ashamed. We're all figuring things out as we go – and finding answers is one of the most beautiful parts of life!

In 2015 I released my first book, *The Healthy Life*. In that book, I highlighted the steps I took to overhaul my life and bring it back into balance. Since the book has come out, I've noticed a few things. People are really starting to embrace the healthy life. They're excited about health, and that makes me smile. They're realising that healthy food can be delicious. But they're also feeling overwhelmed – the health world is absolutely buzzing right now, and it can be information overload. People are confused, and I get it!

While *The Healthy Life* is a handy bible for health and nutrition, now we're going deeper. This book is about resetting your body and finding the solutions to the health challenges you are still facing. Firstly, this book will give you the background information for living a healthy life and help you to understand your body in a new way. Then we connect the dots and lay out an 8-week action plan for you to be your best self ever. To support you on your journey, I've included over 160 of my most delicious, simple recipes.

I'll also be revealing the health issue I've been battling recently. It's been an incredibly difficult time for me, but now that I'm out of the woods, I feel I can speak about it openly – and hopefully you will learn something from my experience.

We'll be delving into the issues that are affecting so many women today: sky-high stress levels; food addiction, bingeing and emotional eating; and uncontrollable sugar cravings. This book also shines the spotlight on dieting, and how it affects everything from your hormones and thyroid function to your self-esteem. Because enough is enough. Guilt is out, balance is in. We're going to take things one week at a time, one step at a time, with a unique plan that's just right for you.

So, let's find out what's 'broken' – whether it's your relationship with food, energy, sleep, or a mind that doesn't switch off. Then, let's fix it with my 8-week action plan that you can start today!

I learned to heal my body and my life. And you can do the same.

Welcome to *Living the Healthy Life*.

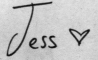

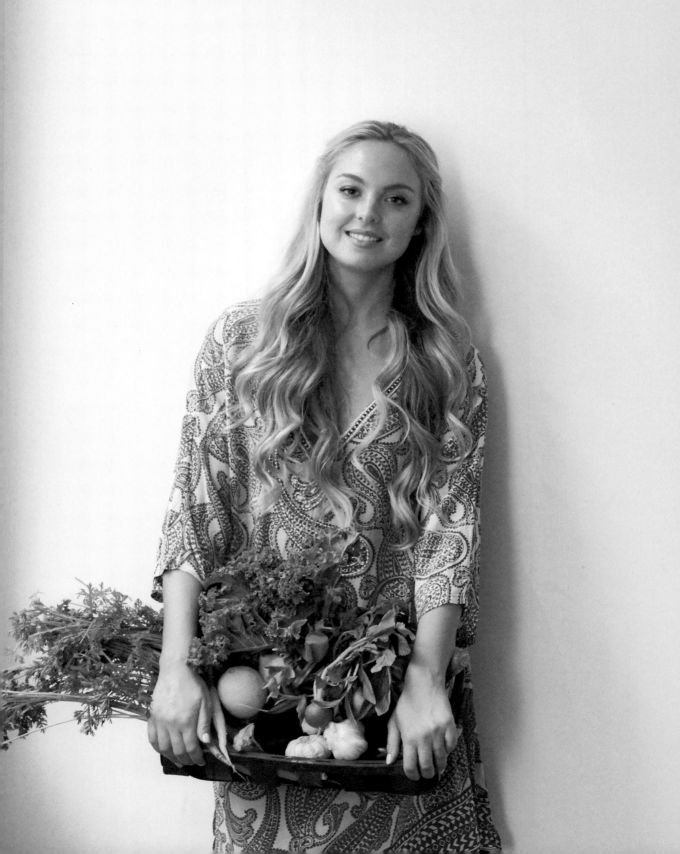

# LIVING
# A HEALTHY
# LIFE

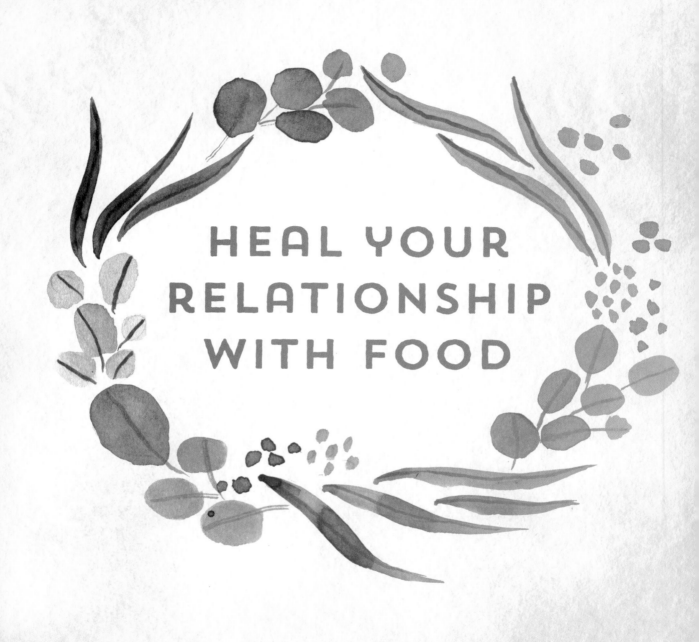

HEAL YOUR
RELATIONSHIP
WITH FOOD

*Recently, I've realised that the connection between food and weight is the filter through which many of my readers and clients view their health. This is a mindset that needs to change. Let's focus on healing your relationship with food, as it is the very foundation of good health and an important step in your healing journey.*

## MY STRUGGLE WITH FOOD

My passion in life is helping women to heal their relationship with food. Because it wasn't so long ago that my own relationship with food was broken and complicated.

There's a moment I remember so vividly. I was just 18 years old and standing in the kitchen one afternoon following my weekly visit to the dietician. She had told me I'd put on 400 grams. Not kilos or pounds, but *grams*.

She wasn't impressed and the interrogation that had followed made me feel like a total failure. She'd put me on a strict diet, which I'd followed to the letter (thank you, A-type personality), but I'd gained weight instead of losing it. 'Didn't you stick to what I told you to do?!' she'd said.

I wasn't overweight. I was trying to be 'perfect'. Losing those last three kilos meant the world to me. Oh, and seeing a dietician was a trend – a cool luxury – amongst my friends. It became a game of sorts. If I lost weight, I was 'succeeding'. If I gained it, I wasn't good enough. It was a toxic cycle.

I came home feeling betrayed by my own body. I was so disappointed with myself. I was studying health and experimenting with different fad diets, yet I couldn't even 'fix' myself. To manage my weight (and, if I'm honest, punish myself), I'd restrict my eating even further to the point of obsession – like so many teenagers today. But the more I deprived myself, the harder my weight was to control.

I was so focused on that stupid number that I'd completely lost sight of the importance of how I was *feeling in my own body*. I felt terrible. I had low energy, low moods and shattered self-esteem. And, of course, this had an incredibly negative impact on my relationship with food and my body.

Then, while I was standing in my kitchen, I had a lightbulb moment. I realised just how ridiculous it was that a few hundred grams (which could have been PMS fluid) could affect my life so much. I realised that my focus on weight was starting to impact my ability to enjoy life. It had to stop.

This was the moment when I decided to heal my broken relationship with food for good. The moment I decided to start jotting down my thoughts and feelings in a blog to show people how I wanted to fight this desire to be perfect. The moment I decided to kick off my journey to a healthy mind and body.

And, slowly, food became my friend. I began to heal my body and shift my attitude. I tuned in to my body for the first time in a long time and figured out which foods worked for me. Key word: me. (We'll go into this later on.)

I said 'no' to diets. I'd had enough. I vowed to never give into them again. I told myself I'd rather live with those couple of kilos than suffer through one more diet. Life is too short. I became an intuitive eater – someone who listens to the signals their body gives them, then responds to them. I began eating mindfully and with gratitude. I immersed myself in studying and understanding the powerful healing nature of food.

I also realised that today's health and fitness standards are just that – standardised. They assume we are all the same. They don't reflect who we are: beautiful, unique and worthy individuals, both physically and emotionally.

I finally realised that no one diet fits all. It was then, and only then, that everything changed for me.

## Why do we strive to be skinny?

Skinny is everywhere – in our magazines, on our TV screens and our news feeds, and walking the runways. It's no wonder we feel immense pressure to be skinny. In the past, being skinny and underweight helped me to feel in control. It gave me a (false) sense of confidence. I thought skinny meant healthy. But now I realise that there is a difference between being health-conscious and being weight-conscious.

Being weight-conscious, I had never felt more lifeless. I was a controlling person, to the point where my own friends and family didn't want to be around me.

Now, I strive to be strong and healthy. I have arrived at a balanced, sustainable weight. I am flexible with myself about my weight. If I gain two kilos, I know that a small fluctuation is normal and healthy. Being health-conscious is my way of making my body happy. I urge you to adopt this attitude. Skinny is out; healthy and strong is in.

## Fear of the scales

Many of my clients and friends are absolutely terrified by the number on the scales. It's a very real fear, and it was for me, too. I would go as far as to say I'm scarred by scales. I'd see that silly number as a reflection of my self-esteem and self-worth. And all that worry didn't do me any good – in fact, it was a huge stressor.

### LIFE TIP

#### Say your affirmations

*Stand in front of a mirror and say this out loud: 'I am enough just as I am. I am beautiful just as I am. I am worthy just as I am.'*

On this healing journey, I want you to give up the scales for at least **three months** and focus on how you feel instead. Of course, it's important to keep track of your health, but there are other ways to do this that don't involve an arbitrary number, like how you feel in your clothes. When you make a decision to live a balanced, active life, your weight will naturally even out and it will be much more consistent. It may go up and down by about two kilos due to fluid, hormonal changes, and dehydration, but this is normal.

Go on, then: give up the scales. I guarantee it'll make a difference to your stress levels and help to bring you balance.

> YOU ARE NOT DEFINED BY YOUR WEIGHT. NOT NOW, NOT EVER.

## HOW TO EMBRACE A POSITIVE FOOD VOICE

Your 'food voice' is what I like to call your healing food friend – that little voice in your head that makes you see sense when you're eating. It guides you to eat wholesome food with balance and kindness. It helps you in times of food anxiety, and it's there to relieve guilt.

Tune in to your food voice when guilt, panic or restrictive thoughts pop up, or when a diet becomes tempting. Your food voice will remind you that your body can handle the foods you eat. It will encourage you to eat mindfully and slowly. Your food voice does not believe in diets or guilt around food. It will never be afraid there won't be enough food.

Your food voice is there – it's up to you to turn up the volume.

Call on your food voice when anxiety rears its ugly head. It will bring reason to the table.

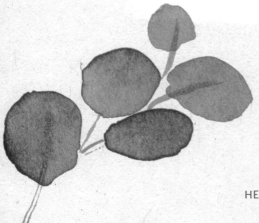

## Have you taken the obsession with food and weight too far?

Do you view food as the enemy? Is it on your mind all the time? Do you feel anxious and guilty after eating? Do you refuse to eat anything 'bad'?

If so, you've developed a complicated relationship with food and you may have disordered eating to some degree. When taken to the extreme, this is called 'orthorexia', and it's far too common for my liking. Orthorexia is an obsessive way of eating that involves only eating foods that one considers healthy. It's a medical condition in which the sufferer avoids specific foods with the belief they are harmful.

Thanks to social media and the amount of information available to us, many young people I meet suffer from orthorexia. It's a relatively new term that I think is the next big concern in the health world – especially amongst teenagers. It seems like every second conversation I have or overhear is about food and fitness.

Yes, we're becoming more health-conscious, and that's great. I'm a proud nutritionist, after all! But some people are taking it to the extreme. I used to be one of them, so I recognise the signs. It's easy to fall into the trap of being obsessive with food, being too careful, and literally being scared to eat unhealthy food. We need to think of food as fuel and nourishment – that's all. It's not the driver of our thoughts. There is so much more to life than worrying about what we're eating all the time.

## Is guilt getting in the way of your healing?

Ah, guilt. It's not fun, is it? Recently, I caught myself having guilty thoughts about food. I was in LA and I woke up feeling guilty about what I'd eaten for dinner the night before. I berated myself for not eating as well as I 'should have'. That word 'should' can haunt you. I think it's a good thing these old thoughts of guilt popped up – they reminded me how overpowering this emotion can be. Guilt makes things seem harder and more exhausting. Feeling guilty about food after you've eaten it prevents healing.

For a healthy relationship with food, you have to give yourself a little freedom and leeway. Some days, you'll eat super cleanly and exercise, and on others, you'll indulge a little and find you're not feeling up to exercise. That's why the 80/20 approach is so important. You have to tune in to your body and listen to what it needs. A night out with your girlfriends and a few glasses of vino or some gelato is good for the soul – so why kick yourself the next morning? A sleep-in or a day on the couch could be just what your body needs to restore – so why beat yourself up about it? Be kind to yourself.

### WHAT TO DO WHEN YOU FEEL GUILTY ABOUT FOOD

Close your eyes, take a big, deep breath, and then let it go slowly.

Guilt manifests itself as heaviness and stress in the body. I believe that when we fill our minds with these 'heavy' thoughts, they weigh us down. The mind is so powerful, and we need to monitor our thoughts.

Let. It. Go. Say 'I trust my body'. Guilt and anxiety come from a lack of trust within your own body.

If this doesn't work, try writing down what you're feeling anxious or guilty about. Transfer the thoughts onto paper and get them out of your head. Alternatively, practise yoga or meditation, this has really helped me.

# OUR BROKEN RELATIONSHIP WITH FOOD

## Emotional eating

This is the practice of consuming large quantities of food – usually 'comfort' or junk food – in response to feelings besides hunger. Experts estimate about 75 per cent of overeating is tied to emotions. Have you ever noticed people reaching for food when an uncomfortable topic of conversation comes up? Or do you find yourself turning to food when you're feeling sad? Food isn't there to solve our emotional problems. It's there to nourish us. As babies, we eat intuitively; we fuss when we're hungry and stop eating when we're full. Then, as we grow up, many of us lose touch with our true hunger signals.

To combat emotional eating, the first step is identifying the underlying emotional issues affecting our relationship with food. The next time you reach for a chocolate bar or order a plate of fries, ask yourself if you're actually hungry, or if there is something else at play. When it comes to emotions, food isn't the answer. Self-love is. Food is food. Why do we give it so much emotional power?

Here's why I believe so many of us develop a complicated relationship with food:

- *Fear of rejection, of not being enough, not being accepted, appreciated or loved.*
- Lack of trust. *When you lack trust in your body, anxiety is the natural result.*
- A need for control. *Food control is so often anxiety-based. Because food is such an integral part of our lives, controlling it allows us to cope with anxiety around family relationships, social groups, our weight and body image. Food brings comfort – in choosing to eat or avoid certain foods, you feel like you have gained control.*
- Societal pressure *to look a certain way.*
- Losing perspective *of what really matters.*
- Guilt *and the belief that we are not enough.*
- Low self-esteem. *You don't feel worthy.*

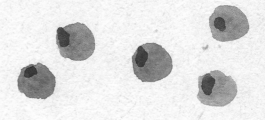

## Is your family contributing to your weight obsession?

Does your family comment on your weight? Or do they diet and constantly worry about their own food or weight? If so, you're likely to start stressing about it too.

When I was six years old one of my family members said to me, 'Wow, you're a big eater!' This comment was repeated many times while I was growing up. I ultimately developed a very complex relationship with food in later years. While I can't blame these comments, they definitely didn't do any good to a vulnerable little girl. Here's what to do if your family is commenting on what you're eating:

- *Have a conversation. You can be assertive without being aggressive and let them know how you feel.*

- *Stand up for yourself. Politely tell them you don't need to know their thoughts.*

- *Let it go and remember everyone is entitled to an opinion, but you don't have to agree.*

- *Be honest about your legitimate dietary requirements. Most people will respect them and want to ensure you're taken care of.*

- *Learn to say 'no, thanks' if you don't want to eat something. Don't worry about pleasing them or meeting their needs.*

- *Figure out what makes you feel good. You may find what you've been told growing up is not the best formula for you.*

## Bingeing – the new epidemic

Bingeing: it's a dirty word for many people. Binge eating can be a truly scary experience, and I believe it has become an epidemic. For those of us who binge, food takes over. They eat more than they know they need. They eat until they feel sickeningly full. And they feel like they can't control it.

Often women fall into patterns of bingeing without realising what they're doing. There can be many causes: stress, anger, fear of not enough food, dieting, deprivation and even happiness. In my opinion, it's the result of having a complicated relationship with food as well as not feeling good enough.

Here's what a typical binge looks like: you start a diet; you fear or deny yourself certain foods. You start missing those foods. One day, you crack. You eat as much as you possibly can until you feel ill. You literally can't stop. The guilt and self-loathing kick in. Then you repeat out of anger at yourself. It really is a horrible, vicious cycle.

The guilt we feel after that binge is worse for our health than any 'bad' food. And it needs to stop.

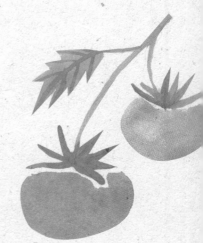

# How do you break the cycle?

You have to relieve the pressure and stop punishing yourself when it comes to food and build up your self-esteem. See page 24 for more support on doing this.

**It starts with forgiving yourself.** Forgive yourself for past behaviours. You fell off the wagon, but you're only human. It's time to get up and remind yourself that we all fall sometimes. Give yourself permission to enjoy the foods you love in moderation.

**Let go of the 'I blew it' mentality.** I see this all the time: clients have high standards when it comes to their eating, so when they eat something that doesn't align with their 'perfect' diet plan, they punish themselves with a binge. It's really important to stop classifying food as good or bad, so that in turn, you can stop describing your eating as perfect or imperfect. This is why you need to eat wholefoods for life and give up dieting.

**Crank up the self-love.** Instead of berating yourself, do something that'll boost your spirits. Perhaps take a walk along the beach or a long, hot bath followed by a few episodes of your favourite TV show? Or indulge by going to bed a little earlier?

**Don't eat as soon as you get home after a busy day.** Shower first. Take a few deep breaths. Go to the kitchen and think about your next step by actually putting your food on a plate. Make each meal pleasurable by always sitting down with your plate of food.

**Try to analyse the binge.** Write in a diary what you were thinking about or feeling before and after it happened. Tune in to your appetite. Connect the dots. For some people, seeing their actions and emotions in black and white can help them to get perspective. Think carefully about your definition of beautiful. For me, it used to be skinny. But now, beauty means waking up healthy, having glowing skin, clear eyes, thick hair, lots of energy and feeling comfortable in my own body. What is your definition of beautiful? Does it need to change? See a therapist if it will help you.

Along with the emotional factor, bingeing can stem from physical needs. To keep your hunger and appetite in check, you need to ensure you're eating enough of the right macronutrients (fats and protein) at breakfast, lunch and dinner, as well as protein-rich snacks. (See page 96 to guide you.) Steer clear of all sugar (even fruit) in the afternoon and have no more than one coffee per day. These are all important parts of reducing the urge to overeat or binge.

## THE 4 PM SNACK

Planning a protein-rich snack at around 4 pm is crucial to balance blood-sugar levels and avoid overeating at dinner.

I treat this snack as a mini meal. I commit to sitting down for 10 minutes in a calm state and eating slowly and mindfully. This has changed my health.

Find my favourite blood-sugar control snacks on page 108.

When you skip meals, or eat non-nutritious meals, you're likely to overeat later in the day because your body is crying out for food. This is why I believe in the importance of the 4 pm snack.

The bottom line is this: when you commit to eating wholefoods with balance, you can give yourself permission to enjoy treats in moderation and without guilt. You'll see how the pressure of being on a restrictive diet will start to decrease. This leads to being in control of food which will result in less bingeing and overeating, and your weight will start to balance out.

## Why do I keep eating even though I'm full?

Being painfully full feels terrible. So why do we eat until we can't fit anything else in? There are several reasons, but it boils down to this – we are disconnected to our bodies. We don't listen to our bodies' needs, or we don't love them enough to listen. Either way, it's not healthy. Overeating can be an emotional or physical reaction.

### Emotional
Something is missing in your life, so you use food to fill the gap. Or something's making you feel uncomfortable or upset, so you use food as a distraction or balm. How to fix it:

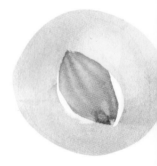

- *Fall back in love with yourself. See page 24 for tips on building your self-esteem.*

- *Uncover old pain in your life. Don't run from it. It's okay to feel sad, angry or down sometimes. See a good therapist – it's a great first step. This really helped me!*

**I HAVE POWER OVER FOOD. IT DOES NOT HAVE POWER OVER ME.**

### Physical
You haven't eaten enough during the day, or you're on a restrictive diet, or your blood sugar is unbalanced due to eating irregular meals or sugary/processed foods. How to fix it:

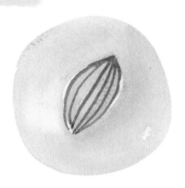

- *Eat regular meals. Aim for five small meals a day, including two snacks to keep your blood sugar in check.*

- *Consume protein and good fats. These are the two most satiating macronutrients, so eat them with every meal. (See page 96 for more.)*

- *Give up dieting for life. The goal is to tune in to your hunger and satiety signals.*

## Body dysmorphia

Body dysmorphia, when a person obsesses about their body image, is a mental illness. The sufferer believes they have a flaw – minor or major – and that flaw causes them significant distress. They feel ashamed of their appearance to the point that it affects their ability to function in day-to-day life. In severe cases, sufferers will undergo cosmetic surgery or excessively exercise to 'fix' their flaw. I used to be obsessed about my weight and the way I looked. Imperfections were not acceptable. I'd look in the mirror 100 times a day and would never be satisfied with my reflection. This had a domino effect on my life, especially my stress levels. I believe having heavy thoughts may lead to a heavier body. We need to feel light in our bodies. If you are at the point of depriving or starving yourself it may be because you are denying yourself the ability to enjoy life because you feel unworthy. I felt this way too so I get your pain. Remember that you are worthy of the most beautiful and abundant life. Try these steps that I used to help heal body dysmorphia or a bad body moment:

- *Let go of the desire to have a perfect body – it does not exist. Change your focus from weight to health.*

- *See a psychologist or cognitive behavioural therapist to help retrain your mind and deal with underlying emotional issues.*

- *Write down the parts of your body you feel grateful for.*

- *Stop comparing yourself to others. We are all biochemically unique.*

- *Try swimming, doing yoga or meditating for 10 minutes to clear your mind. Focus on your breathing. Visualise lightness and goodness flowing into your body.*

- *Replace negative thoughts with positive affirmations. For example, swap 'I look fat' to 'I am light and I trust my body'. This has really made a difference for me. It may take time to get the hang of it, but keep practising.*

## LIFE TIP

*Try my mirror exercise. Every time you see your reflection in a mirror you probably say something negative or critical about yourself. Agree? Perhaps you're not even aware of it.*

*My darling husband taught me this tip: never ever step away from a mirror without giving yourself a compliment. It changes your thoughts, body and life. It has really helped me heal my relationship with my body.*

## WHAT TO DO WHEN THE SHAMING STRIKES

If you're not feeling great about yourself, steer clear of mirrors and go into a forward fold right away. To do this, sit on the floor and lean over your body. Breathe deeply and give thanks for your health and the body parts you like. If you can't think of any, thank your legs for carrying you every day or your heart for beating life into your body. Keep breathing deeply until the feeling passes. Avoid photos, modelling channels and diet books while you're feeling this way.

# HEALING YOUR RELATIONSHIP WITH FOOD

## Dieting stops now

I don't like fad diets one bit. They're not sustainable. How many people do you know who have stuck to a diet for a long time? And by that, I mean more than a few weeks. Whether it's the Dukan Diet or the 5:2 way of eating, diets DO. NOT. WORK. Perhaps you see short-term results, but my concern is that people cannot stick to them. All diets do is complicate your relationship with food, and cause body hatred, stress and feelings of failure, which can be disastrous, not to mention dangerous, in the long term.

Free yourself from dieting and embrace a wholesome way of eating. This is the key to long-lasting health and happiness – and a balanced weight.

Here's how to give up diets forever:

* *Throw out any books/magazines/DVDs that promise to help you lose five kilos in seven days. They offer false hope and make me mad! And unfollow those Instagram accounts that spruik the latest diet trends and products.*

* *If you find yourself being tempted by a diet, remind yourself that the results won't last and you won't be giving your body the love it deserves.*

* *Make a commitment to eat a wholesome, balanced range of food forever. It's the only way of eating that serves you and it's not a passing fad. (See page 96 for more.)*

* *Add 'balance' and 'moderation' to your vocabulary, and delete 'deprivation' and 'restriction'. They've got to go.*

* *Allow yourself small indulgences from time to time. Follow the 80/20 approach – eat well 80 per cent of the time, and eat what you like the other 20 per cent of the time. It's good for your soul and your body will be able to handle it. If you don't give in a little, you'll end up overeating or bingeing. (See page 23 for more on this.)*

* *Listen to your food voice (see page 13).*

* *Bin the scales and stop counting calories. Numbers do not define you. They only add stress to your body.*

* *Finally, subscribe to the idea that your body is your temple. Why on earth would you want to put it through the torment of dieting? It deserves better. Your life is too precious to be consumed by dieting.*

# Be a mindful eater

Dieting requires willpower and is characterised by restriction and deprivation. Dieters are always looking for a quick fix, and food is the enemy. They count calories (numbers!) and succumb to societal pressure to look perfect. But guess what? Perfection doesn't exist.

On the other hand, mindful eaters see food as nourishment. They're flexible with food and trust that their body can convert it into fuel. They eat nutrient-dense, REAL food until they're satisfied, and then they stop. They are able to indulge with moderation, which you will learn how to do. Mindful eaters don't even think about dieting or bingeing because they know neither option is worth the fallout. How good does that sound? My mum is the best example of this!

Healthy living is meant to be simple, not complicated. Food is here to take care of our bodies' needs. Too many people view food as 'good' or 'bad', asking: 'Will this make me thin or fat?' This is not healthy and creates so much stress within the body. I'm passionate about putting an end to this extreme and obsessive mentality around food and weight. Help me to spread the message.

Mindful eating means eating with awareness. Here's how to do it:

- Choose nourishing foods most of the time but also give yourself room for indulgence. (See page 96 for more.)

- Make each meal a pleasurable experience. Slow down, sit down and eat away from distractions. Take a big breath before you start your meal. Put your fork down in between each bite, and chew, chew, chew! Really savour every morsel before swallowing. Food is meant to be enjoyed.

- Stop the vicious cycle of all or nothing. If you make a 'bad' food choice, let it go. Don't write the rest of the day off.

- Say positive affirmations when you eat. These will help to release negative thoughts and overcome anxiety around food. My favourites are: 'My body is about to be nourished with so much goodness', 'This plate of food is so good for me' and 'I trust that my body can break this down'.

- Keep a symptoms diary. This is like a food diary, except you write down how you feel before and after each meal. Are you genuinely hungry, or are you eating out of boredom or habit?

## THE ART OF STRESS-FREE EATING

1   Take three long deep breaths and relax your entire body.

2   Remove distractions from your environment including phones, TVs or computers.

3   Look at the food and simply say: 'Thank you for this plate of goodness'. Feel how lucky you are to have access to foods that help you thrive.

4   Try your best to remove all judgement about what you are about to eat – instead, focus on slowly enjoying each mouthful. Let go of the negative self-talk: 'This food isn't healthy', 'This food will make me fat'. Replace this with positive affirmations, 'It's okay to indulge. My body can handle it.'

5   Pay attention to your food and how you feel during and after eating it – this is the best guide to knowing which foods make you feel good. When you start to be present with food, you taste and enjoy it more, which will make you feel much more satiated after eating. Remember, food is to be enjoyed.

6   After your meal, state: 'Thank you for nourishing my body'.

## Find a unique eating plan that works for you

We've been led to believe there is a certain diet that works for all of us. It's absurd! We're biochemically unique. Your nutritional needs are very different to that of your friend, sister, cousin and mother. On top of that, we compare our diet to everyone else around us. Sadly, this has caused many women to damage their relationships with their bodies. It needs to end! We need to tune in to our own bodies and what we need as individuals.

I've found that when I eat what I like in moderation, my body responds with good health. So listen to your body and give it exactly what it needs. For example, I've realised gluten makes me tired, so I choose not to eat it. I've also discovered that eating five small, balanced meals a day works best for my metabolism, energy levels and mental clarity. To find your unique eating plan, follow these steps:

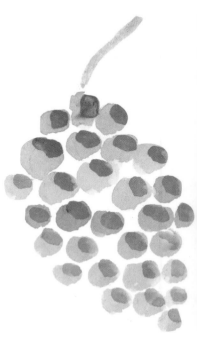

* *Forget what your friend, mum and Instagram are telling you.*

* *Educate yourself about food and nutrition, with the help of reputable sources.*

* *Design your own lifestyle and experiment until you find what works for your body. How often do you need to eat? When are your energy levels highest? Adjust your eating and exercise habits accordingly. Take note of how you feel about each meal. If you're tired or bloated every time you eat lentils, cut them out for two weeks and see if you feel any different. I also suggest eliminating gluten, refined sugar and processed dairy for a trial period. Most people feel better when they do this.*

* *If you're looking for guidance, visit an integrative health practitioner who views the body as a WHOLE and values the mind–body connection.*

The good news is you don't need to be regimented with your eating. When you discover the foods that work for you, you'll understand that not every meal should be the same. And not every meal will be perfect.

The aim is to listen to your appetite and feed your body what it needs. Sometimes, you won't have access to healthy foods (like when you're travelling), and that's okay. Just do your best with the choices available to you. Trust that your body can handle this.

In the same vein, you don't need to be so rigid with food. Don't be that person who pushes around the food on their plate at a dinner party or refuses to eat anything at a wedding. Be versatile. Be free. Be a flexible eater (a flexitarian).

Tune in to your emotional wellbeing and eat according to that. For example, did you wake up feeling teary today? Eat delicious, warming foods as opposed to cold, raw foods to heal. (See page 86 for more on this.)

## Indulgence and the 80/20 mindset

People often ask me, 'Jess, do you ever indulge? Do you ever just eat an ice-cream?' Of course I do! I actually go out of my way to eat imperfectly, because I believe being too regimented with your eating is unhealthy. As a nutritionist, my world is very health-focused and so I'm conscious not to be too strict or fussy. On the weekends, I indulge a little without the worry or guilt, and my body loves it. The key is indulging with mindfulness and moderation.

I can't tell you how many people I meet who won't eat something 'naughty' because they're scared they'll spiral out of control and binge. Think about little kids: as soon as they can't have something, it's all they want! We may think we've grown up, but we all have weak spots. It's not a bad thing; it's human nature. Playing the game of mental negotiation will get you nowhere and only make you more stressed in the long run.

Once or twice a week, I enjoy a scoop of good-quality gelato, a couple of glasses of red wine, a little frozen yoghurt or a few pieces of chocolate. I give myself *permission* to eat my treat without guilt. This is the trick as guilt adds stress to your body.

I can do this because I trust my body. Will one indulgent meal cause a skin breakout? Or significant weight gain? Will it derail my good habits? No. What matters is how I eat MOST of the time. This means eating cleanly 80 per cent of the time, and allowing myself to eat imperfectly for the remaining 20 per cent. This keeps me balanced and on track, and I never feel deprived so I rarely overeat.

Does this mean you can go crazy and eat all the junk food you crave? Nope, that's not my point. Healthy indulgence means being able to eat these foods in moderate amounts, while still loving yourself. No stress, no guilt. Next time you want a treat, ask yourself if there's a healthier alternative. My recipe section is a good place to start – honestly, the sweet treats in there taste better than the traditional versions!

If that doesn't tickle your taste buds, sit down with your favourite treat. Eat it mindfully, and give thanks. Release the guilt. Trust that your body can handle it and take care of you.

## THREE STEPS TO HEALTHY INDULGENCE

1 *Plan to indulge. If you're going to a birthday party or dinner with friends, there's no need to restrict your eating that day so that you can go 'all out'. Just be mindful. It's important to eat satiating meals that day to keep your blood sugar stable. Also, if you're prepared and excited about the indulgence, you're less likely to feel guilty. Permission granted!*

2 *Watch your language. Avoid terms like 'cheat meal' or 'giving in'. You're not cheating on anything or anyone. You're not giving in; you're in control and have made a conscious decision to indulge. You're just being human!*

3 *Eat your treats in moderation. Remember, this is not your only meal for the day, so don't overdo it. You can have some more tomorrow if you wish because you are no longer depriving yourself.*

*Tag #JSHealthTreatYourself to be part of this gorgeous, one-of-a-kind community of healthy eaters!*

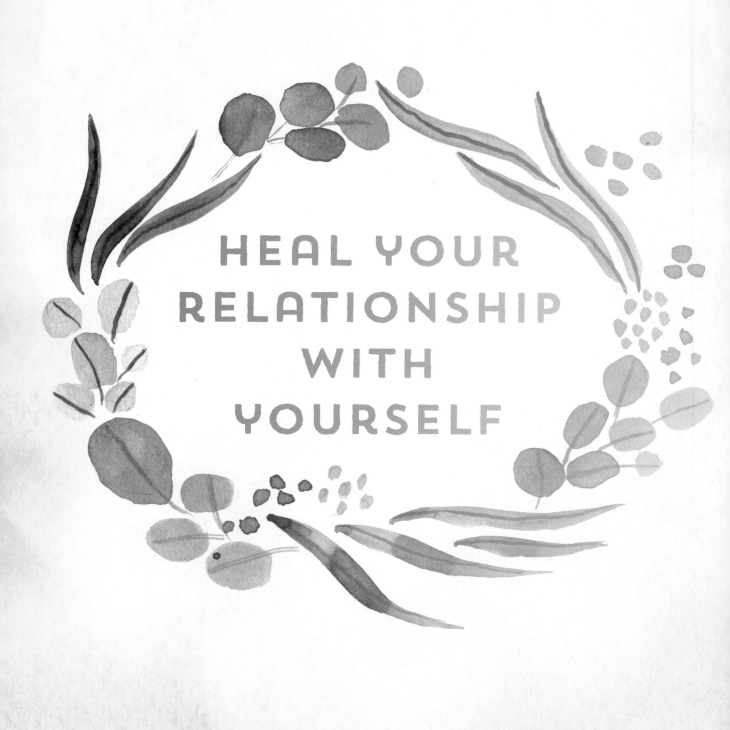

HEAL YOUR
RELATIONSHIP
WITH
YOURSELF

*It's time to put yourself first. To live a healthy life, you need to start by healing your relationship with yourself. You're going to uncover the sources of tension, build your self-worth, become grounded and centred, and start living in a space of gratitude. You'll also be reconnecting with yourself, as self-love is the foundation of health, wellbeing and healing your relationship with food and your body.*

# IDENTIFYING SOURCES OF NEGATIVITY

Uncovering and coming to terms with the source of your negative relationship with yourself probably sounds like a horrible activity. But then, so is living with a broken relationship with yourself. You have the strength and power to work through your issues and emerge stronger and happier than ever. I'm with you!

When you're ready, dig deep and try to uncover where this pressure and negativity is coming from. Did your parents instil it in you? When did you lose your love for yourself? When did the trust in yourself break? What are you trying to control? Were you never given praise or validation growing up? Can you trace it back to your A-type, perfectionist personality?

See if you can go one step further and figure out why you have these beliefs about yourself. There may be a few reasons why you might not be feeling good enough – identifying them is the first step. This process might be painful but uncovering the root of your negative relationship with yourself will give you the clues as to how to heal your relationship with food and your body.

## RELIEVE THE PRESSURE

We are so good at putting immense pressure on ourselves to be everything at once: perfect mothers, sisters, friends, career women and partners – while always maintaining the perfect body, of course. This pressure can also be a huge trigger for bingeing and dieting.

So, how can we relieve this kind of pressure once and for all? Begin by knowing and accepting that you're *not* expected to do it all. It's okay to ask for help, and it's okay to disappoint people sometimes.

Forgive yourself for anything you're feeling guilty about and commit to respecting yourself and your body from today onwards.

## Forget about the 'what ifs'

Coulda, woulda, shoulda. When you're always thinking about what might have happened, you're essentially living in the past. Before I started my healing journey, I was definitely someone who dwelled on the past. And all it did was stop me from feeling joy and gratitude, and rebuilding my self-worth because I was always thinking about where I went wrong.

But I've since realised that we're all human. We all make mistakes. The important thing is that we live, learn and move on. The silver lining of messing up is that we grow so much in the process. For many people, the 'what if' and the 'coulda, woulda, shoulda' thoughts revolve around food. What if I had eaten better last night? I shouldn't have eaten that frozen yoghurt. I shouldn't have had that glass of wine. I should have gone to the gym instead of sleeping in. Who cares?!

You did it, but it's now in the past. Don't beat yourself up. If you can learn something from it, that's great, but what's most important is to move forward and let it go. Be kind to yourself and learn for next time. Don't give up on yourself, you are too precious for that.

## Stop apologising for who you are

How many times do you say 'sorry' in a day? Women are particularly inclined to do this (I know I'm guilty!). The word is starting to lose ALL meaning!

I spent so much of my life doubting myself and apologising. I was my own worst critic. I'd find myself apologising for having a big personality, or for being too sensitive, too intense, too expressive, too anything … It was exhausting.

Something clicked a while ago, and I decided I was fed up with apologising for the person I am. Why should I? I'm not everyone's cup of tea, and that's fine. I am who I am. And there's no reason why I should have to say sorry for my emotions. I'm entitled to them.

If you're also saying sorry more than you should, stop. Easier said than done, I know, but practice will make it a habit.

## YOU DON'T NEED TO DEAL WITH THIS ON YOUR OWN.

I will tell anyone who listens to see a therapist. I'd shout it from the rooftops if I could. There is absolutely no shame in asking for help – in fact, it makes you a very intelligent human being. We all need help sometimes, and for some reason, it can be easier and more comforting to talk to a stranger.

I see a psychotherapist. In my sessions, we uncover pains and struggles from my past in order to heal current emotions and patterns of behaviour. Seeking professional help was one of the best decisions I ever made and, if you're able to, I'd encourage you to seek out this support too.

## Know it's okay to be vulnerable

Vulnerability can be a gift. My vulnerability enables me to talk more openly to my clients about their struggles. Don't be afraid of yours. Being vulnerable allows us to feel more connected to ourselves and the people around us. It relieves the pressure to be perfect, and helps us to accept ourselves just as we are. Don't be afraid of feeling or saying that something is hard. Life is hard sometimes. Being honest and open about your struggles is healing in itself.

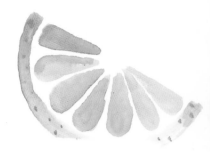

## Stop with the comparing

I used to compare myself to everyone. It was exhausting. Now I've learned that comparison makes you feel stuck. It can kill your shine. The next time you catch yourself comparing, stop and swap the thought. Think of something you're proud of or grateful for, like your family, friends, work, or a personal achievement.

And remember, there is enough for everyone. Why do we think that if he/she has something, we can't have it too? We can all be successful. We can all be happy.

'COMPARISON IS THE THIEF OF JOY.'

– Theodore Roosevelt

## Break out of the victim mentality

I was a victim for years. I always felt that the world was against me. And thanks to this mindset, everything was a struggle. I was sad and lonely. I didn't love myself; instead, I criticised and compared myself to everyone around me. I tried to find love and approval in the wrong places. I always thought, 'Why me?' and 'When will it be my turn?' I blamed everything on everyone else.

It's challenging to adjust your mentality from negative to positive. It's tough to shift from being a pessimist to an optimist, but it's the best investment you can make for your health.

### IN YOUR WORDS

*I love that Jess doesn't shy away from sharing her struggles around food, and for someone like me, who has suffered from disordered eating, it is so refreshing and inspiring! Finally a book that isn't just about shedding weight but gaining self-esteem, happiness, energy and control over those pesky fad diets! Thank you Jess for writing what is so needed. Thank you for your bravery, and your commitment to helping other women live healthier and happier lives.*

TARA O (FACEBOOK), TALKING ABOUT THE HEALTHY LIFE

# HOW TO GET YOUR SPARKLE BACK

Not only is confidence oh-so-sexy, but it's oh-so-healing, too! You know those people who light up a room as soon as they walk in? What do you notice most about them? Is it their toned thighs or tight tummies? No – it's their confidence! Happy, confident people radiate from within. They have that glow we all know and love. Here are some ways you can achieve that confidence for yourself:

* *Focus on the parts of your body that you do love. Say 'thank you' for them every time you look in the mirror. Do this daily until it becomes a habit. (See page 19 for my mirror exercise.)*

* *Stop comparing yourself to others.*

* *Unfollow Instagram accounts that make you feel inadequate. Do it now!*

* *Book in to see a therapist. Just talk about what's going on; let it all out.*

* *Tune in to the goodness within you. Start acknowledging how valuable you are as a human being and how appreciated you are as a family member or friend. Your loved ones may not tell you all the time, but know you are appreciated and needed.*

> **YOUR BODY LISTENS TO YOUR THOUGHTS. MAKE THEM GOOD ONES.**

## PRACTISE GRATITUDE

We often get so caught up in the daily grind that we forget to pause and reflect on how amazing our lives are. We forget to count our blessings. And in times of hardship, we forget that this, too, shall pass.

When you feel grateful you instantly feel less stressed and your body heals faster. This is what I do every day to help me reconnect with my body. Every morning, take five minutes to give thanks. Close your eyes, breathe deeply and think of the things, people and parts of your body you are grateful for.

Here are some examples. Don't just say it, feel it!

* *Thank you for my family and friends.*

* *Thank you for my clear mind.*

* *Thank you for my good digestion.*

* *Thank you for my strong body.*

* *Thank you for my work.*

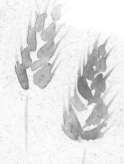

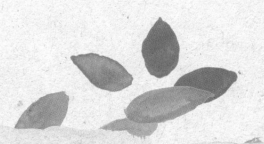

## CHANGE YOUR
## THINKING RIGHT NOW

* Tell yourself every single day that you are worthy of the best life – because you are! Whenever you revert back to old habits and put yourself down, pause and think: 'I am worthy'. Say it until you feel it.

* Talk to yourself as you would a three-year-old. Would you tell the little you that you were fat, stupid or ugly? No way. Be kind.

* Praise yourself on the reg. Start to acknowledge all the things you do, rather than the things you don't. You do enough!

* Practise swapping negative thoughts for positive ones. Do this so often that it becomes a habit.

* Remind yourself that every challenge you've faced has been a stepping stone to get you to the best point in your life. The best is yet to come. Believe it.

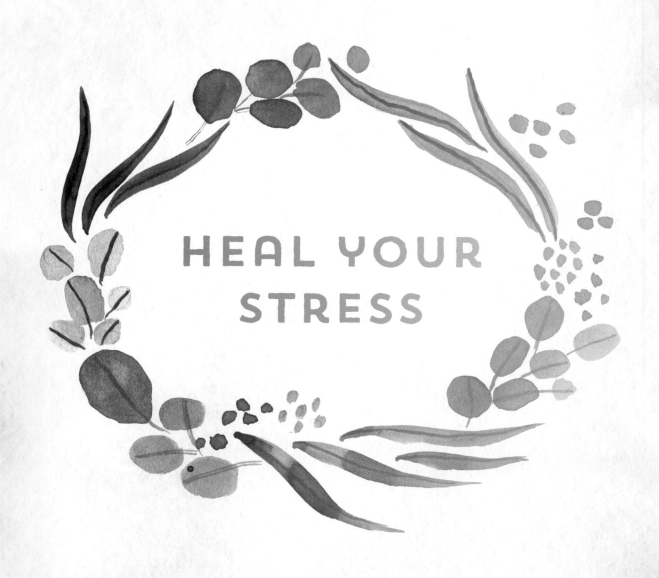

HEAL YOUR
STRESS

*As a nutritionist, I believe food is instrumental to our health and happiness. However – and this is a big call, I know – I also believe stress can undermine all our good eating and exercise habits; and that it is the root of most health conditions. If you're stressed, your body simply can't enter a state of true health and wellbeing. It just can't function at its best when it's under enormous amounts of stress.*

# THE IMPACT OF STRESS

Stress is inevitable. It's part and parcel of the modern-day lifestyle. It would be unfair and unrealistic for me to say, 'You need to live a stress-free life,' because that's just not going to happen. In fact, a little bit of stress is healthy – it keeps us motivated. But too much stress affects your energy, hormones, weight, mood – the list goes on. We'll be exploring these aspects later on.

I'd love to help you to be honest about your stress and your stressors. Then, using the healing tips in this chapter and in the 8-week action plan, help you find options and solutions to help heal your stress. You can do it! I'm supporting you all the way.

## Stress and adrenals

'Stress' and 'adrenal exhaustion' are two terms that often go hand in hand.

Your adrenal glands sit on top of the kidneys, and they're chiefly responsible for releasing hormones in response to stress. They also regulate blood sugar, maintain the body's energy levels and produce hormones like adrenaline and cortisol.

Ongoing stress – whether it be emotional, environmental or physical – and high levels of cortisol are disastrous for the adrenals. When overworked adrenals crash, the result is adrenal exhaustion – which comes with all kinds of fun symptoms like exhaustion, chronic fatigue, anxiety, intense sugar cravings, lack of motivation etc.

All stress is the same to the body. It can't tell the difference. The physical effects of stress can include hormone or blood-sugar imbalance, impaired thyroid function, weight gain around your middle, poor digestive function, poor sleep and tiredness on waking, low motivation and increase incidence of emotional and binge eating.

## How our nervous system works

The parasympathetic nervous system is responsible for the body's 'rest and digest' function. It works to bring the body to a state of calm. On the flipside, the sympathetic nervous system is responsible for the body's 'fight or flight' response. It controls how we react to perceived threats.

These two systems work like yin and yang, and they need to be in balance in order for your body to respond to stress well.

When we are stressed, the sympathetic nervous system steps in and our cortisol levels shoot up. It shuts down all systems that aren't essential for survival, like digestion. This goes back to the caveman days, where we couldn't exactly stop for a bathroom break when a lion was chasing us down.

When the 'danger' is gone, the parasympathetic nervous system takes over to counterbalance those responses and bring us back to neutral. Our heart rate steadies and muscles relax.

The problem is, these days, we're stressed – and unnecessarily so – to the point where our sympathetic nervous system never stops working. We're in a constant state of stress, and it's not healthy. I believe societal pressure to look a certain way can contribute to us being so stressed that our bodies can't cope.

## Stress and hormones

Stress directly affects the synchronicity of your hormones. If you're stressed, your hormones will be out of whack. When your cortisol levels are constantly high, they affect the production of sex hormones, slow down thyroid function and cause blood-sugar imbalance. They also make it hard for your body to create those 'feel good' hormones, like serotonin. Ever wondered why you're feeling stressed AND sad? That's the reason!

The first step to rebalancing your hormones is to minimise stress.

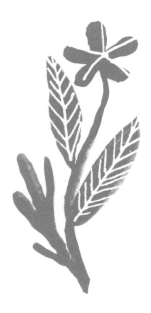

### IS STRESS AFFECTING YOUR PERIOD?

The short answer is: it may be. Stress disrupts the balance of your reproductive hormones, and, in turn, your menstrual cycle. If your periods are light, irregular, or not coming at all, it's time to make adjustments to your life.

- *Take a break from excessive and intense exercise. Trust me, it works!*

- *Don't be afraid to include good carbs and good fats in your diet.*

- *Breathe. Make a conscious effort to relax. Schedule it in. (Go into the Stress-Free Zone on page 34.)*

## Stress and weight battles

High-cortisol levels are linked to lower thyroid function and weight gain, especially around the stomach area. Cortisol also throws off our blood-sugar levels, which triggers cravings and overeating. On the other hand, low-cortisol levels occur when your stress levels have been high for so long and then crash – aka adrenal fatigue. This can also make it hard to manage weight, as your energy levels lower and you start to crave sugar. Low or high cortisol can also impact healthy thyroid function.

From an emotional point of view, I believe that when we worry and stress about our weight – like so many women and men do – we are more likely to gain weight because worrying spikes our cortisol levels.

When your body is stressed, your digestion slows down. The blood diverts away from the digestive tract to other parts of the body, as part of the 'fight or flight' response mentioned on the opposite page.

So, one of my biggest tips is to always eat in a calm environment. Never eat while you're in a stressed state because you won't digest that food as well. Most people don't chew their food properly when they're stressed, and this puts a huge strain on the digestive tract. Studies have shown that those diagnosed with IBS (irritable bowel syndrome) have higher cortisol levels compared to those who don't. Interesting!

## Stress and rushing

Rushing causes stress – both emotional and physical.

When I went to therapy, the number one piece of advice I was given was to SLOW DOWN in order to heal my life. Rushing is usually caused by panic. When you rush around, you don't breathe slowly and deeply, which is so important for restoring your nervous system and adrenal-gland function. Rushing can actually impede your hormonal system. When you rush, you are not present in that moment. When you rush, you miss things happening in your own life.

Let's start focusing on the now.

### NUTRIENTS FOR COMBATING STRESS

Try these supplements with the guidance of a health practitioner.

- *B complex*
- *Vitamin C*
- *Magnesium powder at night*
- *Adrenal herbal supplements recommended by a naturopath (these really helped me).*

**THIS ALL LEADS ME TO MY MOTTO: A RESTED BODY IS A HEALTHY BODY.**

## THE STRESS-FREE ZONE

To combat your stress, I suggest you enter what I call the Stress-Free Zone (#JSHealthSFZ) every single day for 10–20 minutes. This means no phone, computers, emails or social media. Spend this time taking a nap or a bath, meditating, reading, or going for a walk outside. This is your time to heal and your body will thank you.

---

## HOW TO DEEP BELLY BREATHE

1   Place one hand on your tummy, and the other on your chest.

2   Open your mouth and sigh. As you do, allow your shoulders and upper body to relax.

3   Close your mouth and pause for a few seconds.

4   With your mouth still closed, inhale slowly through your nose and into your diaphragm until your stomach pops out. Pause for a moment.

5   When you're ready, exhale slowly.

*Aim to do 10–20 of these daily. I do mine in the morning, before breakfast.*

*Alternative nostril breathing is brilliant for relaxing the nervous system (see page 87).*

*Also try putting your legs up against the wall for 10 minutes. This is where you put your backside against the wall and throw your legs up against it. Then close your eyes and breathe deeply. It really relaxes you!*

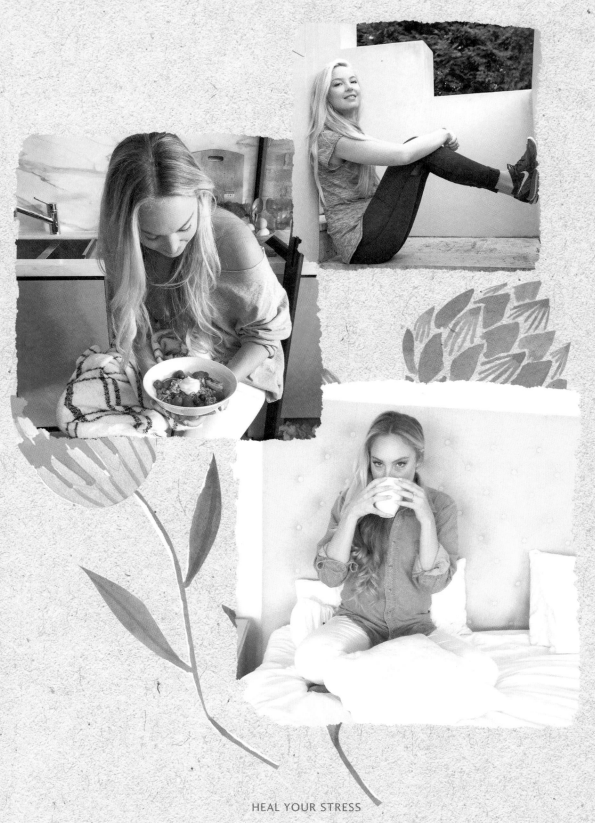

HEAL YOUR STRESS

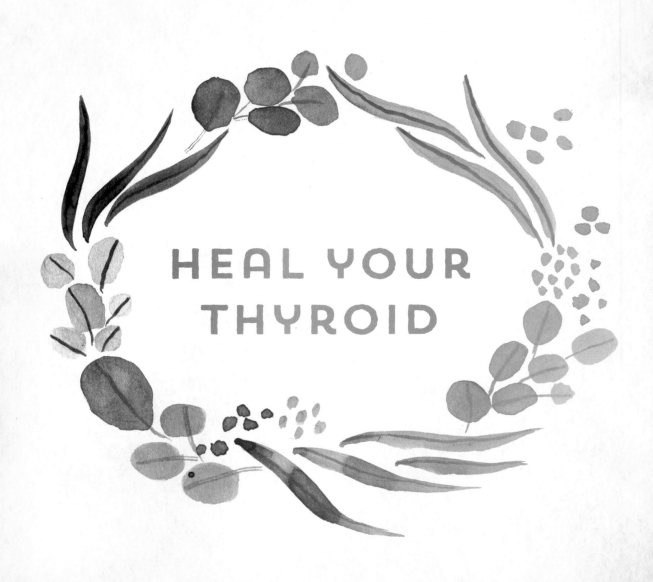

HEAL YOUR
THYROID

*I want to focus on a part of the body that you might not know much about. If your thyroid isn't functioning well, you're likely to feel awful: exhausted, unmotivated, foggy and not your usual self. Even if your thyroid isn't a problem, you can still focus on ways to nourish and protect your thyroid to keep it functioning in peak condition.*

# GET TO KNOW YOUR THYROID

The thyroid is a butterfly-shaped gland in the neck, just below the Adam's apple. It takes nutrients and converts them into two key thyroid hormones: thyroxine (T4) and triiodothyronine (T3). The thyroid also needs selenium to convert the T4 into T3. These thyroid hormones then get released into the bloodstream, where they flow through the body to control metabolism. It is important that thyroid levels stay balanced for good metabolic function.

Your thyroid is controlled by the pituitary gland – a tiny gland in the brain. When your thyroid-hormone levels drop, the pituitary gland begins producing TSH (thyroid *stimulating* hormone), which – as the name suggests – sends a signal to the thyroid to start making more hormones, stat. Once this happens, the clever pituitary gland decreases its TSH production to bring everything back into balance. (On a blood test, normal TSH levels for an adult range from 0.4–4.0 mIU/L, however it is widely considered that a TSH reading less than 2.5 mIU/L is ideal – a sign that your thyroid hormones are balanced.) However, there are other factors that influence TSH levels, leaving us with issues resulting from having too many or not enough thyroid hormones.

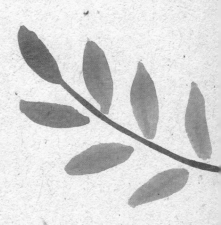

## What are the different types of thyroid conditions?

The two most common thyroid conditions are hypothyroidism and hyperthyroidism. Their symptoms can be subtle, but the sufferer definitely feels their effects as they go about their daily life.

Hyperthyroidism is an overactive thyroid, resulting from too much T3 and T4 in your body. Symptoms include irritability, sweating, anxiety, hair loss, irregular periods and weight loss.

Hypothyroidism is an underactive thyroid, resulting from not enough T3 and T4 in your body. Symptoms include fatigue, difficulty concentrating, muscle and joint pain, heavy periods and weight gain.

# TESTING AND TREATMENT

With the help of a GP and an endocrinologist, you can undergo a range of tests to determine your thyroid function. Every thyroid case is different and will require individual treatment, so it's important to be guided by your doctor and to tune in to your own body. Often TSH and T4 tests are only requested when looking at thyroid function, but I don't believe this is enough. I also recommend asking your doctor to test T3 levels as well as levels for important nutrients like zinc, selenium, iodine, vitamin D and iron, even if you're out of pocket from some of these tests.

If you're found to have hypothyroidism or hyperthyroidism, a range of treatment options are available to you, including hormone treatment, and diet and lifestyle adjustments, or a combination of both. Consult with your healthcare professionals.

## THINGS THAT CAN AFFECT THYROID FUNCTION

* *Genetics.*

* *Stress: high cortisol levels can impair the conversion of T4 to T3.*

* *A high intake of iodine (including iodine supplements) without enough selenium.*

* *Environmental toxins such as radiation, and heavy metal exposure such as mercury toxicity.*

* *Deficiency of minerals such as selenium, iodine, zinc and iron.*

* *Abnormal pituitary gland function.*

* *Low vitamin D levels.*

* *High oestrogen states such as pregnancy, added oestrogen from contraceptives, or an inability to break down oestrogens combined with gut or liver problems, can all affect thyroid hormone production.*

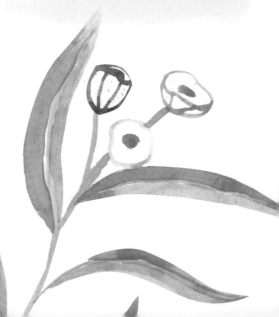

# MY SECRET BATTLE WITH THYROID DISEASE

In 2014, I was away in South Africa for six weeks when I started noticing symptoms that were very unusual for me. I had a puffy face, fluid retention around the thighs, heart palpitations, so I went to do my annual blood tests. My TSH had jumped up (it should be below 2.5, mine was 4.4) and my thyroid antibodies were on the rise. I was diagnosed with Hashimoto's Thyroiditis, an autoimmune disorder that is four to ten times more common in women than men. Hashimoto's is usually associated with hypothyroidism, an underactive thyroid condition, but sometimes first presents itself in an overactive state. Basically, it's when your own immune system starts attacking your thyroid gland and your body is in a state of inflammation.

I was dumbfounded. I couldn't believe that this was happening to me, considering how healthy my lifestyle was. I was devastated that I, a nutritionist and health-nut, had developed a health condition. It knocked my self-esteem massively.

The worst part of the diagnosis with Hashimoto's was that I felt like no one could help me. I wanted to treat the trigger, or underlying cause, but it was unclear as to what exactly that was in my situation.

There were a few possibilities, but no definites, which drove me mad. The major change I'd recently gone through was removing my IUD, a contraceptive device that would have caused my oestrogen and progesterone levels to shift. I'd also been taking a high dose of iodine supplements, because a urine test had detected low levels. (Little did I know that iodine can worsen thyroid function when taken in excess without sufficient amounts of selenium.) In addition, I'd picked up a gut parasite while on holiday in South Africa, which may have triggered the immune attack. Finally, a blood test showed I had high mercury levels, thanks to overdoing the cans of tuna growing up.

I was initially placed on Thyroxine, a synthetic thyroid hormone, but it wasn't making me feel any better. The doctors then added compounded T3 to the mix to boost

## TOP THYROID RESOURCES

These are the websites I found to be the most reliable and useful when I needed some thyroid questions answered.

*Thyroid Pharmacist: thyroidpharmacist.com*

*Sarah Wilson: sarahwilson.com*

*Wellness Resources: wellnessresources.com/health_topics.php*

*Chris Kresser: chriskresser.com*

*Stop The Thyroid Madness: stopthethyroidmadness.com*

*Natural Endocrine Solutions: naturalendocrinesolutions.com*

*Dr Mark Hyman: drhyman.com*

my T3 levels. I was still exhibiting symptoms so I made changes to my diet, eliminating dairy and caffeine. I saw more doctors and made the change to a thyroid extract that was recommended by an integrative doctor. But my thyroid antibodies were still rising and I still didn't feel like myself.

I was then advised to switch back to Thyroxine and compounded T3, and I went back and forth on different treatments for months. I was panicking, so I sought out far too many different opinions. Every doctor had a different opinion and I tried them all and my treatment became a MESS. I tried everything in the hope that my energy would bounce back and my weight would rebalance back to normal, but nothing happened. Changing medications so frequently didn't help matters. I was desperate, hence the constant changes. I just wanted to find the answer.

While all this was going on with my body, I was an emotional wreck – I was anxious and disheartened. I felt the medication was controlling my body and life. I was planning my wedding at the time, and I was terrified I wasn't going to look or feel my best. The thyroid drama brought up my old demons of not feeling good enough, thin enough, perfect enough. Now I had a 'disease', so I wasn't in 'perfect health' and this was a huge battle for me to overcome. As a nutritionist and health practitioner, I knew all the tricks of the trade, yet my own health was compromised. I just couldn't accept it, and the extra pressure only worsened my condition. My thyroid condition was all I thought about.

## What I did next – the ultimate healing treatment

I buckled down and did my own research. I tuned in to my body. I simplified the information and I began doing everything I could to heal and restore my thyroid. I started a strict thyroid protocol (see page 44), which I created based on everything I'd learned. My thyroid antibodies began dropping and my levels rebalanced.

My (one!) doctor and I then made a decision to go off thyroid medication for a period of time to see if my thyroid could work on its own again. The medication wasn't helping and we were beginning to think that my body didn't want or need it anymore.

As my thyroid antibodies had dropped, I had probably dealt with the underlying cause, which meant it was a safe time for me to go off medication.

## Fast-forward to today . . .

My blood results are now normal, and my thyroid is functioning as it should. My energy has returned and my weight has balanced out. I am currently off thyroid medication while being carefully monitored. This does not suggest for one second that stopping thyroid medication is right for everyone. This is just my story. I may need to go back on it again – who knows. My doctor and I are keeping close and careful tabs on my thyroid function.

While my body is back on track, I'm still working on the mind element. I sometimes feel uneasy or anxious about the fact that I'm off medication after being reliant on it for so long. I'm also working on getting my self-esteem, confidence and trust in my body back to the high levels they were before this battle. I know this will take time – it's all part of the healing process.

I've learned a number of lessons from this battle. Most importantly, you can't always be in perfect health – 'perfect' just does not exist. All in all, it's a happy ending and I am so, so grateful.

## MY THYROID MEAL PLAN

*The meal plan on the following page brings together some of the key principles of the protocol that helped heal my thyroid. Here's an overview of the plan; for the full protocol, see page 44:*

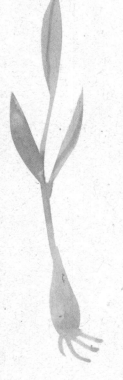

- *Eat brassica veggies, like broccoli, kale, cauliflower and brussels sprouts, well-cooked – avoid them raw.*
- *Add seaweed and dulse flakes to soups and salads.*
- *Enjoy three to four brazil nuts each day for your selenium hit.*
- *Sprinkle Himalayan or Celtic sea salt onto your meals.*
- *Avoid grains for four weeks – especially those that contain gluten.*
- *Eat lots of warming cooked foods, which are very soothing for the thyroid.*

- *Avoid dairy for four weeks, but do enjoy dairy alternatives such as coconut milk, almond milk, coconut milk yoghurt and coconut water.*
- *Limit your intake of fish that is high in mercury, such as tuna. See seafoodwatch.org/seafood-recommendations/consumer-guides for good low-mercury options.*
- *Stick to one coffee per day, before 10 am.*
- *Avoid all soy products for four weeks, and preferably long-term (a little tamari sauce is okay).*
- *Use lots of herbs and spices to flavour your meals.*

# THYROID MEAL PLAN

| | MONDAY | TUESDAY | WEDNESDAY |
|---|---|---|---|
| **EXERCISE**<br>Listen to your body. | Yoga. | Brisk walk for 30–40 minutes. | Interval training. |
| **BREAKFAST**<br>A good time to have your one daily coffee with or after food.<br>Try using a dairy-free milk alternative such as coconut milk/almond milk (or simply have black coffee). | 1–2 slices Gluten-free Green Bread (see page 156) with 1–2 poached or boiled eggs and sautéed kale/spinach. | Gluten- and grain-free cinnamon granola (see 'No Recipe Granola' on page 140) with almond milk or Greek-style yoghurt, fresh berries and a serve of pea or rice protein powder. | JSHealth Protein Smoothie (see page 147). |
| **MID-MORNING SNACK** | Carrot sticks with 2 tablespoons hummus or tahini. | Green apple with a smear of almond or peanut butter and a sprinkle of cinnamon. | 2 JSHealth Sugar-free Protein Balls (see page 269). |
| **LUNCH** | Shredded Chicken San Choy Bau (see page 224). | Teriyaki Salmon Bowl (see page 206). | Leftover Green Detox Soup (see page 196) with 1–2 boiled eggs. Sprinkle with dulse seaweed flakes. |
| **MID-AFTERNOON SNACK** | 2 nori rolls filled with sliced veggies and avocado, then drizzled with tamari. | Veggie sticks with 2 tablespoons tahini or hummus. | Carrot and cucumber sticks with 2 tablespoons tahini or hummus. |
| **DINNER** | Healthy Fish Tacos (see page 225). | Green Detox Soup (see page 196), Harissa Chicken with Cauliflower Steaks (see page 211, omit yoghurt) and steamed green beans with olive oil and Himalayan pink rock salt. | Cauliflower & Brazil Nut Soup (see page 192) and Moroccan Chicken Skewers (see page 210) with a green salad and baked sweet potato. |
| **SUPPER** | Caffeine-free herbal tea of your choice. | Caffeine-free herbal tea of your choice. | Caffeine-free herbal tea of your choice. |

*Cauliflower &
Brazil Nut Soup
(see page 192)*

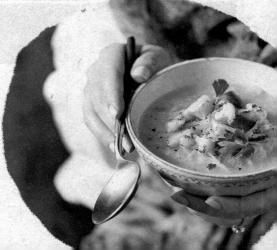

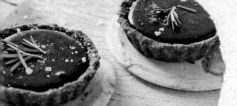

*Salted Chocolate &
Rosemary Tarts (see page 282)*

| THURSDAY | FRIDAY | SATURDAY | SUNDAY |
|---|---|---|---|
| Brisk walk for 30–40 minutes. | Interval training. | Yoga or Pilates. | Rest day or light yoga. |
| Vegan Breakfast Salad (see page 177). | JSHealth Protein Smoothie (see page 147). | Vegan Breakfast Salad (see page 177). | 2-egg omelette with ¼ avocado, sautéed greens and 1 slice of Gluten-free Green Bread (see page 156). Or Apple Crumble Pancakes (see page 172). |
| Carrot sticks with 2 tablespoons hummus or tahini. | 3–4 brazil nuts and a handful of carrot sticks. | 2 bliss balls (see pages 266–9). | 3–4 brazil nuts and 70 g berries. |
| Chop Chop Tuna Salad (see page 185): swap the tuna for wild salmon or lentils. | Energy Chop Chop Salad (see page 185) with your choice of protein. | Shredded Chicken San Choy Bau (see page 224). | Roasted chicken with cumin-spiced cauliflower, rocket and avocado. |
| 2 nori rolls filled with sliced veggies and avocado, then drizzled with tamari. | A handful of raw nuts and carrot slices. | Carrot sticks with almond butter. | 2 nori rolls filled with sliced veggies and avocado, then drizzled with tamari. |
| Shredded Chicken San Choy Bau (see page 224). | Fish with Baked Asparagus (see page 221), Truffle Cauliflower Purée (see page 242) and a green salad. | Baked herb-crusted chicken with Fried Kale with Almonds (see page 236). | Tuna Pasta Bake (see page 205). |
| Caffeine-free herbal tea of your choice. A gluten- and dairy-free treat (see pages 248–87) or 2 pieces of 85% dark chocolate. | Caffeine-free herbal tea of your choice. | Caffeine-free herbal tea of your choice. A gluten- and dairy-free treat (see pages 248–87) or 2 pieces of 85% dark chocolate. | |

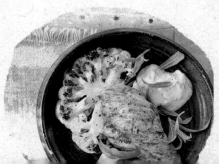

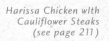

*Harissa Chicken with
Cauliflower Steaks
(see page 211)*

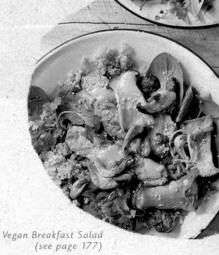

*Vegan Breakfast Salad
(see page 177)*

# MY THYROID PROTOCOL

## GUT HEALING

- I embarked on a 4-week gut cleanse using a strong anti-microbial supplement with oregano, garlic, Chinese wormwood etc. to get rid of the parasite, as they can trigger autoimmune disease. (Ask a health practitioner to guide you with this, or follow the gut cleanse protocol in my first book, The Healthy Life.)
- I eliminated gluten for three months. Strictly.
- I eliminated dairy for three months.
- I increased my stomach acid with the help of apple cider vinegar, lemon water and bitter greens. This helps your gut to fight against unwanted toxins/bugs.
- I took glutamine powder to heal my gut lining – I added it to my daily smoothie.
- I took multi-strain probiotic and Saccharomyces boulardii, which is a probiotic that helps to fight candida and promote the growth of good bacteria.
- I took a turmeric supplement, which reduces inflammation in the gut, heals the liver and boosts the immune system.

## LIVER HEALING

- Every month, I went on my 3-day Liver Reboot (see page 58), which involves cutting out caffeine, alcohol, dairy, meat and sugar.
- I minimised my alcohol consumption to special occasions only.
- I reduced my caffeine intake to one coffee a day before 10 am, and took it without milk for three months.

## ADRENAL HEALING

- I went to sleep by 9–10 pm, and got eight hours every single night.
- I took magnesium powder (magnesium dyglicinate) before bed.
- I took vitamin C every day.
- I turned all social media and technology off by 8 pm when I could.
- I put my legs up against the wall every night for 10 minutes.
- I said NO to people and social arrangements when I needed to lay low. I just had to do it for myself.
- I took an adrenal healing herbal formula as recommended by a naturopath.

## MY THYROID HEALING EATING PLAN

I began an anti-inflammatory diet to support my immune function and gut health.

- I had no gluten or dairy for three months.
- I limited brassica vegetables (e.g. cauliflower, broccoli, kale) unless cooked VERY well. Some research suggests that when eaten raw they can leach iodine from the body, which is necessary for thyroid function.
- I eliminated soy products.
- I used lots of herbs and spices in my cooking, such as turmeric, parsley and coriander.
- I had lots of good fats – fish (low-mercury options), avocado, virgin organic coconut oil, nuts, seeds etc. I added olive oil to my foods and drizzled flaxseed oil onto my salads.

- *I ate plenty of antioxidant-rich foods, like berries, greens, nuts, seeds, sweet potatoes etc.*
- *I had protein at every meal – organic and good quality. Tyrosine is an amino acid found in protein that is key in the production of thyroid hormones.*
- *I ate more warming foods as opposed to raw foods.*
- *I had iron-rich foods – lamb, chicken, seeds, lentils, greens etc.*
- *I made concoctions to increase my stomach acid: juice ½ lemon in warm water every morning, and 1 tbsp apple cider vinegar in a glass of water before each meal.*
- *I enjoyed slow-release, gluten-free carbs, like brown rice and sweet potato, which are important for thyroid function.*

## SUPPLEMENTS

Always ask a practitioner for advice – the below are rough guidelines that I did for six months which worked for me. I supplemented with a small amount of iodine (200 mcg) with selenium (150 mcg) as my iodine levels were quite low. Patients who are on thyroid medication may be getting enough iodine through their medication. It is best to supplement according to an iodine urine test. I also took zinc, fish oil, vitamin D, iron and the gut healing supplements on the opposite page.

## CHELATION OF MERCURY

I got my mercury removed via DMPS suppositories. This would only be necessary for people with high mercury. Usually, integrative doctors can do this or recommend a place that does. The suppositories basically bind to the mercury and sweep it out of the body. Alternatively, you can chelate it intravenously. It's not the most pleasant experience (you don't feel great after), but it worked for me.

## THERAPY

Emotionally, I needed to get a grip on my panic and learn how to trust my body again. Old insecurities were starting to arise that I needed to take care of, so I saw a therapist once a week.

## MEDICATION

As mentioned, I'm off all medication while being carefully monitored. My TSH levels are in the correct range, and I feel much better. However, every case is different. I believe thyroid medication that contains both T3 and T4 is best. If you're dealing with a thyroid condition, remember that the doctors will only put you on medication if you really need it, and they'll take you off it if they're confident your body can do its job on its own.

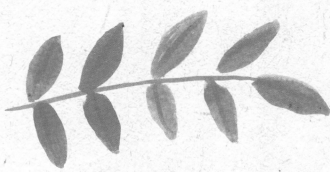

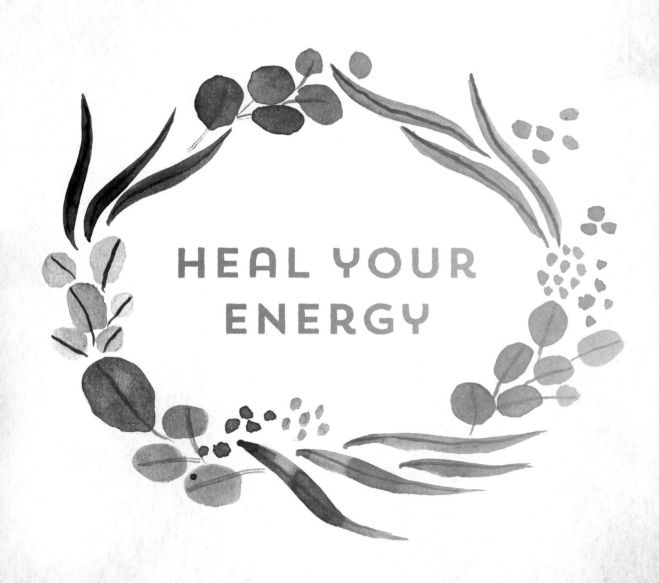

HEAL YOUR ENERGY

*Your body is always talking to you. You just have to stop and listen. When I ask my clients how they are, most of the time the response is, 'Good. But exhausted.' When you feel tired, everything feels hard. You feel heavy. Life is quite literally a drag. There are many reasons why fatigue can creep up on you – here, I'll teach you how to heal those bodily systems for long-lasting energy.*

# GETTING YOUR ENERGY BACK

## Energy and the digestive system

By now, you've probably realised that much of health comes down to digestion. When your digestion is poor, it has a domino effect on the rest of your body. Basically, your digestive system takes the food you have eaten and metabolises it to give you energy. The small intestine gets to work funnelling those nutrients into the bloodstream so your body can use them as fuel. You know how you feel human again after eating a meal when you're starving? That's the principle at work. The problem is many of us aren't digesting our food well enough for our bodies to extract those nutrients for energy. Processed foods and refined carbs have become staples in modern-day diets. They're making our digestive systems sluggish and leaving us with that 'heavy' feeling in our stomachs. In addition, the microbiome (gut bacteria) has a huge impact on energy.

The aim is to eat foods that produce good bacteria, keeping the gut happy and healthy. Refined foods, sugar and alcohol all do their best to eat away at the good bacteria in the gut, leaving us with an imbalance. That's why I recommend adding lots of greens to your diet, ensuring you get enough fibre, and popping a probiotic every day (with the guidance of a health practitioner). Doing this will give your gut a hit of good bacteria, and help to bring it back into balance. (See page 52 for more on this.) Also see the Energy Meal Plan on the next page to see if it makes a difference.

### NEED A BURST OF ENERGY RIGHT NOW?

Try cutting out sugar and gluten for a trial period of four weeks. For many people, it's the biggest energy zapper there is. See page 98 for alternatives.

## Energy and the adrenals

We live in a fast-paced, stressful world, so it's not surprising that many of us are low in energy. But when we're tired for a long period of time, the damage goes further than just making us feel sleepy or cranky. Our adrenal gland function can be compromised, sending us into what is known as 'adrenal fatigue', which is a deep, deep fatigue. You feel like you need to sleep all the time. You wake up tired. You often get a second wave of energy at around 11 pm. Exercise is the last thing on your mind. Your happiness and motivation diminishes. And your sleeping patterns become erratic – you sometimes wake up at 2 am, or 4 am, or maybe both. You crave salty and sugary foods more than ever. Your appetite decreases, but when you're hungry, you'll overeat or binge. Your weight can become harder to manage. You are irritable – even though you don't mean to be.

There are some simple habits you can adopt to 'nourish' your adrenal glands and keep them functioning properly.

Limit your caffeine intake to one per day – preferably before 10 am and never after 3 pm. Commit to regular breathing practices. Get eight hours of sleep, and try to be in bed by 10 pm. Reduce or cut your sugar intake. Ask your nutritionist/naturopath to prescribe some delicious adrenal tonics – they do wonders!

## Energy and the thyroid

When your thyroid function slows down, you'll feel deeply tired – as if someone has turned off the light switch. If you're dealing with low energy and suspect your thyroid may be to blame, ask your doctor to test your thyroid levels and especially your T3 levels. (See page 36 for more on this.)

## Other factors that affect energy

There are many other lifestyle factors that can affect your energy levels. Tailoring your exercise habits to suit your lifestyle is important. My advice is to exercise for energy, not until exhaustion. In my opinion, less is more. As always, you need to tune in to your body to find out what works for you. If high intensity interval training energises you, go for it! If you finish yoga feeling on top of the world, do a few classes a week. Listen to your body, and give it what it needs. You'll have fewer stress hormones pumping through your body, and more energy. (See page 80 for my thoughts on exercise.)

Your emotions may play a part. If you're feeling fatigued, reflect on who you're surrounding yourself with. To be healthy and happy, it's really important to spend time with people who lift you higher, not drain the living daylights out of you. (See page 90 for more on this.)

### VITAMINS FOR ENERGY

With the guidance of a health practitioner, these supplements may be useful in boosting your energy:

- *B complex*
- *Magnesium – it's also fantastic for supporting stress*
- *Iron (get your iron levels checked first)*
- *Zinc*
- *Fish oil and/or flaxseed oil.*

Nutrition may be a factor, too. Eat a wholesome, balanced diet with good iron levels to give you all the energy you need to live a healthy, healed life. Check out page 96 for a complete nutrition plan – it's all about going back to basics and fuelling your body with the foods it needs to survive and thrive.

A healthy liver is vital to maintain blood-sugar levels, metabolise carbs, fats and proteins, store vitamins and minerals, regulate hormones and eliminate toxins. When the liver is clogged up thanks to things like alcohol, caffeine, sugar, pollution or medications, it can't do its job properly.

And that toxic build-up can make you feel awful. Fatigue is a common symptom of an overworked liver. For high-energy levels, your liver needs to be working optimally. To figure out if your liver needs a good cleanse, check out page 58.

Last but not least, are you getting enough sleep? Prioritise quality sleep for better energy levels. We all know how refreshed we feel after a good night's sleep, and that should be the norm. Flick to page 60 for the lowdown on sleeping soundly.

# MY ENERGY MEAL PLAN

*See the following page for my 7-day energy boosting meal plan. See page 96 for my recommended serving sizes. The golden rules for eating for energy are:*

- *Avoid all gluten (except oats) for four weeks.*
- *If you feel tired after eating eggs, cut them out for now.*
- *Enjoy good fats at every meal, such as avocado (stick to ½ per day), nuts, seeds, olive oil, virgin organic coconut oil and tahini.*
- *Don't be afraid of good carbs but stick to gluten-free, if possible.*
- *Include protein in each meal.*

- *Make some breakfast bars (pages 164–7) and bliss balls (pages 266–9) each week. You will be prepared with wholesome snacks that will lift your energy when you need it.*
- *Stick to one coffee per day max. Have it before 10 am and drink it with or after food.*
- *Eat good quality grass-fed and organic red meat twice a week to maintain your iron levels.*
- *Give up refined sugar and artificial sweeteners. Use stevia or cinnamon to sweeten your food instead.*

# ENERGY MEAL PLAN

| | MONDAY | TUESDAY | WEDNESDAY |
|---|---|---|---|
| **EXERCISE**<br>Listen to your body. Try jogging, yoga, Pilates, walking, interval training or weight training. Remember to mix it up and allow 1–2 rest days every week. | 30 minutes of your favourite exercise. | Rest day or 30 minutes of your favourite exercise. | 30 minutes of your favourite exercise. |
| **BREAKFAST**<br>A good time to have your one daily coffee with or after food. | JSHealth Protein Smoothie (see page 147). | Apple Pie Oats (see page 152). | Cinnamon, Cardamom & Orange Zest Bircher Muesli (see page 148). |
| **MID-MORNING SNACK**<br>A good time to have a fresh, fruit-free green juice. | Breakfast bar (see pages 164–7). | Green apple with a smear of almond or peanut butter and a sprinkle of cinnamon. | A handful of raw almonds. |
| **LUNCH** | Pesto Chicken Bowl with Broccoli & Pumpkin Seeds (see page 184). | Energy Chop Chop Salad (see page 185) with fish, chicken, lentils or egg. | Brown Rice Bowl with Smoked Trout & Avocado (see page 184). |
| **MID-AFTERNOON SNACK** | Choc Cinnamon Yoghurt (see page 262). | 2 bliss balls (see pages 266–9). | JSHealth Protein Smoothie (see page 147) without fruit. |
| **DINNER** | Lemon Herb Fish in a Bag (see page 227) with Coconut & Rosemary Wedges (see page 240). | Green Detox Soup (see page 196) and Healthy BBQ Chicken (see page 210) with sautéed broccoli/kale. | Shredded Chicken San Choy Bau (see page 224). |
| **SUPPER** | Caffeine-free herbal tea of your choice.<br>2 pieces of 85 % dark chocolate (optional but avoid if you are sensitive to cacao/caffeine). | Caffeine-free herbal tea of your choice. | Caffeine-free herbal tea of your choice. |
| **SYMPTOMS / EMOTIONS**<br>How is your energy? | | | |

*Lemon Herb Fish in a Bag (see page 227)*

HEAL YOUR ENERGY

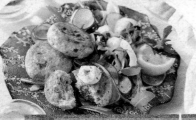

Salmon & Quinoa Cakes with Lemon
& Tahini Yoghurt (see page 228)

| THURSDAY | FRIDAY | SATURDAY | SUNDAY |
| --- | --- | --- | --- |
| 30 minutes of your favourite exercise. | 30 minutes of your favourite exercise. | 30 minutes of your favourite exercise. | Great for a rest day or some light yoga stretches in your living room. Remember to sleep more – no guilt attached! |
| JSHealth Protein Smoothie (see page 147). | Tahini Banana Granola Toast (see page 160) or a Choc Tahini Energy Bar (see page 166) if you're on the go. | 1–2 slices Gluten-free Green Bread (see page 156) with 1–2 poached or boiled eggs and sautéed spinach/kale. | Chia, Blueberry & Banana Breakfast Muffin (see page 143). |
| Breakfast bar (see pages 164–7). | Carrot and cucumber sticks with 2 tablespoons hummus or tahini. | 120 g berries with a sprinkle of cinnamon. | A handful of raw almonds. |
| Chop Chop Tuna Salad (see page 185) with dressing of choice (see pages 294–7). | Salmon & Quinoa Cakes with Lemon & Tahini Yoghurt (see page 228). | Thai-style Fried 'Rice' (see page 247). | Brown Rice Bowl with Smoked Trout & Avocado (see page 184). |
| 100–200 g Greek-style or coconut milk yoghurt with cinnamon and stevia. §§ Top with crushed almonds. | 2 brown rice cakes with a smear of almond butter or tahini and a sprinkle of cinnamon. | Carrot and cucumber sticks with 2 tablespoons hummus or tahini. | 2 bliss balls (see pages 266–9). |
| Chilli & Rosemary Steak with Sautéed Greens (see page 227). | Chicken & Ginger Stir-fry (see page 210) with brown rice or quinoa. | Bolognese with Zoodles (see page 212) with sautéed greens of choice and/or quinoa (optional). | Thai-style Fried 'Rice' (see page 247) with grilled chicken or fish and sautéed greens of choice. |
| Caffeine-free herbal tea of your choice. | Caffeine-free herbal tea of your choice. | Caffeine-free herbal tea of your choice. A gluten- and dairy-free sweet treat (see pages 248–87) or 2 pieces of 85 % dark chocolate. | Caffeine-free herbal tea of your choice. |

Cinnamon, Cardamom & Orange
Zest Bircher Muesli (see page 148)

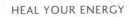

HEAL YOUR ENERGY

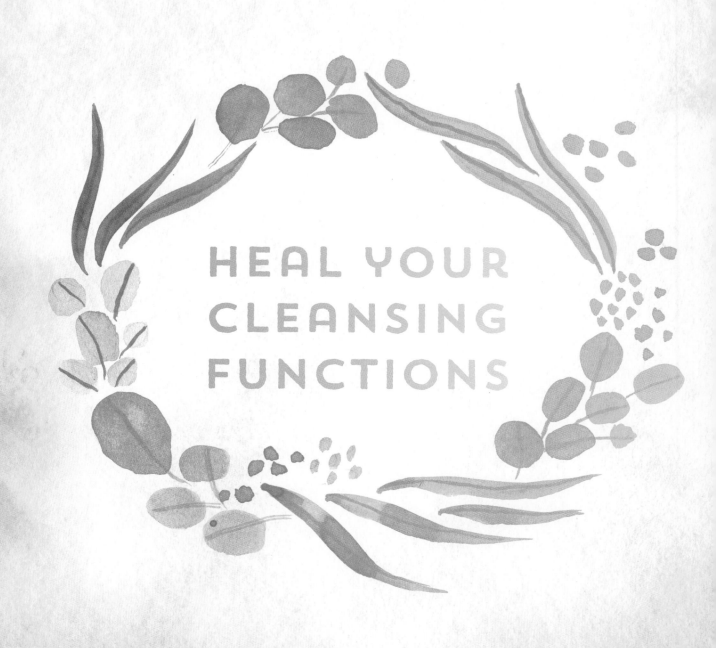

HEAL YOUR CLEANSING FUNCTIONS

*The gut and liver are the two MOST important organs when it comes to healing your body. A healthy gut is the cornerstone to overall health, and a healthy liver equals a 'clean' body.*

*While our body naturally cleanses itself, it does need help every now and then. Thanks to the modern-day environment, we are dealing with a higher toxic load than ever before: think pollution, heightened stress and processed foods. This puts pressure on our bodies' organs, and sometimes we need to step in and help move things along.*

## YOUR DIGESTIVE SYSTEM

Your digestion indicates the state of your health, and also determines how well your body can heal. This is because your gut is where you absorb the necessary nutrients for your body to function and flourish. If there are blockages or issues with your gut, your body won't get the proper fuel it needs.

As a nutritionist, it's frustrating to see just how many people are struggling with gut health. Clients come into my clinic and complain about being bloated, constipated, having irregular bowel movements, or dealing with reflux. They feel like they can't eat anything without having some sort of reaction. Poor digestion can lead to a host of health issues like exhaustion and even adrenal fatigue. Plus, digestive issues cause stress, which causes more digestive issues. It's a vicious cycle.

The first step to healing your gut is undertaking a 4-week gut cleanse. It will involve tweaking your diet and the way you cook a little. Are you ready to feel lighter? Clearer? More energetic? This will help.

For the next four weeks, eliminate the following from your diet:

- Gluten.
- Dairy.
- Refined sugar – including healthy sweeteners like honey. See below for natural sweeteners to enjoy.
- Chewing gum. It can really unsettle your stomach, not to mention bloat you like crazy!
- Soft drinks – including diet soft drinks.
- Artificial sweeteners. They are toxic to the body.
- All processed foods – anything out of a packet.

And here's what you can enjoy in your 4-week cleanse:

- Olive oil, virgin organic coconut oil, ghee. They are soothing for the gut.
- Herbs and spices – think turmeric, cumin, parsley, coriander and mint.
- Warming foods – soups, casseroles and slow-cooked foods are all winners.
- Protein at every meal.
- Prebiotic- and probiotic-rich foods. Eating apple cider vinegar, kombucha and fermented foods is the easiest way to do this. I add 2 tablespoons of fermented veggies to my dinner daily.
- Greens, greens, and more greens! They are the most cleansing foods out there.
- Berries, papaya and lemons are the best fruits for gut healing. Limit to two serves a day.
- Natural sweeteners – cinnamon, vanilla and stevia.
- Good fats.

Other tips:

- Eat fruit on an empty stomach only. First thing in the morning or as a mid-morning snack is best.
- Drink in between meals, not with meals.
- Only eat raw food during the day. So that means no salad with dinner – go for cooked veggies instead. Cooked foods can be easier to digest when your gut is strained.
- Eat slowly and mindfully. Flick to page 21 to learn how to be a mindful eater.
- If your digestion is poor, consider supplementing your cleanse. (See opposite page.)
- Oats – soaked and cooked for optimum digestion.
- Slippery elm, flaxseed and chia seeds.
- Organic dairy – only if you digest lactose well.
- High-fibre foods: fruit, vegetables, legumes, oats, chia seeds, flaxseed and psyllium husk.

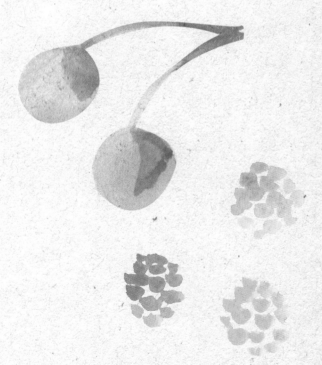

## Gut healing supplements

With the help of a health practitioner, think about aiding your cleanse with these supplements.

- *Glutamine powder – I like to add this to my smoothies to help reduce bloating and promote overall gut health.*

- *Multi-strain probiotics – including Saccharomyces boulardii.*

- *Fish oil.*

- *Turmeric.*

- *Aloe vera juice.*

- *Digestive enzymes – these will help your body to break down food properly.*

## How does dieting affect your digestion?

One of my biggest gripes with diets is they often eliminate good fats, which are necessary for your body to absorb nutrients from food. Yes, really! They also lubricate the digestive tract, making it easier for food to move through it smoothly. That's why people on low-fat diets tend to suffer on the digestive front, particularly with constipation.

Eat good fats in moderation, but do eat them. Repeat after me: fat is not the devil!

### A NOTE ON PROBIOTICS

Before popping any probiotics, I recommend a full gut profile test. There are so many strains of probiotics on the market, and this test will determine the status of your gut bacteria so you'll know which strains you need more or less of.

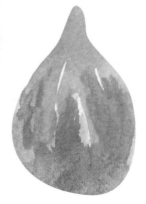
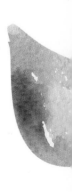

## Tips to reduce bloating

- Cut out gluten, sugar and refined dairy – they can be difficult to digest and cause bloating. Give them up and you'll soon see and feel the difference.

- Drink lemon water each morning, or a shot of apple cider vinegar before meals – this kickstarts the metabolism and produces healthy stomach acid, both of which can reduce bloating.

- Avoid diet drinks, soft drinks and fizzy alcoholic drinks. Bubbles = bloating!

- Take digestive enzymes with each meal.

- Eat papaya each morning – it contains an enzyme that soothes the digestive system.

- Eat fruit on an empty stomach only. If you eat it after other food, it may cause gas.

## What to avoid if you suffer from reflux

- Acidic foods and drinks – such as oranges, tea and coffee.

- Alcohol – especially wine.

- Chocolate, spearmint and peppermint.

- Carbonated drinks.

- Garlic and onions.

- High-fat foods, including full-fat milk.

- Gluten grains, such as wheat, rye, barley and processed oats. Big one!

## Try these to keep you 'regular'

- Take magnesium citrate/glycinate every night before bed. I love to use a product called Natural Vitality, Natural Calm magnesium. It is vegan and well-absorbed.

- Sip on strong chamomile tea (two teabags in hot water) before bed – it relaxes the digestive tract.

- Enjoy 1–2 tablespoons chia seeds daily – I like to throw them into smoothies or make a chia pudding.

- Add 1–2 tablespoons psyllium husk to your smoothies or take it in supplement form (your dosage should be guided by a health practitioner).

- Squeeze lemon into your water to increase stomach acid and boost digestion.

- Deal with your stress. (See page 30 for more on this.)

- Eat more fibre – think leafy greens, brown rice, oats, beans and legumes.

- Drink my fibre tonic on page 306.

### FUN FACT

Banana can be one of the main culprits of constipation. If you're backed up, try cutting it out for a couple of days.

- *Avoid white and refined carbs.*
- *Try acupuncture – it works a treat.*

## The lowdown on candida overgrowth

Candida overgrowth. It's something many people suffer from, but rarely talk about. Candida is a fungus that's actually brilliant for the body – in proper amounts, that is. Everyone has it. It helps with digestion and nutrient absorption, but when it grows out of control it can break down intestinal walls and get into the bloodstream, with toxic results. This can, in turn, cause leaky gut syndrome and a bunch of other health issues. You can't see candida overgrowth, but it has plenty of symptoms. I've seen many of them in my clinic, including bloating and gas, autoimmune conditions, low energy and thrush.

Here are my top nutritional tips to kill candida:

- *Candida thrives on sugar, so you have to starve the bug for four to six weeks, minimum. Eliminate all refined sugar, sweeteners and dairy, and limit fruit to one serve of berries per day. See page 105 for alternatives.*
- *Enjoy bitter foods like lemon, grapefruit, rocket, radicchio lettuce and dandelion. These help to combat sweet cravings.*
- *Cut out alcohol for four weeks. It's not easy I know, but the results will be worth it.*
- *Take cleansing herbs with guidance from a naturopath. Oregano, garlic, Chinese wormwood and black walnuts are really great at killing candida.*
- *Use Saccharomyces boulardii probiotics for four to six weeks under the guidance of your health practitioner.*
- *Eat fermented foods daily (1–2 tablespoons with each meal). Most health-food shops sell them or you can make your own.*
- *Add a few drops of grapefruit seed extract to your water, or take it as a supplement. It acts as an anti-microbial in the body.*

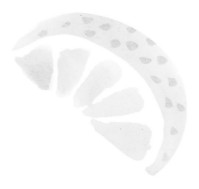

# HEALING YOUR LIVER

When the digestive system is strained, it automatically puts pressure on the liver. That's why you need to heal them together.

Your liver is in charge of detoxifying your body. It's great at flushing out what is no longer needed. That's why I don't really believe in harsh or extreme detox trends. That being said, I've found that when I'm feeling a little rundown or tired, a short-term cleanse gets me back on track to feeling my best. So here's what I do believe in: seasonal cleansing. I believe that when we give our liver a break from certain foods, drinks and environmental stress for a period of time, our body heals faster. Energy and motivation return in huge bursts. Find out for yourself with my 3-day liver reboot which I do every two months.

For three days in a row (usually Monday to Thursday morning), eliminate sugar (even natural kinds), alcohol, red meat, caffeine, dairy and anything processed. Eat lightly and cleanly for these three days. Tune in to your stress levels and try to reduce them even more. (See page 30 for more on this.) Focus on consuming:

* *Greens at every meal!*
* *Veggie-based green juices.*
* *Lots of warming soups.*
* *Coconut water.*
* *Wholesome grains (preferably gluten-free): brown rice, oats, quinoa.*
* *White fish and wild salmon.*
* *Beans and legumes (like lentils).*
* *Low-sugar fruits: berries, lemon, green apples, grapefruit, papaya.*
* *Root vegetables: sweet potato, pumpkin, beetroot.*
* *Nut and coconut milks in moderate amounts.*

* *Good oils: virgin organic coconut oil and olive oil.*
* *All herbs and spices – the more the merrier! Parsley, turmeric and coriander are the most cleansing of the lot.*
* *Wholesome condiments: lemon juice, organic Dijon mustard, tahini, tamari.*
* *Himalayan pink rock salt and ground black pepper.*
* *Organic eggs and chicken.*
* *Drink 2 litres of filtered water a day, but not at meals.*
* *Dandelion root tea or herbal teas of your choice instead of coffee.*
* *Sparkling water, or lemon or coconut water instead of diet soft drinks.*

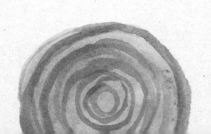

Boost the results of your cleanse with the help of these cleansing vitamin supplements. (Ask a practitioner for guidance on the right dosage for you).

- *Liver tonic – with milk thistle, dandelion root, turmeric, amino acids, brassica sprout powder (really powerful) and so on. (Most health-food shops sell good tonics)*
- *I normally ask my naturopath to make liver herbs in liquid form for me.*
- *Magnesium oxide, magnesium citrate/glycinate (before bed).*
- *Psyllium husk (1–2 tablespoons/day with lots of liquid, or throw it into smoothies).*
- *Chlorophyll in water – sip throughout the day.*
- *Grapefruit seed extract in water.*

## An ideal day on the 3-day Liver Reboot:

### BREAKFAST

Slim-Down Tonic (see page 306).

Protein smoothie with rice/pea protein, berries, greens, stevia, ground cinnamon, ice and almond milk
OR fresh papaya drizzled with lime and a dollop of coconut milk yoghurt, sprinkled with ground cinnamon and homemade sugar-free granola/mixed seeds
OR poached eggs with sautéed greens and avocado.

### SNACK

Carrot sticks with hummus
OR a handful of raw nuts
OR a small bowl of berries
OR a fresh green juice (no fruit).

### LUNCH

Salmon, avocado and quinoa salad
OR a brown rice bowl with pesto and a poached/boiled egg.

### SNACK

Celery sticks with almond butter/ hummus
OR brown rice cakes smeared with almond butter and a sprinkle of ground cinnamon or smashed avo and rock salt.

### DINNER

Green Detox Soup (see page 196).

Grilled fish, tempeh or lentils with sautéed greens of choice.

### AFTER DINNER

A herbal tea of choice.

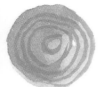
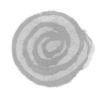
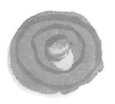

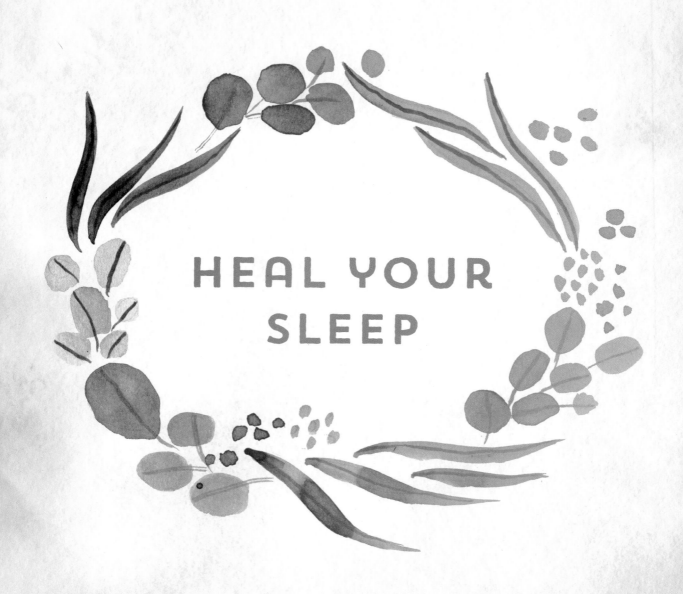

HEAL YOUR
SLEEP

*Getting more sleep is the simplest and easiest way to heal your body. We all know how amazing we feel after a good night's sleep: energised, refreshed, clear and ready to take on the day. Getting quality sleep accelerates healing; it's the body's time to repair and recharge without distractions.*

# OPTIMISING YOUR SLEEP

There are many diet and lifestyle factors that may be preventing you from getting a good night's sleep.

- *You're consuming caffeine in the afternoon – this includes coffee, green tea and black tea.*

- *You're drinking alcohol, such as red wine, which revs up the liver in the lead-up to bedtime.*

- *You're eating refined sugar, or not enough protein, at dinnertime.*

- *You're highly stressed and your mind is full of thoughts, or you suffer from anxiety.*

- *Your pituitary gland is not functioning as well as it should, meaning your hormones are unbalanced.*

- *You're exercising at night, and going to bed with adrenaline coursing through your veins.*

- *Your room is too noisy, bright or warm.*

- *Your face is glued to screens right up until the time you go to bed.*

- *You're on too much thyroid medication. (See page 36 for more on this.)*

- *You're taking fat-burning supplements (e.g. green tea extract powders).*

Basically, all of these things stimulate the body or brain at a time when they should be preparing for rest.

## TOO MUCH COFFEE?

A year ago, I increased my caffeine intake to two coffees a day as an experiment, and I started waking up at random times during the night. See, that first coffee perked me up for the day, but the afternoon coffee gave me a second wind of energy when I didn't need it: at night. This is a common scenario, yet many people can't understand why their sleep is broken. If you're drinking more than one coffee a day, try cutting back and try consuming coffee only in the morning.

# Now, onto the fun part: solutions!

❋ Starting from right now, you need to prioritise sleep. Do whatever you can to get into bed at a decent time (say 10 pm) so that you can sleep for at least seven to eight hours. If you have to wake up early the next day, make an effort to turn the lights off a little earlier than usual the night before.

❋ At night, you need to relax and unwind, signalling to the mind and body that it's almost time for bed. To do that, set up a nightly routine full of deliciously sleep-provoking rituals. In the hour or so before bed, dim the lights, put lavender oil on the pillows and light a candle or burn essential oils. Keep a notepad on your bedside table and jot down any pesky thoughts that come into your mind while you're trying to wind down. Take away computers and distractions so the room is a technology-free zone, and ensure the room temperature is comfortable. Ideally, your bedroom should be dark and cool.

❋ Restorative yoga can do wonders for relaxing the mind (and slowing down that never-ending thought stream). If you can't get to a class, that's okay – just lay out a mat or towel in your living room and hold a few poses. I use doyogawithme.com online classes.

❋ Chat to a health practitioner about taking supplements to help you sleep. Magnesium citrate or glycinate or zinc may help. Adrenal tonics with calming herbs – like passionflower, magnolia and withania – can also be beneficial. If you're still struggling to sleep, melatonin may also be an option.

## FOOD AND SLEEP

The connection between food and sleep is real. Here are the dos and don'ts:

### DO

❋ Eat protein at night. This can really help with sleep and blood-sugar regulation.

❋ Consume good fats to balance out your hormones (see page 99).

❋ Give your liver some loving (see page 58).

### DON'T

❋ Drink alcohol before bed. This is particularly important if you're waking up in the middle of the night – that's your liver shouting at you.

❋ Consume cacao if you're struggling with sleep. It's fine to have a little in your healthy sweet treats, but don't go overboard.

❋ Eat refined sugar – even fruit after midday – it spikes your blood sugar, which can disrupt sleep.

## HELP! I WOKE UP AND NOW I CAN'T GET BACK TO SLEEP

The worst thing you can do is lie there, counting sheep, watching the clock, trying desperately to fall asleep. That just causes more anxiety and restlessness. You need to get up and do something. Try the following tips:

- *Put your legs up against the wall for 10 minutes while breathing deeply.*

- *Go into a forward fold.*

- *Warm up some almond or coconut milk with ground cinnamon and sip it slowly.*

- *Write down any thoughts in that notepad by your bed.*

- *Listen to some calming music or a sleep podcast.*

- *Do what's called 'yoga nidra'. Lie down and breathe while focusing on each body part, working from your toes up to your head.*

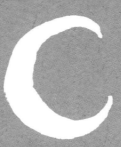

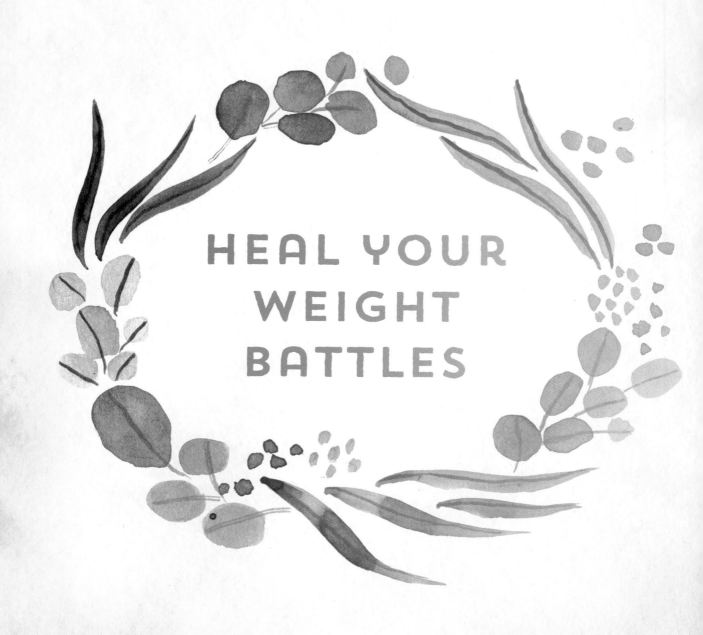

HEAL YOUR WEIGHT BATTLES

*Embrace a wholesome diet (without extremes) and your healthiest, natural weight will follow. Nourish and strengthen your body to arrive at a balanced weight that is right for you. This isn't about crazy weight loss or reaching your 'goal'. It's about finding a sweet spot that you can sustain without stress.*

# ENDING THE BODY BATTLE

So many of us battle our bodies to achieve our 'goal weight'. I see so many beautiful, strong, healthy people obsessing about those 'extra' two kilos that they think they need to lose. So many of my clients have been caught in a tormenting cycle of dieting. If there were a diet that worked perfectly, we would all be on it, right? And weight wouldn't be such a huge issue like it is for so many of us. But there isn't a 'perfect diet' that suits one and all, and the diet mentality needs to stop.

It's time for us all to embrace and accept our bodies and our weight and let go of the battle for perfection. The first step in healing your weight battles is to accept and love your body and stop fighting it. Throw out the scales. Stop thinking about your weight as an arbitrary number because we are all unique. Make your aim a healthy, strong body and mind. As long as your weight is relatively stable and in a healthy range, just let it be. Changing your mindset around your weight is difficult and might be confronting but it really is the key to a healthier you. (See page 14 for more on starting the process of healing.)

If you are beginning your health journey and your weight is significantly above a healthy range, I have compiled some tips for healthy weight management. But keep in mind that, as you embrace a healthy, balanced way of eating and lifestyle, your weight will naturally balance out anyway.

## BE REALISTIC ABOUT YOUR WEIGHT GOALS

You are not going to be the same weight you were when you were 16. Your body is a little older now. Perhaps you are at an age when you are getting ready to have kids or perhaps you are going through menopause. Your body is changing to cater for those needs. Start adjusting your weight goals. Be kinder to yourself.

## 'Calories in vs calories out' is BS

All calories are not created equal. Instead of counting calories, we need to focus on the *quality* of calories. Where are the calories coming from? Our bodies burn calories from wholefoods far better than they do those from processed 'fake' foods.

How your body burns energy depends on a range of factors: your hormones, stress levels, blood sugar, thyroid function, genes and more. We are all biochemically unique. We're not robots with the exact same machinery. The way I burn off a slice of cake is very different to how you would burn it off because we are all different. That's why I don't buy into the calorie-counting game. It doesn't make sense and adds stress to your body. One diet doesn't fit all, and one calorie calculator doesn't fit all either! If you've got the app on your phone – delete it. And nourish, fuel and listen to your body instead. You have all the tools you need within you.

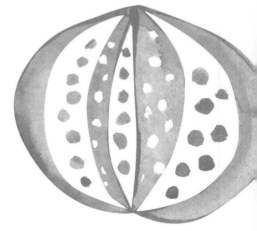

## Natural eating

Eat naturally. Balanced wholefoods, eaten with mindfulness and moderation, is the best way to balance your weight. Remember, dieters think about food all the damn time. They're preoccupied with it, and they have an emotional connection to it.

Natural eaters, on the other hand, don't classify food as 'good' or 'bad'. They simply see it as a source of nourishment. They enjoy eating, but they also know when to stop. They're connected to their body, and they don't play into that whole deprivation game. Because life is for living!

Natural eaters:

- *Eat in tune with their body.*

- *Eat small amounts of everything.*

- *Never deprive themselves but indulge with moderation.*

- *Don't feel guilty after eating.*

- *Don't believe in diets.*

- *Listen to their bodies and exercise moderately.*

*'Calories are NOT created equal. The same number of calories from different types of food can have very different biological effects. If you still think a calorie is just a calorie, maybe this will convince you otherwise. In a study of 154 countries that looked at the correlation between calories, sugar and diabetes, scientists found that adding 150 calories a day to the diet barely raised the risk of diabetes in the population – but if those 150 calories came from soft drinks, the risk of diabetes went up by 700 per cent.'*
– Dr Mark Hyman

# How to eat for healthy weight management

If you are genuinely looking to reduce your weight – for your health, not because of some idea of perfection! – then here are a few suggestions:

- Avoid high-carb or sugar-loaded breakfasts – they often trigger cravings for caffeine or sweets in the afternoon, which can lead to overeating or bingeing. Plus, many people find they're starving an hour or two after eating a sugary breakfast. So cereals and toast with jam are out!

- Eat protein with every meal, especially breakfast. Think eggs, protein shakes, cottage cheese/Greek yoghurt, and nut butters.

- Eliminate gluten-containing foods and all refined white carbs.

- Eat everything in moderation. Small portions are key. I would rather you eat the foods you love in small amounts than deprive yourself.

- Fill up half your plate with greens at every meal.

- Consume enough fibre to keep you feeling fuller for longer and to flush out excess oestrogen. Good sources include psyllium husk, chia seeds, oats, beans and legumes. You could also supplement with Glucomannan powder.

- Include a portion of fat with your lunch to balance your blood sugar. Avocado, seeds, tahini, olive oil and hummus are great options.

- Eat regular meals to avoid overeating.

- Enjoy alcohol only on special occasions or weekends.

- Be careful with overeating nuts. Nuts can actually slow down digestion and energy for some. My recommendation is no more than 4 tablespoons of nuts a day.

- Eat more foods from the brassica vegetable family (like broccoli and kale) as they help clear excess oestrogen from the body. Be sure to cook them well! Alternatively, consider using a broccoli sprout powder – you can find this at health-food shops.

- Avoid all refined vegetable oils. Replace with olive oil or virgin organic coconut oil.

- Give up sugar, for life. I recommend Sarah Wilson's I Quit Sugar program. My nutrition plan will also help you find sugar alternatives. (For tips on banishing sugar cravings, see page 105.)

- Avoid carb-heavy foods at dinnertime – you just don't need a burst of energy when you're winding down your day.

- Only eat organic chicken and meat.

- Be mindful when eating out. (See page 112 for more of my tips on eating out.)

- Ask your healthcare professional for guidance with these supplements: B complex, fish oil, fibre blends, probiotics, and thyroid support formula containing zinc, iodine and selenium.

## Gut health and inflammation

One of the first steps in trying to manage your weight is to heal your gut. You need to absorb the nutrients from food to allow your body to function effectively. Many people are not digesting and absorbing their food because of a compromised digestive system. This impacts the metabolism and energy levels.

When you eat processed foods, sugar and alcohol on a regular basis, you're feeding the bad bacteria in your gut. In particular, antibiotics and alcohol mess up the gut micro flora, as do artificial additives and preservatives. This imbalance of good and bad bacteria influences metabolism.

If you're struggling to lose weight, it could be due to inflammation, which can be caused by stress, environmental toxins, autoimmune conditions, gut issues, food and medications. You need to tackle inflammation holistically, by looking at your stress, diet, lifestyle and gut health. Start by healing your gut as on page 54 and giving up sugar and gluten.

## Exercise is a key part of weight management – just not too much.

From clinical and personal experience, I can tell you that over-exercising can do more harm to your weight than good. When you work out too much, your cortisol levels can spike if you don't balance your body out with rest. Then when you stress about working out your cortisol levels increase too. And high cortisol makes it harder for you to burn off fat. It's too busy trying to balance out your parasympathetic and sympathetic nervous systems.

That's where rest comes in. A rested body is a healthy body – and it is incredibly important to commit to resting daily. When it comes to weight loss, studies show that 20–30 minutes of high intensity interval training three to four times a week is effective. But most importantly, do what works for YOU. I believe yoga is brilliant for weight balance as it relaxes the nervous system. Make your focus on a strong, rested, healthy body, not a skinny one. See page 80 for more on working out.

### HEALTHY GUT FLORA

A new study in the *Journal of Biological Chemistry* found that overweight mice who were given a micro flora transplant from slimmer mice lost weight. The study proved that gut flora can ward off weight gain and diabetes. It makes perfect sense to me: for a healthy, balanced body, your gut needs to be in tip-top shape. So one of the first steps in trying to manage your weight is to heal your gut.

### YOUR LIVER

Your liver is a fat-burning organ. When it's clogged up by substances such as caffeine, alcohol, sugar and processed foods, you will no doubt struggle with your weight. Try my 3-day Liver Reboot on page 59. It's a short and simple cleanse that will do wonders in healing your liver, which in turn will help make your weight much easier to manage.

### YOUR THYROID

Your thyroid is the driver of your metabolism, so if you have an underactive thyroid, you can gain weight. (For more on managing thyroid issues, see Heal Your Thyroid on page 36.)

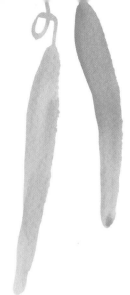

## Balancing your hormones

If you can keep your hormones in check, you're far more likely to be able to maintain a steady weight. Here are a few tips for balancing your hormones:

- *Take care of your stress levels (see page 30). This is the key to restoring hormonal balance.*

- *Cleanse your liver (see page 58). Your liver processes all of your hormones and when it's clogged up from excess alcohol, caffeine or medication, it can cause your hormones to go out of sync.*

- *Cap your coffee intake to one a day, and drink it before 9 am.*

- *Take a break from booze for four weeks, then enjoy it on weekends and special occasions only after that.*

- *Think carefully about which contraception you want to use. Chat to your doctor about your contraceptive choices.*

- *Regulate your insulin and glucose levels for balanced blood sugar.*

- *Check your oestrogen levels. Oestrogen dominance can make it difficult to lose weight. The symptoms include sore/swollen breasts, irritability, fluid retention, low mood, heavy menstrual flow and PMS. If you get tested and discover you have excess oestrogen, decrease it by eating more fibre and brassica veggies (make sure they're cooked well), and taking a 4-week break from dairy or swap to organic dairy.*

- *Normalise your leptin levels. Leptin is an appetite-control hormone that signals to your brain when you're full. Too much insulin can block the leptin hormone, making it easy to overeat. That's why people with high-sugar diets tend to overeat – they literally can't control when to stop. To bring your leptin back into balance, work on eating more protein at each meal. Also, stop eating when you're 80 per cent full (as opposed to stuffed), and wait 20 minutes before reaching for more food.*

- *Be careful with dairy. Swap to organic sources and eat no more than two serves a day.*

- *Work on balancing your thyroid function. (See page 36 for a full lowdown.)*

### SLEEP

You need sufficient sleep for your body to restore, heal and burn fat effectively. Sleep deprivation affects those hormones that control appetite, plus leaves you too tired to make good choices. I get you! Getting eight hours of sleep can really help with weight. (See page 60 for more on this.)

# MY HORMONE BALANCING EATING GUIDE.

*This is my tried-and-tested meal plan to help balance your hormones. Try to commit to this way of eating for 14 days and see how you feel. If you feel amazing – which I think you will – continue this for 30 days.*

- *Avoid processed/packaged food – not good for your hormones!*

- *Swap processed dairy for organic dairy.*

- *Stick to one coffee per day max. Have it before 10 am and drink it with or after food.*

- *Start your day with 30 minutes of exercise, yoga or meditative breathing and drink lemon water or herbal tea – avoid coffee and overly intense exercise as you wake up. Do this for a trial period and see how you feel.*

- *Make sure to have breakfast within an hour of waking.*

- *Don't drink alcohol.*

- *Remove refined sugar for 14 days – and then reduce it altogether for life!*

- *Use free-range organic eggs.*

- *Be strict about including greens in every meal.*

- *Eat only organic poultry and meat.*

- *Eat sustainably caught fish, especially wild salmon – avoid tinned tuna.*

- *Avoid all artificial sweeteners – use stevia liquid or granules, or try cinnamon for flavour.*

- *Drink 2 litres of filtered water each day.*

- *Eat lots of cooked brassica veggies: broccoli, cauliflower, kale, brussels sprouts.*

## LIFE TIPS

*See page 105 to learn how to deal with sugar cravings.*
*If you're too busy for breakfast; make one of my breakfast bars (see pages 164–7) or Bircher muesli the night before (see page 148).*

Enjoy good fats at every meal, such as avocado (stick to ½ per day), nuts, seeds, olive oil, virgin organic coconut oil and tahini.

Avoid all diet/soft drinks.

Have 1 tablespoon of apple cider vinegar mixed in water before each meal as this can lower insulin levels.

Try these supplements: broccoli sprout powder, B complex, zinc, magnesium, fish oil or flaxseed oil — all under the guidance of a health practitioner.

Reduce exercise — focus on yoga, Pilates or walking, and enjoy one or two rest days each week. Avoid boot camp, spinning or intense workouts for 21 days.

Get lots of rest — just see how amazing you start to feel.

Avoid eating from plastic containers. Use stainless steel containers or glass jars.

Swap refined vegetable oils for olive oil or virgin organic coconut oil.

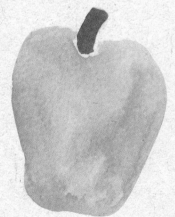

## SERVING SIZES
### (SEE PAGES 102 AND 103 FOR MORE):

Protein: about 150–200 g of fish/chicken/meat/Greek yoghurt

Good fat: 1–2 tablespoons

Good carbs: a fist size

At every meal, your plate should be ½ greens and veggies, ¼ protein, ¼ good carbs (or gluten-free whole grains/beans/legumes) and 1–2 tablespoons of good fat.

## PROTEIN REPLACEMENTS FOR VEGANS/VEGETARIANS:

- Lentils
- Chickpeas
- Eggs (for vegetarians)
- Goat's cheese (for vegetarians)
- All beans (add some brown rice to make it a complete protein)
- Tempeh or tofu in small amounts (I prefer you to have tempeh)

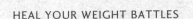

# HORMONE-BALANCING MEAL PLAN

| | MONDAY | TUESDAY | WEDNESDAY |
|---|---|---|---|
| **EXERCISE** | Yoga, Pilates or walking. | Rest day or yin yoga. | 30-minute light jog or interval training. |
| **BREAKFAST** <br> A good time to have your one daily coffee with or after food. | Vegan Breakfast Salad (see page 177) on gluten-free toast or Gluten-free Green Bread (see page 156). | Oatmeal (see page 152) with almond milk topped with mixed seeds, berries and a serve of pea or rice protein powder. | JSHealth Protein Smoothie (see page 147). |
| **MID-MORNING SNACK** <br> A good time to have a fresh, fruit-free green juice. | Carrot and cucumber sticks with 2 tablespoons hummus or tahini. | Green apple with a smear of almond or peanut butter and a sprinkle of cinnamon. | 120 g berries and a handful of pumpkin seeds. |
| **LUNCH** | Brown Rice Bowl with Smoked Trout & Avocado (see page 184). | Shredded Chicken San Choy Bau (see page 224). | Cumin-spiced Lentils with Shaved Brussels Sprouts (see page 202) with grilled chicken or fish. |
| **MID-AFTERNOON SNACK** | A handful of raw nuts and veggie sticks. | Carrot and cucumber sticks with 2 tablespoons hummus or tahini. | Two brown rice cakes with a smear of almond butter or tahini and a sprinkle of cinnamon. |
| **DINNER** | Moroccan Chicken Skewers (see page 210) on broccoli mash and a green salad with a serve of brown rice (optional). | Lemon Herb Fish in a Bag (see page 227) with sautéed garlic greens of choice. | Green Detox Soup (see page 196) and a salmon stir-fry with greens of your choice. |
| **SUPPER** | Decaf chai tea with almond or coconut milk. Sweeten with stevia or cinnamon. | Chamomile tea. <br> 2 pieces of 85% dark chocolate (optional, but avoid if you are sensitive to cacao/caffeine). | Decaf chai tea with almond or coconut milk. Sweeten with stevia or cinnamon. |
| **SYMPTOMS / EMOTIONS** <br> Tell me how you feel. | | | |

Cauliflower, Labneh & Harissa Salad (see page 180)

Green Detox Soup (see page 196)

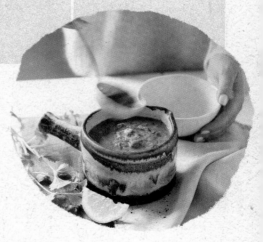

HEAL YOUR WEIGHT BATTLES

| THURSDAY | FRIDAY | SATURDAY | SUNDAY |
|---|---|---|---|
| Yoga, Pilates or walking. | Rest day or yin yoga. | 30-minute walk in nature. | Yoga. |
| Gluten-free Green Bread (see page 156) with 1–2 poached or boiled eggs and sautéed spinach or kale. | Mum's Coconut & Mango Chia Overnight Oats (see page 153). | Vegan Breakfast Salad (see page 177) on gluten-free toast or Gluten-free Green Bread (see page 156). | Avocado Asparagus Toast (see page 160) with a poached or boiled egg. |
| 2 bliss balls (see pages 266–9). | Green apple with a smear of almond or peanut butter and a sprinkle of cinnamon. | A handful of raw almonds and veggie sticks. | 2 bliss balls (see pages 266–9). |
| Energy Chop Chop Salad (see page 185) with fish, chicken or egg. | Pesto Chicken Bowl with Broccoli & Pumpkin Seeds (see page 184). | Cauliflower, Labneh & Harissa Salad (see page 180) without labneh, with chicken and ¼–⅓ avocado and dressing of choice (see pages 294–7). | San Choy Bau (see page 224) with tuna. |
| Carrot and cucumber sticks with 2 tablespoons hummus or tahini. | A handful of raw nuts and veggie sticks. | JSHealth Protein Smoothie (see page 147) without fruit. | 2 brown rice cakes with a smear of almond butter or tahini and a sprinkle of cinnamon. |
| San Choy Bau (see page 224) with mince or lentils. | Bolognese with Zoodles (see page 212). Swap mince for chicken, fish, or lentils, if desired. | Fish with Baked Asparagus (see page 221). | Cajun-spiced salmon with Crispy Brussels by Cayley (see page 238) and a green salad. Or a green veggie omelette for a lazy Sunday dinner. |
| Peppermint tea. | Chamomile tea. 2 pieces of 85% dark chocolate. | Decaf chai tea with almond or coconut milk. Sweeten with stevia or cinnamon. | Peppermint tea. |

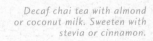

*Decaf chai tea with almond or coconut milk. Sweeten with stevia or cinnamon.*

*Mum's Coconut & Mango Chia Overnight Oats (see page 153)*

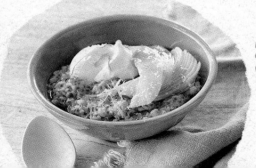

HEAL YOUR WEIGHT BATTLES

# What about weight gain?

There is so much focus on weight loss, with little attention on those who need to put on weight. I thought it would be useful to include some weight-gain tips here.

Firstly, you need to uncover why you are underweight and struggling to reach a healthy weight. Are you nutrient deficient? Do you have a low appetite? Perhaps you have a complicated relationship with food and have taken dieting too far? Or maybe you have a medical condition that makes gaining weight hard? All of these potential issues must be taken seriously. I encourage you to seek professional help from a therapist, doctor or nutritionist to help you to identify your weight issues. If you have anorexia or bulimia, you most definitely need professional advice – this book is not enough.

Once you have identified what's behind your inability to gain weight, begin adding the required nutrients to your diet. The goal is to gain weight by eating wholesome and nutritious foods. No calorie-counting allowed.

Skinny and emaciated is not the goal – healthy and glowing is.

## TIPS FOR GAINING WEIGHT IN A HEALTHY WAY

- *Add more good fats (avocado, nuts, organic dairy), oils (coconut and olive oil) and wholegrains (sourdough, rye or Ezekiel breads) to your diet – your body needs these to heal.*

- *Eat protein at each and every meal, such as eggs, oily fish or meat. If you're struggling to do this, invest in a high-quality protein powder without the nasty additives. A nutritionist can help you with this.*

- *Don't skip meals or snacks. I recommend two snacks every day, plus a small dessert after dinner.*

- *When it comes to exercising, take it slow. If you're underweight, over-exercising is counterproductive.*

- *Enjoy rest days, and when you need to exercise for your mind, choose brisk walking or yoga. No running, spinning or strength training until you reach a healthy weight.*

- *Avoid anything 'fat-free' or 'low-fat' – they are not the healthiest options.*

- *Enjoy slow-cooked meats such as lamb.*

- *Have a designated treat every day. It can be a healthy treat. For example, dark/raw cacao chocolate, banana nice-cream, one or two slices of my healthy banana bread, a muffin topped with almond butter, nutella bliss balls, some good-quality gelato or a couple of brownies.*

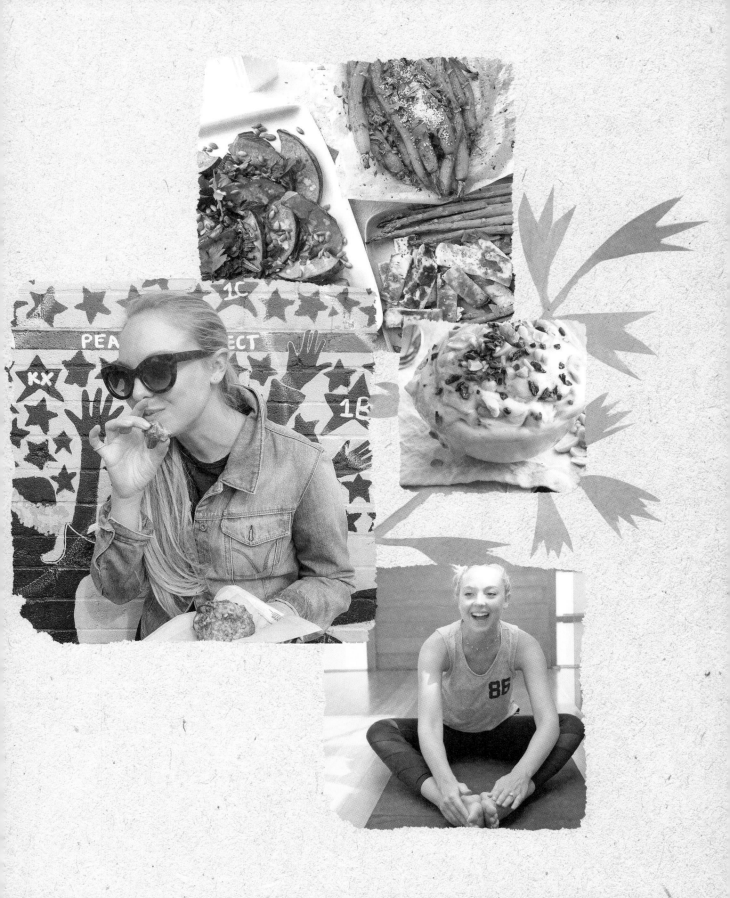

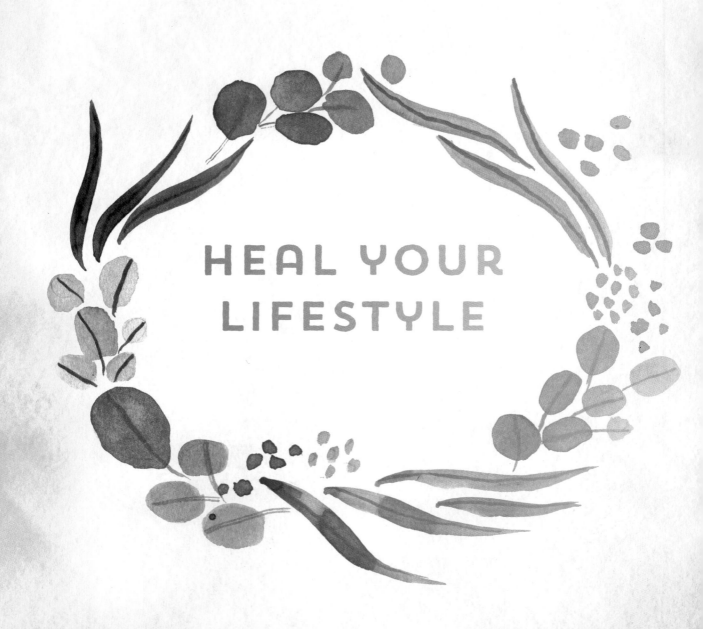

HEAL YOUR
LIFESTYLE

*Healthy living isn't a short-term phase – it's a lifestyle, so we're going to focus on the elements of your lifestyle: routines, working out, career and travelling. In the past few years, I've created a healthy way of life that is sustainable – that means I can keep it up now and forever. Gone are the days of diets and workout routines that promote intensity, restriction and deprivation.*

*You have to prioritise YOU, and spend some time discovering what works for YOUR life. You are never too busy to love yourself.*

## EMBRACE STILLNESS

We live in an extremely chaotic and fast-paced world, and it's detrimental to our health. To counteract the craziness going on around us, we need to find stillness in our days. When I don't spend time by myself being quiet and still, my world starts to feel more rushed. Stillness creates space and balance.

Let's try to let go of this 'doing' addiction, and schedule some self-love into our diaries. It doesn't matter if you have 20 minutes a week or 20 minutes a day to spare, every little bit counts. Me-time is essential for a healed life.

I encourage you to *take it slow* some days. If you wake up and don't feel up to the day ahead, that's okay. Just do everything more slowly: eat slower, speak slower, and breathe deeper. Give yourself permission to leave the tasks that can wait till tomorrow.

### DO MORE OF WHAT MAKES YOU HAPPY

Happiness and health go hand in hand. You only live once, so make the most of it! Sure, we all need to work, but play is just as important. Instead of making chaos and stress the leaders of your life, focus on doing things that make you happy.

Write down five things you wish you could do more of, and commit to doing two of those this month! Because life is meant to be LIVED.

# THE IMPORTANCE
# OF DAILY ROUTINES

I'm often asked, 'What is the number one change people can make today for a healthier life?' My answer is simple: set yourself up with a healthy daily routine.

## Mornings

Mornings can be frantic in most households but if you can carve out a little time for yourself, you'll be starting your day off with an extra spring in your step. Before I started healing my body, I'd wake up tired, then immediately check my phone in bed, feeling the anxiety well up in my stomach. Exercise was the last thing I felt like doing, but I'd still push my body with a hardcore workout that I hated. I'd then make myself a low-calorie breakfast – egg whites and black coffee with sweetener, or maybe some 'non-fat' yet artificially sweetened yoghurt. As I picked at my food, I'd think, 'life is so hard'. The day had barely started, and I was already stressed and down. Thank goodness that stage of my life is over. Here's what my morning routine looks like now:

### 6.30 AM: WAKING
I have a strict no-phone rule. Instead, I take a few deep belly breaths and centre myself by saying a few positive affirmations.

### 6.35 AM: MEDITATION
I give thanks or do the JSHealth Body Love Scan exercise on page 127.

### 6.45 AM: TONGUE SCRAPE
This ancient Ayurvedic practice removes built-up bacteria and toxins in the mouth, and is believed to boost mental, physical and spiritual health. You can find tongue scrapers at most health-food stores.

### 6.50 AM: HYDRATE
Enjoy a warm lemon water with a pinch of cayenne or ginger. This alkalises the system and fires up digestion.

### 7.00 AM: EXERCISE
Depending on what I feel like, I'll go for a walk, do yoga, or enjoy a bit of weight training or high-intensity interval training.

### 7.45 AM: COFFEE
My favourite ritual of all! I normally have my one piccolo a day with full cream milk, or almond milk if I'm taking a break from dairy.

### 8.00 AM: BREAKFAST
Eggs with avocado, a protein smoothie, or a bowl of porridge are on high rotation.

### 8.30 AM: SHOWER
I switch between hot and cold water to get my blood flowing.

### 9.00 AM: WORK
With my morning routine complete, I begin my working day. Only now will I respond to texts and emails.

Your morning routine might not be as long as mine, but try to prioritise some time for yourself if you can and you'll feel focused, calm, and ready to tackle the day's tasks.

## Nights

How you end your day is just as important as how you start it. After a long day dealing with work, family and all your obligations, health may be the furthest thing from your mind! While it's essential to unwind, and fine to watch your favourite show, plonking yourself in front of the telly for hours isn't the healthiest thing in the world. It makes you tired but wired – the exact opposite of what your body needs at that time of day.

That's why it's a good idea to establish a healthy night routine in the lead-up to bed. Not only will this help to reduce stress, but it will also set your body up for a quality sleep.

> YOU WORK HARD ENOUGH DURING THE DAY. AT NIGHT, FOCUS ON YOURSELF.

* *Prepare a wholesome dinner at home. Think simple: protein and greens.*

* *Savour your meal. Eat it slowly and mindfully, enjoying the time with your family/partner/yourself. Chat about or reflect on your day.*

* *After you've cleaned up, switch off your electronics. This includes your phone and all forms of social media! My phone is switched off strictly by 8 pm.*

* *Make a cup of herbal tea. Chamomile is great, or try my healthy chai latte: roobois chai tea with warm almond milk, ground cinnamon and stevia. Yum!*

* *Soak in a bath with essential oils and Epsom salts to relax your muscles and mind.*

* *Put your legs up on the wall for 10 minutes and take a few deep belly breaths or go into the Stress-Free Zone (see page 34).*

* *Jump into bed and read a book, or snuggle up to your partner!*

* *Turn the lights out at a reasonable hour.*

I realise that not all of these things are realistic every evening – but pick and choose the rituals that work for you. I promise you'll feel the difference.

### IN YOUR WORDS

*Jess, thank you for actually teaching and explaining why and how to use different foods. I've used your healthy eating guide for a month now and the difference has been astounding. More energy and no bloating or guilt.*

STEPH

# WORKING OUT

Do you often think you should be spending more time at the gym?

I don't blame you – we are bombarded with fitness messages, so it's not hard to start second-guessing yourself. I used to exercise intensely twice a day and I still found it very difficult to control my weight. I see the same with my clients in the clinic and my friends too.

From my personal and professional experience, I believe we should be exercising moderately, not intensely. Less exercise, more rest. Of course, I encourage you to move your body every day, but not to the point of exhaustion or obsession. Exercise is a fantastic stress-reliever, and it helps to keep our cardiovascular and nervous systems in tip-top condition, but there's no reason to overdo it. In my practice, I ask my clients to tone down their exercise for a 1-week trial. They are so afraid to do it but once they add more yoga, walking and rest days, they walk into my office the next week saying they have more energy and their clothes feel looser!

I suggest that 30–45 minutes of exercise a day is enough. I love yoga, Pilates, barre, weight training and HIIT, because they all incorporate resistance, which increases muscle mass and revs up the metabolism. It's also good to embrace incidental exercise, so opt to take the stairs, and catch up with friends over a brisk walk instead of coffee and cake.

If you're strung out on stress and pushing yourself to exercise hard, have a 'let yourself off the hook' week. Swap one of your intense exercise sessions this week for a restorative yoga class or walk, and enjoy one or two rest days. Go to the end of this chapter for my body blitz gym routine.

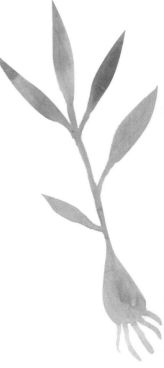

## THINK YOU CAN RUN OFF YOUR EATING SINS?

It doesn't work that way. There's no point punishing yourself. Your body wants to be treated with love, not cruelty. You don't need to 'work off' your indulgences. Your body can handle it. Balance is the key.

## My typical week in workouts looks like this

MONDAY: HIIT. Run on treadmill for 20 minutes + weight training for 20 minutes.

TUESDAY: Yoga (vinyasa flow).

WEDNESDAY: Walk in nature.

THURSDAY: HIIT. Run on treadmill for 20 minutes + weight training for 20 minutes.

FRIDAY: Yoga (either vinyasa flow or a restorative yoga class).

SATURDAY: Walk in nature with friends or my husband.

SUNDAY: Rest day or restorative yoga.

As you can see, I balance out my high-intensity sessions with gentler forms of exercise. The key is to be active and move your body every day, and enjoy rest days when you need them. Remember, it's important to rest!

# CAREER

Many of my clients have rewarding jobs in fields they are passionate about, but I also see far too many people miserable in their work. Your work doesn't have to mean 'everything' to you, but if you lie awake at night worrying about work, or you feel unmotivated, down, tired or hopeless about your job, that needs to change.

* *You shouldn't end up with chronic stress or insomnia over a job.*

* *You don't need to give up your health for your career.*

* *You should wake up MOST days feeling good (not every day – that's unrealistic).*

* *You don't need to work yourself into the ground to be at the top of your game.*

* *You can work balanced hours and still be successful and productive.*

* *You are more productive when you take time to rest and repair.*

* *You are not defined by your job. Your identity is so much more than that.*

If any of this is striking a chord with you, take the time to assess your career situation and think about the potential for a change. Too many people feel stuck but the power is yours to change your life.

# TRAVEL

Keeping healthy while travelling can be challenging – I often find my anxiety about food increases as I don't have control over what kind of food will be available. Here are my top tips to stay healthy while on the move.

* *Get plenty of rest – aim for eight hours of sleep a night.*

* *Switch off from email and social media at some point each day.*

* *Practise meditation to zen out.*

## HOW TO TREAT JETLAG NATURALLY

* *Stay hydrated – you need to be drinking 2 litres a day.*

* *Avoid alcohol on the flight and for the first couple of days in your new destination*

* *Use an eye mask to sleep. Light destroys melatonin production, the hormone that helps you sleep.*

* *Avoid caffeinated drinks and drink chamomile tea at night to aid sleep and relaxation.*

* *Carry nutritious snacks with you.*

* *Travel can upset digestion, so I always pack digestive enzymes and probiotics. I also use psyllium husk or ground flaxseed with lots of water to keep everything moving.*

* *Use valerian root tablets or magnesium to help you relax and fall asleep.*

- *Don't worry too much about formal exercise when travelling, but keep moving. Walking, biking and jogging is always a great way to sightsee.*

- *Try to spend at least 10 minutes a day alone. Switch off, practise some deep breathing, and journal about your experiences that day.*

- *Practise yoga. You need very little space for this — you can easily do sun salutations and warrior poses, or work your core with planks and crunches in your hotel room.*

- *If old insecurities pop up, lie down — if you can — place a hand on your stomach and imagine love and kindness flowing into your body. Think about the parts of your body that you like and replace negative thoughts with positive ones.*

# USING THE POWER OF MANIFESTATION TO HELP CHANGE YOUR LIFE

*I'm not an airy-fairy health preacher — far from it. But I do believe in the power of visualisation and manifestation to help you achieve your goals. When I started healing my life and shifting my mentality from negative to positive, things changed. My worldview altered. I began envisioning the future that I wanted. I firmly believed to my core that I could do and achieve whatever I put my mind to. I felt sure that I could turn my dreams into reality — and slowly but surely, with a lot of hard work, I am doing just that. Knowing you CAN do something (if you really want to) is essentially what manifesting is all about. It's seeing the glass half full. It's about putting your self-belief into action to achieve your dreams. It's not about wishing. It's about creating a positive mindset, opening yourself up and following through with all your energy to get what you want. Here are the steps that I take to visualise and manifest:*

## Step one: have a dream

Build your self-worth. You need to know you deserve everything you desire. You have power and a purpose. Once you realise this, your universe will shift for the better. You have the ability to create the life of your dreams. Work through some of the tips in Heal Your Relationship with Yourself on page 24 to boost your self-esteem, self-confidence and, ultimately, self-worth.

### Step two: channel all your positive thoughts and energies into your dream

Saying positive affirmations puts you in a positive frame of mind. By the law of attraction, if you tell yourself you're going to have a good day, in all likelihood you will!

Create five affirmations for yourself. Make sure they're in the present tense to keep that good energy pulsating. They don't work in past or future tense. For instance, instead of saying, 'I want a fulfilling career,' say, 'Thank you for my fulfilling career'. Even if they're not true just yet, saying them on a repetitive basis will help your mind to figure out ways to change that. Sometimes you have to fake it until you make it. Here are some examples:

'I am living my dream life.'

'Thank you for my dream job.'

'Thank you for my health and energy.'

'I attract love.'

'I am thankful for my body.'

'The universe is on my side.'

### Step three: create a vision board

Collect photos and drawings of the things you want in your life, or the person you'd like to become. These could include photos of friends and family, places you'd like to travel to and your dream car or house. It could also include your business goals or inspirational quotes. There are no rules, so get creative!

Once you've collected all these bits and pieces, assemble them onto a foam board or pinboard. Then, put the board somewhere you'll see every day, like your office or bedroom.

The idea is that when you surround yourself with positive images of who you want to become, what you want to have, where you want to live, and the things you're grateful for, your thoughts and actions are geared towards making those desires a reality.

### Step four: do my manifestation dance (if you like)

It sounds weird, I know, but lately I've been taking my manifestation to a whole new level. It's a dance. Literally. I open my arms out wide and shout out positive affirmations to the universe. I twirl around and sometimes I even put music on. Please give it a go!

### Step five: work hard to make that dream come true

Now that your mind and energies are aligned towards your goal, and you know that you can do it, free yourself to pursue your dream with everything you've got. You need to feel the dream and desire. Fall asleep every night thinking and feeling good thoughts about your dream. Don't doubt yourself because it stops the law of attraction from working. Swap the doubt with positivity. Believe in yourself!

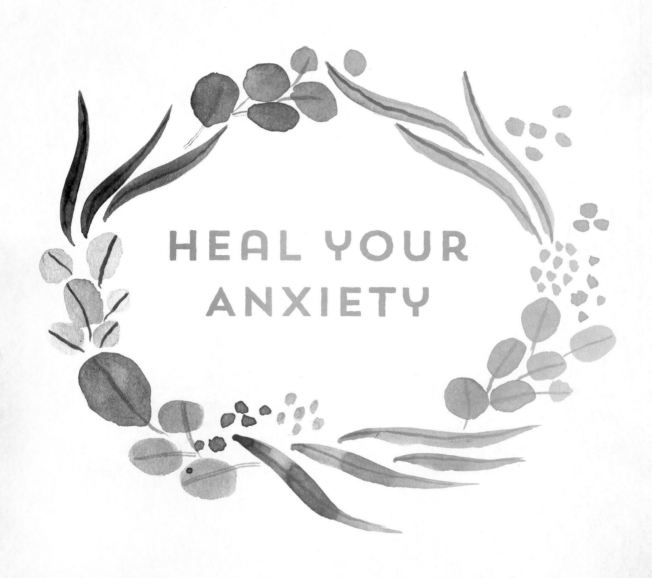

HEAL YOUR
ANXIETY

*Anxiety is a condition that affects so many people. It is different to stress, which we will address later on. There are many ways to deal with and ultimately heal anxiety, including therapy, diet and lifestyle modifications, yoga, medication and natural supplements. As with all things health-related, you need to tend to anxiety in a holistic manner, and address both physical and emotional symptoms. Work your way through the suggestions here – they helped me, and hopefully they'll help you too.*

## THERAPY

Anxiety can be a real battle, but you don't need to fight it alone. To manage your anxiety, enlist help, starting with your GP and a referral to a good therapist. Don't be afraid of this process. A therapist can help you to uncover the roots of your anxiety, develop strategies to cope with it and alter your thinking patterns to keep your worries to a minimum.

Depending on the severity of your symptoms, your doctor may prescribe medication to help treat your anxiety. Anxiety is like any medical condition; there is no shame in taking medication when it's needed. Consult with your healthcare professionals and figure out what is right for you.

Anxiety has been a key topic in my therapy sessions. One technique I've learned for managing anxiety is to ground myself by saying affirmations. When you feel anxious, you can blow things out of proportion. You overthink. Saying affirmations helps bring you back to reality and makes you appreciate what you have. It also calms the mind, therefore alleviating anxiety. Here are some of the affirmations that have been amazing at easing my anxiety:

- *'This will pass.'*
- *'It will all work out the way it's supposed to.'*
- *'The answer will come to me.'*
- *'I'm doing the best I can.'*

**PLEASE, IF YOU'RE STRUGGLING WITH ANYTHING, ENLIST AN EXPERT FOR HELP. DON'T HESITATE.**

# MODIFY YOUR LIFESTYLE

## Change your diet mentality

Nourishing your body can help to fight anxiety. Give up the diet mentality. Instead of cutting out entire food groups, think about eating wholefoods that'll help to ease anxiety.

For instance, when you're feeling anxious, ditch cold, raw foods and turn to warming foods: think curries, stews, soups and stir-fries. These foods are incredibly nourishing and soothing – for both the body and soul! At the same time, enjoy protein, good fats and greens at every single meal. Carbs are also needed as they produce the 'feel good' hormone, serotonin.

Drink more water – eight glasses a day if possible. Dehydration can cause fatigue and agitation.

During anxious periods, avoid caffeine, refined sugar and alcohol. The aim of the game is to calm and relax the mind and body, and all these substances do is stimulate. They affect energy levels and sleep, and a lack of sleep inevitably worsens anxiety.

Avoid processed foods, which cause inflammation, and artificial sweeteners (these contain aspartame which has been linked to mood disorders).

## Exercise right

Whether you're dealing with mild or severe anxiety, it's important to mix endorphin-releasing activities with restorative exercise. In other words, you need a blend of the yin and yang types of movement.

When I'm feeling anxious, I choose yoga, brisk walking or nothing at all. I've found that when I put pressure on myself to do a hardcore workout, my anxiety worsens.

Some people feel amazing and calm after doing high-intensity exercise like spinning or running. If that sounds like you, go for it – but just make sure you balance out your week of workouts with some low-intensity forms of exercise. If you're not sure if your workouts are making your anxiety better or worse, I'd advise sticking to yoga, Pilates and walking for a 2-week trial period, and then reassessing your anxiety levels.

## Practise yoga

Yoga is phenomenal for managing anxiety. It connects you to your breath, which relaxes the nervous system. It also connects the body and mind, restoring the adrenal glands and bringing a sense of peace to the soul. I know it sounds airy-fairy, but it's the best way to explain it: when your mind, body and soul are in sync, you'll feel good.

Finally, and perhaps most importantly, yoga gets you out of your own head – even just for an hour. Plus, yoga classes always end with *savasana*, the resting pose (literally lying down for five minutes). This alone can decrease anxiety.

## Meditation

Meditation is incredible for anxiety – again, it's all about slowing down that mental chatter. It doesn't need to be fancy, or follow specific rules. Just sit in a quiet spot, close your eyes and focus on breathing. You can do this for as few as five minutes a day to feel the difference. Try the JSHealth Body Love Scan (see page 127).

## Consider natural supplements

There are some powerful natural remedies out there for anxiety. Before taking anything, chat to a health practitioner to find out what is suitable for you.

Here are the supplements that have worked for me and some of my clients dealing with anxiety of varying levels:

- *B Complex*
- *Fish oil*
- *Zinc*
- *Magnesium glycinate powder.*

Herbal concoctions can also be incredibly effective. Ask a naturopath about blending the likes of passionflower, magnolia, withania and lavender. Also, one of the cheapest and easiest ways to combat anxiety is to sip on chamomile tea. It soothes the system and is especially good to drink before bed.

### JUST BREATHE

In many cases, simply connecting to your breath will help to ease any anxiety you're feeling. There are a few ways to do this:

- *Deep belly breathing exercises (see page 34).*

- *Alternative nostril breathing. Press against one nostril with your finger so it closes, take a deep breath in through your nose, then exhale. Release and repeat with the other nostril, alternating until you feel calmer.*

- *Go into child's pose, and stay there for as long as you need.*

## Is social media giving you anxiety?

Social media is amazing. It allows us to share moments, to document our experiences and to connect to a greater community. But it also has its downfalls. Have you ever found yourself stressing about how many likes or comments your latest post will get? Do you compare yourself to the seemingly perfect images posted online? So many of us get caught in the trap of measuring our bodies, lives and self-worth against people we don't even know.

But guess what? Social media is like a museum – it only shows the carefully curated parts of a person's life. The parts they want us to see. The best parts. There will always be someone who appears to be thinner, richer, smarter or more successful than you. There will always be someone who appears to have more or do more than you.

It doesn't matter. Social media is about appearances, not reality. What matters is that you believe in YOU, and that you value YOUR self-worth. The number of 'likes' or comments you get does not define you. The most important relationship in life is the one you have with yourself.

If social media is giving you anxiety, detox from it. Just take a break. Deactivate your accounts for a week and take some time to do the things you really love. See how you feel at the end of the week. Readjust your mindset about the images you see and enjoy the fun of social media without the anxiety. Only follow accounts that lift you up.

## IN YOUR WORDS

*It's so unlike me to email someone I don't even know, but I HAVE to thank you for the tremendous change you have helped me make in my life. Before reading your book, The Healthy Life, I had no idea I even had a bad relationship with food and my body. You have opened my eyes up so much as to how easy and effortless living a healthy, balanced lifestyle can be. I never realised how much of a difference taking time for myself, adding yoga into my routine and loving my body more could contribute to becoming a holistically healthier person. I am no longer afraid of food! I never thought I would feel so free and positive when it comes to making food choices. I am so so grateful for you. You have changed my life.*

MICHAELLA

# HOW TO IMPROVE YOUR MOOD

We all have 'off' days. Days where we don't feel up to life. It's normal. Sometimes I wake up feeling sad for no good reason, but it's okay because I know it will pass.

To keep your mood stable, give your body and mind a little daily love. Get a good night's sleep, and drink water all day. Incorporate good fats, good proteins (amino acids create mood-boosting chemicals) and complex carbs in your diet – they boost the feel-good hormones. Go into the Stress-Free Zone for at least 10 minutes (see page 34), and try to get outside in the sunshine (or watch the rain falling) if you can.

When you're down in the dumps, here are some more things you can do to lift your spirits:

* *Go for a swim. In the ocean, if possible. It clears the mind better than anything else.*

* *Walk with your puppy (or ask to borrow your friend's pet). I don't know about you, but being around animals makes me happy!*

* *Grab your headphones, pump up the music and go for a walk/jog.*

* *Listen to relaxing music.*

* *Watch a feel-good movie or watch a few episodes of your favourite TV show.*

* *Soak in a warm bath.*

* *Write in a gratitude journal.*

* *Meet your bestie/mum/someone you can relax around for a cup of tea.*

* *Treat yourself to a Thai foot massage.*

* *Say affirmations such as, 'I am good enough' and 'I love and accept myself.'*

* *Finally, remove the pressure to do it all. For that day, choose to do less and be fine with it. Just do the bare minimum and know that tomorrow you'll have the energy to do more.*

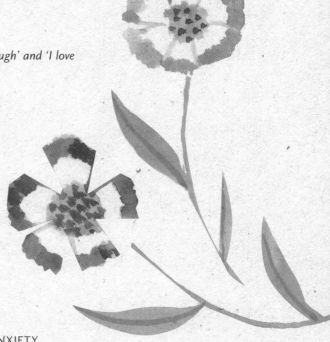

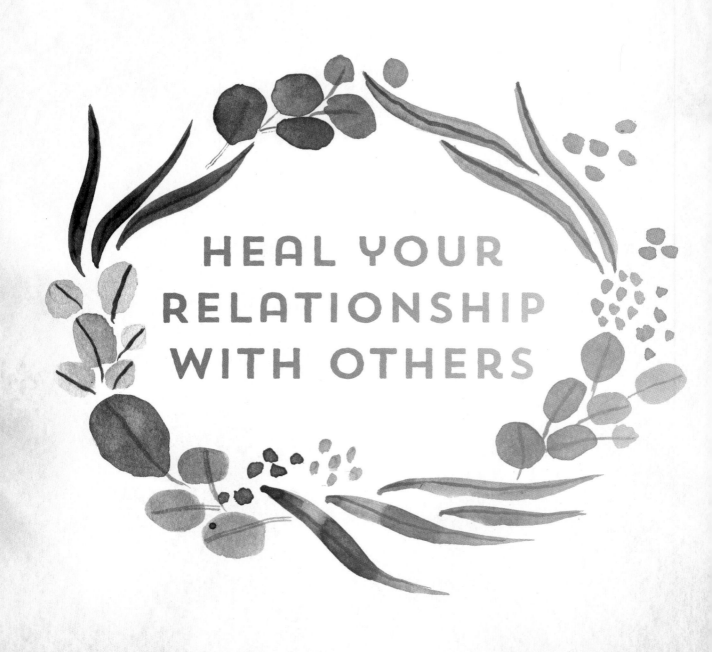

HEAL YOUR
RELATIONSHIP
WITH OTHERS

*Never underestimate the power of the human connection. In this section, I will help you connect with others and heal your relationships with those around you, prioritising the relationships that support you and containing the ones that hurt.*

# NOURISH YOUR GOOD RELATIONSHIPS

When life gets busy, it can be hard to make time for loved ones. Sometimes I find socialising and scheduling time for friends and family to be an extra chore. Sometimes the thought of catching up with people in the midst of an insanely crazy week is overwhelming. I'm sure you can relate.

So if I'm in the middle of a huge project (like, oh, writing a book) and can't commit to or don't feel like a night out, I'll arrange to see my friends and get things done at the same time. For example, we might head to yoga and grab a quick juice afterwards, or go for a coastal walk.

Whenever I put in face time with family and friends, I feel happier. It's worth the investment to keep the good people in my life, even when I'm busy. But having said that, don't feel bad about saying no to social arrangements and gatherings when you need to. When you're tired, stay in and give your body the rest it's craving. Listen to your body and know when it's time to get out and see your loved ones and when it's time to give your body a break. I have learned to say no personally. It has brought balance to my lifestyle and I've created space in my life for me. So when I say yes to social engagements, I arrive with excitement and energy, not exhaustion.

Remember you can't make everyone happy all the time. The key is finding a happy balance. Be aware of others, and don't be selfish. But take care of yourself first. Set boundaries with people. Give up the need to please.

# TOXIC FRIENDSHIPS

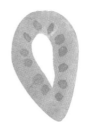
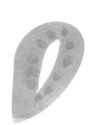

As we grow up and progress through life, our friendship circles change. People drift away, and that's completely natural. But what happens if a toxic person sticks around?

You know the kind of person I'm talking about: someone who makes you feel crappy when you're with them or after they've left. It could be for a range of reasons. Maybe they're selfish and don't care about anyone else. Maybe they're all about take, take, take, with very little give. Maybe they're miserable to be around.

Whatever it is, if you dread being around someone, it's likely a toxic friendship. One that's not serving you. And it's time to break up with that person.

First up, think carefully about who is dragging you down or making you feel angry/frustrated every time you see them. If they're a family member or someone you can't really cut, consider gentle ways of putting up boundaries. Perhaps you can see them less often? Or you could tell them you're focusing on yourself for a while and won't have as much time to see them. With some people, simply saying 'no, thanks' to an invitation may work well. Even though it may feel awkward, just remember that you're doing what's best for YOU. You're doing this for your health – and I don't say that lightly.

If there's a specific person you just don't want to see anymore, slowly but surely start to distance yourself from them. Take their calls less, or say no to catch-ups. They'll eventually move on. If you're confident, you can also tell them kindly and gently that you need some time off from the friendship due to your healing journey. You know this person better than I do – choose whichever strategy you think they'll accept.

On a less intense note, what do you do when you don't want to necessarily break up with someone, but you're feeling overwhelmed by the amount of social contact? This is easier. Only respond to messages and calls when you have the energy. Tell your friends you're using your phone less or doing a little 'tech detox' (everyone loves and respects a detox) – they'll get used to it.

## IN YOUR WORDS

*You are such an inspiration and you have helped me so much in healing my relationship with food. Throughout high school I was surrounded by such a gorgeous group of friends who, like with many girls that age, were pressured to be thin. Many of them suffered from eating disorders. I knew that food should not take over your life but it did not stop the pressure I felt to be thin. I decided to buy your ebook and it was life-changing. I am now healthier and happier than ever. I do not feel deprived in the slightest. I have realised that healthy living is my passion and I would love to be able to help people the way you have helped me.*

LAURA

# RELATIONSHIPS AND LIFESTYLE CHANGE

You're on a mission to live a healthy, healed life and you're also in a relationship. Can the two go hand in hand?

The answer is yes. The key is acceptance, compromise and communication – just like everything in relationships! Talk to your partner about your new healthy lifestyle and ask for their support. I know some partners who get annoyed by their partner's lifestyle. To be frank, it's not fair. Your partner should want you to be the happiest and healthiest that you can be and should be supportive and not critical of your efforts to improve your health and wellbeing. Your partner needs to accept your decision to live healthily and hopefully they'll decide to join you in your endeavours.

If your partner isn't looking to make changes to their lifestyle, however, you can't force them. Perhaps your partner already feels good about their health and lifestyle and doesn't feel the need to make changes. Whatever their reason, that's their call – no matter what your opinion is! Remember that everyone is unique.

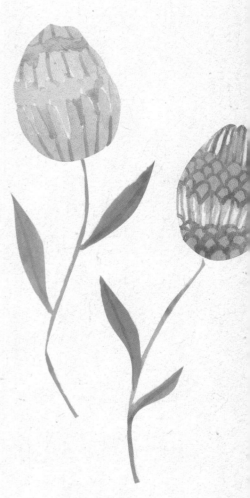

You can still make the changes that you feel will benefit you. Go to yoga. See a therapist. Turn off your phone and go to bed early. When it's your turn to make dinner, cook the nutritious food that you want to eat. When you go out together, be empowered by making healthy choices and don't feel pressured by them (they shouldn't be pressuring you anyway).

There are lots of ways your partner can support you. Perhaps they could do some more housework or run some of your errands to enable you to have more time go to yoga or exercise more often. They can respect your wish to avoid processed food by agreeing not to have it in the house – they can still eat what they wish when they're out. Talk about positive activities you can enjoy together: a walk, swim or time spent in nature, or just resting at home together (social media off!). Talk to your partner and come up with ways for the two of you to support each other and your choices.

As your partner sees how much happier and healthier you become with your new lifestyle, they'll probably come round of their own accord. But if they don't, you can still continue on your journey together through love, communication and acceptance.

# RECOVERING FROM A BREAK-UP

If you've been hurt in the past, it can be difficult to open up your heart to people again.

But when you live life with a closed heart, you aren't allowing amazing people, experiences and opportunities to flow in.

Love is what makes the world go around. Love is what makes every human being feel connected to the planet and to each other.

Open your heart up in order to heal.

Yes, having an open heart can lead to heartache. But heartache is part of living.

Don't be afraid to get hurt. You are worthy of love and being loved. No one – not a family member, friend or ex-partner – can ever take that away from you.

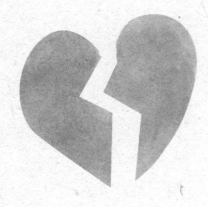

## HEALING A BROKEN HEART

Break-ups are hard. They hurt. And they're meant to – this person occupied a huge space in your life, and now they're gone. It's probably a good thing, but you still need to take steps to heal, otherwise the break-up will be detrimental to your health and wellbeing.

- *Do things that make you feel fulfilled and happy. Your passions will remind you that your life is full, with or without that person.*

- *Keep your distance. You broke up for a reason, so cut communication from this point on.*

- *Hold on to your dignity. Otherwise, you'll lose self-esteem and self-confidence, and go into a cycle of hating yourself when your ex doesn't respond. This is exactly what you don't want.*

- *Protect yourself emotionally. Spend time with people who love you, and say positive affirmations daily.*

- *Accept it is happening. Don't fight the journey; treat it as a learning curve.*

- *Forgive. Easier said than done, I know.*

# DON'T HOLD GRUDGES

Someone did something really bad to you, and you can't – or won't – let it go. Sound familiar?

We're all guilty of holding grudges from time to time. But what you hold on to emotionally, you hold on to physically. So, emotional baggage will affect your physical body. You'll feel heavy.

Therapy, yoga and meditation may help with this, as well as taking a big step back from that situation or person. Space is important. Creating distance seems to ease tension, especially with family members.

Keep the following mantras in mind:

- *You cannot change people.*

- *You are not responsible for other people's pain, struggles and insecurities.*

- *You are in charge of your own feelings and thoughts – stop trying to control everyone else's.*

- *You are doing the best you can. And, usually, so are they.*

- *Everyone is going through something. Dissolve your anger into empathy. Be kind.*

## BE KIND, ALWAYS

Have you heard the saying, 'You don't know someone until you've walked a mile in their shoes?'

I love it.

When you find yourself reacting to something or someone, take a step back. Sure, people can be irritating and frustrating, but being reactive only creates stress for YOU, not the other person. Instead, try to understand where that person is coming from and why they may be acting in a certain way. If you can't understand, just choose to accept that you're different, and wish that person well. There's no point trying to change or 'fix' people.

Everyone struggles at some point, and the people around them have the ability to lift them up and make their journey that little bit easier.

Judge less. Be that person who makes a difference. Be kind, always.

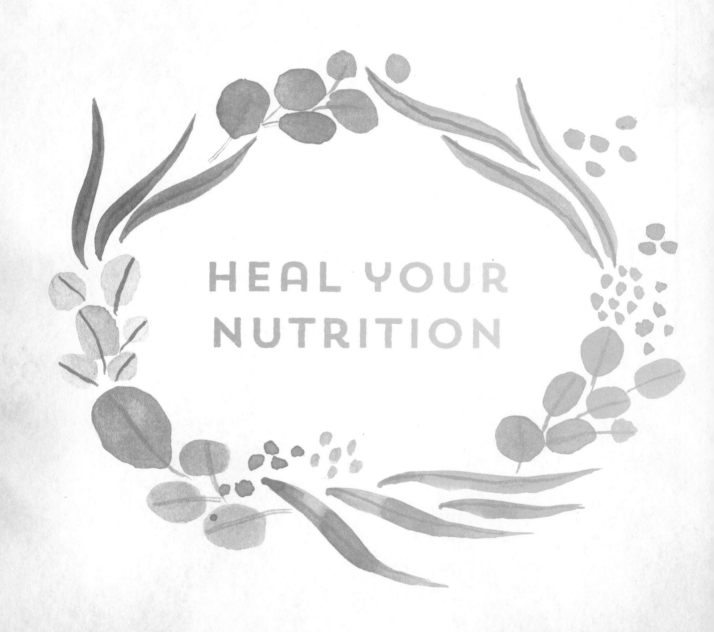

HEAL YOUR
NUTRITION

*Don't just feed your body; fuel it. Here, we're going to focus on nourishing your body with top-quality nutrition. Hopefully by now you have the tools to heal your relationship with food and you have a new appreciation for the joy and positive wellbeing that good eating can bring.*

# MY FOOD PHILOSOPHY

I believe in fuelling and nourishing my body with REAL wholefoods. That means clean, unprocessed foods that are as close to their natural state as possible. I choose to eat nutrient-rich foods that heal my body.

The way I eat looks like this most of the time – this is what works for me:

- *No refined sugar or gluten.*
- *Gluten-free grains.*
- *Good fats (in moderation).*
- *Organic dairy.*
- *Plenty of high-quality animal protein, sustainably caught fish, beans and pulses.*
- *Fruit in moderate amounts – preferably low-sugar options such as berries or green apples.*
- *Loads of colourful, particularly green, veggies.*
- *Lots of herbs and spices to jazz up my meals.*

I also follow the 80/20 approach. Eighty per cent of the time I follow the above, and 20 per cent of the time I eat anything I want – in moderation.

## GOOD FOOD HABITS

- *Stop fad dieting. Make a decision to quit.*
- *Eat through the rainbow – this means colourful fruits and veggies.*
- *Drink water all day long.*
- *Eat slowly and mindfully.*
- *Buy local and organic produce where possible.*
- *Be kind to yourself when it comes to food.*

# NUTRIENTS

Good health comes down to finding the right balance of macronutrients and micronutrients in your body. Everyone has a unique optimal balance, and tuning in to your body's needs will help you find yours. The three macronutrients required in large amounts are protein, fats and carbohydrates.

## Protein

Protein is crucial for the healthy growth and development of muscles, blood, skin, hair, nails and organs. Increasing your daily intake of protein will increase your energy and satiety as well as speed up your metabolism and help produce healthy hormones. Aim for one palm-sized portion at every meal. When buying fish and seafood, use the Marine Conservation Society's website, www.mcs.uk.org, to find out what types of seafood are caught in a way that's beneficial to the earth and your health. Avoid sausages and deli or smoked meats.

Having protein within the first hour of waking up is essential for optimal health, so I make a protein smoothie most mornings. In terms of protein powder, opt for a whey, rice or pea protein. If you suffer from digestive issues or lactose intolerance, choose pea or rice protein. Many powders on the market are full of junk so ensure you choose one that is free from artificial sweeteners, colours and preservatives, is gluten-free, naturally sweetened (with stevia), low carb (below 3 g), high in protein (around 20 g per serve) and non-GMO.

### ANIMAL

- Organic free-range eggs (1–2)
- Seafood and fish: wild Alaskan salmon, Atlantic salmon, ling, mackerel, seabass, sardines, trout, Arctic cod and haddock (150–200 g) – smaller white fish are better to avoid mercury
- Tinned or bottled tuna (90–150 g) – maximum twice per week to limit mercury levels
- Prawns (90 g)
- Oysters (6)
- Mussels (450 g, shell on)
- Free-range and organic poultry and game: chicken, turkey, duck (100–150 g)
- Grass-fed lean red meat: lamb, veal, beef, pork (150 g)

### VEGETARIAN

- Beans and legumes: lentils, chickpeas etc. (100 g)
- Tofu and tempeh – I prefer tempeh (100 g)
- Hummus/tahini (2–3 tablespoons)
- Dairy products: organic natural yoghurt, goat's/sheep's milk yoghurt, goat's cheese (100–200 g)
- Nuts and seeds (4 tablespoons)

### WHEY

- Whey/rice/pea protein powder (30 g)

If you suffer from any digestive havoc or if you are vegan or vegetarian, avoid whey and stick to pea/rice protein.

# Fats

After years of 'fat' talk, modern nutritional science is finally telling us fat isn't the problem. Good fats are absolutely vital for good health and wellbeing. They make hormones, protect organs and reduce inflammation. You won't get fat from eating fat. In fact, eating a moderate amount of good fat will keep you fuller for longer.

Omega-3 and omega-6 are known as 'essential fatty acids'. Our bodies can't produce these on their own, so we must get them from food. Most people don't get enough omega-3 especially if they avoid healthy fats and fish, which can lead to fatigue, depression and hormonal imbalance. Eating the right amount of fatty acids will give you hormonal equilibrium, better mood, lower blood pressure and improved heart health. Up your intake of omega-3 by eating oily fish, flaxseed, egg yolks, walnuts and dark leafy green veggies.

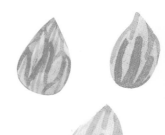

## GOOD FATS YOU CAN ENJOY:

- *¼–½ avocado*
- *1 tablespoon cold-pressed extra-virgin olive oil or virgin organic coconut oil*
- *4 tablespoons mixed nuts and seeds*
- *1 tablespoon nut butter*
- *1 tablespoon tahini*

## FATS TO AVOID:

- *Vegetable fats that have been extracted from various seeds: rapeseed oil, soybean, corn, sunflower, safflower and groundnut oil commonly found in processed, packaged and deep-fried foods – even 'healthy' muesli bars*
- *Margarine and spreadable butter*

## RAW NUTS AND SEEDS

Nuts and seeds are high in essential vitamins and minerals and contain the kind of essential fatty acids that are vital for good health. Choose unroasted and unsalted varieties. It's best to soak all nuts and seeds or buy 'activated' ones. Enjoy 4–8 tablespoons of nuts and seeds once a day only, especially if you are trying to balance your weight.

## HOW TO SPOT TRANS FATS

If you want to be healthy, trans fats are the ones to avoid. Found in virtually all processed, packaged, fried and baked foods, artificial trans fats (or trans fatty acids) are the result of adding hydrogen to liquid vegetable oils to make them more solid. They're industrially-made and the furthest thing from natural. The body doesn't recognise trans fats or know how to break them down. Over time, trans fats build up in the system and, in some cases, start to cling to artery walls, causing problems like heart disease and increased cholesterol. To avoid trans fats, stick to fresh wholefoods, and put down anything that lists 'partially hydrogenated fats' on the label, even protein bars at health-food shops.

# Carbohydrates

Repeat after me, carbs are not the devil! They are actually the body's chief source of energy in the form of glucose, when eaten in moderation. But to sustain energy it's better for our bodies to absorb glucose slowly. That's why it's important to go for complex rather than simple carbs; as simple carbs are likely to cause a blood-sugar spike and subsequent drop which affect energy and weight control.

## COMPLEX CARBS

(Eat in moderation)

* Rye bread, sourdough and spelt bread (1 slice)
* Mountain bread wraps (1–2)
* Pumpernickel/Ezekiel bread (1 thin slice)
* Organic rolled oats (30 g, uncooked)
* Oat bran (25 g, uncooked)

## GLUTEN-FREE GRAINS

* Brown or wild rice (100 g, uncooked)
* Quinoa (85 g, uncooked)
* Millet, amaranth or buckwheat (about 100 g, uncooked)
* Gluten-free noodles: buckwheat, kelp, konjac, soba and black bean (about 100 g, cooked)
* Corn thins (3–4)
* Brown rice cakes (2)

## SIMPLE CARBS

(To Avoid)

* White bread
* White rice
* Pastries
* Crisps
* Chocolate bars
* Refined sugar and cereals

## WHAT ABOUT GLUTEN?

Gluten is a protein found in grains. The main sources of gluten are bread, cereal, cakes, biscuits and crackers. Sources of hidden gluten include gravies, soups, sausages, bottled sauces and some marinades. Gluten intolerance or sensitivity occurs when a person has a reaction after eating a food containing gluten.

If you don't know if you're sensitive to gluten, cut it from your diet for three to four weeks, and then reintroduce it. If you feel better off gluten (or worse when you bring it back), then it's likely causing problems. Consult with a healthcare professional and see my first book, *The Healthy Life*, for more tips on being gluten-free.

# VEGETABLES

The best advice I can give you about nutrition is: eat more greens! Have at least 450 g of veggies a day and lots of greens at each meal if you can. Green veggies are high in nutrients and fibre and will keep you full. Opt to steam, stir-fry, grill or pressure-cook your veggies, or eat them raw – just don't microwave them.

## BEST-OPTION VEGGIES
(Load up on these low carb veggies with each meal)

- Asparagus
- Aubergine
- Brassica veggies: brussels sprouts, broccoli, cauliflower, cabbage, kale. These need to be cooked well as they contain goitrogens, which can mess with the thyroid.
- Cabbage
- Celery
- Courgettes
- Cucumber
- Fennel
- Peppers
- Dark leafy greens: pak choi, Swiss chard
- All lettuces
- Mushrooms
- Onions, garlic, leek
- Radish
- Rocket
- Tomato
- Green beans
- Seaweed

## STARCHY VEGGIES
(Limit these higher carb veggies to 75 g per meal)

- Carrots
- Sweet potato
- Pumpkin
- Yams
- Beetroot
- Parsnip
- Peas
- Organic sweetcorn

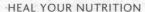

# FRUIT

Since fruit is a starch, limit yourself to two serves a day. The correct serving sizes are listed in brackets in the table below; typically, one serve = one medium-sized piece of fruit or about 70 g berries. I love to have a handful of raw nuts with fruit to balance out the sugar.

## BEST-OPTION FRUITS
(These are low GI aka good for your blood sugar!)

- *Granny Smith apples (1)*
- *Berries: strawberries, blueberries, raspberries (70 g)*
- *Goji berries (4 tablespoons)*
- *Figs (2–3)*
- *Citrus fruits: lemons, grapefruit, oranges (1)*
- *Papaya (1 medium-sized)*
- *Kiwi fruit (2–3)*
- *Passionfruit (2)*
- *Stone fruit: nectarines, plums, peaches (1)*

## FRUITS TO EAT MODERATELY

- *Dates (2)*
- *Small banana (1)*
- *Small mango (1)*
- *Grapes (1 small bunch)*
- *Cherries (6–8)*
- *Watermelon (1–2 wedges)*
- *Lychees (6–8)*

## AVOID

- *Dried fruits – high in sugar and sulphur preservatives*
- *Fruit juices – unless homemade*
- *Stewed fruits, unless homemade*

To nourish your body with the highest quality food, try to buy organic and locally grown produce. If you don't have access to organic fruits and veggies, at least buy the most seasonal, freshest ones you can and wash them thoroughly.

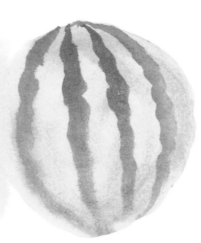
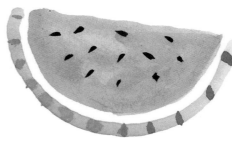

# DAIRY AND DAIRY SUBSTITUTES

When it comes to dairy, it's all about the quality. Dairy is a good source of protein and calcium. If you can tolerate dairy/lactose, feel free to enjoy organic versions.

So many yoghurts and milks these days have added sugar and preservatives. Check the labels and choose organic and natural alternatives that aren't sweetened. Sweeten your yoghurt with stevia, ground cinnamon or a little raw honey.

## CHEESE

- *Goat's cheese (2–3 tablespoons)*
- *Cottage cheese (2–3 tablespoons)*
- *Ricotta (2–3 tablespoons)*
- *Other white cheeses (2–3 slices)*

## YOGHURT

- *Organic natural/Greek-style yoghurt with no added sugar (100–200 g)*
- *Goat's/sheep's yoghurt (100–200 g)*
- *Coconut milk yoghurt (100 g)*

## OTHER

- *Organic or A2 cow's milk (250 ml)*
- *Organic butter (1 teaspoon)*
- *Whey protein*

## DAIRY SUBSTITUTES
(Great for cleansing or gut healing)

- *Almond milk (250 ml)*
- *Rice milk (250 ml)*
- *Hemp milk (250 ml)*
- *Coconut milk or coconut milk yoghurt (250 ml)*
- *Cashew cheese (found at health-food shops)*

## WHAT ABOUT SOY?

Most soy products, like soya milk and tofu, are GMO, which can depress thyroid function, mess with hormones and slow down digestion. However, fermented soy products contain beneficial bacteria for the gut, and the fermentation process destroys the anti-nutrients in soy. So, enjoy miso, natto, tempeh and tamari (wheat and gluten-free soy sauce). If you have an underactive thyroid, cut out ALL soy products, even fermented ones.

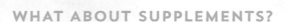

# FIBRE

Fibre is in charge of keeping the digestive system moving and is great for weight balancing. Fibre stabilises blood sugar, lowers cholesterol and cleanses excess hormones from the body. Aim to get 30–40 g of fibre a day through wholegrains (e.g. oats), dark leafy greens, fruit, nuts, flaxseed, chia seeds and psyllium husk.

# WATER

H2O is by far the best drink to keep your body hydrated and healthy. Aim for 1.5–2 litres of filtered water a day, and start with two glasses first thing in the morning.

## WHAT ABOUT SUPPLEMENTS?

I used to be a self-confessed supplement junkie. At my nutrition practice in Sydney, I prescribed good supplements based on very sound research and some of these supplements did prove to help my clients.

But when it came to my personal life, I overdid it. Each day I was taking fish oil, magnesium, probiotics, vitamin C, B complex, zinc, selenium, vitamin D, iron… I'm a perfectionist, so I thought all these vitamins would help to keep me in perfect health. Before long, I lost touch with one of my favourite mottos: use foods to heal first.

When I tried to stop taking vitamin supplements, I felt incomplete – like I had to take them every morning otherwise 'something would happen'. Looking back, it was like an addiction.

I decided to go off supplements for one week, just to see what difference it made. I continued eating beautiful wholefoods and I discovered I had so much more energy without the supplements! It was crazy.

Now I take vitamins based on my bloodwork and health state. I am careful and specific with what I take.

So, this is my advice: ensure you are eating nutrient-rich wholefood. If you still have nutrient deficiencies or issues with digestion, it may be appropriate to take supplements – as guided by a health practitioner. Never self-prescribe. Always ask for help and guidance.

# SUGAR

If you want to improve your overall health, the single best thing you can do is cut down on refined sugar. It is inflammatory to the body, encourages weight gain and spikes your insulin levels, which can result in depression, obesity and/or sugar addiction. It irritates the gut and feeds bad bacteria, wreaking havoc on the digestive system. It also messes with your hormones and mood.

Artificial sweeteners are even WORSE. Avoid chemicals such as saccharin, aspartame and sucralose. They cause a toxic build-up in the body and trigger your sugar cravings. Also steer clear of high-fructose corn syrup.

## Natural sweeteners

Great news! There are some natural sweeteners that will tempt your taste buds. Enjoy the following in moderation (no more than 1–2 teaspoons a day): raw honey, pure maple syrup, rice malt syrup and coconut nectar.

For natural sweeteners that won't spike your blood-sugar levels and will help stop sugar cravings, choose from my personal favourite spices and flavourings: stevia granules and liquid, ground cinnamon, vanilla bean/powder and grated nutmeg.

## HOW TO BANISH SUGAR CRAVINGS NOW

- *Sip on lemon tea morning and night (½ fresh lemon squeezed into warm water).*

- *Add more bitter foods to your diet – think rocket, lemon, grapefruit, dark leafy greens, organic Dijon mustard and dandelion root tea.*

- *Reduce caffeine and alcohol as they can trigger cravings.*

- *Swap regular chocolate for dark/ raw cacao chocolate.*

- *Add more good fats and protein to your diet. Enjoy them at every meal.*

- *Avoid sugar in the afternoon, as it can trigger post-dinner cravings. Instead have a protein-rich afternoon snack around 4–5 pm.*

- *Cut out all refined white carbs. Only eat wholegrains – preferably gluten-free ones.*

- *Be careful with fruit. Stop at two serves a day, and opt for low-sugar types like berries and green apples. Eat before midday and pair fruit with a good fat or protein such as a handful of nuts.*

- *Always eat a protein-rich breakfast.*

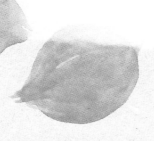

## HEALTHY LIVING DOESN'T HAVE TO BREAK THE BANK

'But Jess, eating healthily is SO expensive. I can't keep this up!'

This is a common complaint. And while I completely understand the importance of spending within your means – especially if you're a university student or if you have a family – I can tell you it is possible to eat healthily on a budget. Here are my tips:

- *Prep a meal plan. That way, you'll only buy what you need, and nothing will go to waste.*

- *Shop with a list. In the same sense, having a plan of attack before you go to the store will help to keep you on track. It's easy to fall victim to clever marketing when we stray from the items that we actually need.*

- *Love leftovers. Make extra dinner to eat for lunch the next day. Not only does it save a lot of time, but it saves money, too!*

- *Buy in bulk and go to your local farmers market. Try buying nuts, grains and protein in bulk – you'll save so much money.*

- *Cut back on alcohol. Booze is expensive, and you can save a significant amount of money by cutting back on it.*

## THE LIMITED LIST

I avoid or limit the following foods:

- high-sugar fruits: *grapes, watermelon, dates, dried fruits and fruit juice.*
- limit tinned food: *fresh is best!*
- stock cubes *(unless organic) or pre-made stocks; best to make your own.*
- factory-farmed *eggs, chicken, turkey, pork, beef, veal, sausages, smoked/deli meats, tinned meats.*
- factory-farmed fish *(max twice a week): tuna, salmon, swordfish.*
- soy products: *tofu, soya milk, soybeans.*
- processed dairy products: *cow's milk, powdered milk, cream cheese, butter, margarine.*
- pre-packaged foods: *even the low-fat/diet ones or health bars.*
- high fructose corn syrup *and agave syrup.*
- refined sugar and artificial sweeteners: *white and brown sugar, lollies, chocolate, ice-cream, energy bars, jellies, jams.*
- wheat products: *bread, pasta, noodles, cookies, cakes, pies, cereals, waffles, pitta bread, bran, couscous (although I enjoy gluten-free bread, pasta and cereal).*
- All processed spreads *except 100 per cent almond butter, peanut butter and tahini.*
- All commercial condiments, *as they are packed with sugar and preservatives: packaged salad dressings, tomato/BBQ sauce, relish, chutney. (See page 58 for some healthy alternatives.)*
- deep-fried and microwaved *foods.*
- gluten-free diet products *made with cornstarch, rice starch or potato starch; these are incredibly processed and high in sodium.*
- diet/soft drinks *– try sparkling mineral water or homemade vitamin water (see page 304) instead!*
- alcohol: *limit to weekends and special occasions.*

## SUPERFOODS

Boost your smoothies, oats, yoghurt and salads with a tablespoon of these superfoods:

- *Raw cacao powder or nibs*
- *Bee pollen*
- *Maca powder*
- *Mesquite powder*
- *Spirulina*
- *Chia seeds*
- *Flaxseed*
- *Goji berries*
- *Acai berry powder*
- *Macqui berry powder*

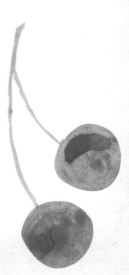

# THE JSHEALTH EATING FORMULA

*Every main meal contains a complex carbohydrate, a quality protein, a good fat and lots of greens.*

My plate is usually made up of one-quarter protein, one-quarter gluten-free grains or starchy veggies and half greens. As for snacks, they always contain some kind of protein to keep my blood sugar stable and cravings at bay. I also drink 1.5–2 litres of water daily.

You get to eat a lot using my eating guide. The aim is to eat five small meals a day – three 'main' meals and two snacks – to get your metabolism firing and keep cravings at bay. You may find that four meals suits you better, and that's fine. Once you're back in tune with your body, you'll know how often and how much you need to eat.

## HOW TO CONTROL PORTION SIZES

- *Serve your meals on a smaller plate.*
- *Eat slowly and chew each mouthful 10–20 times. You'll be less likely to want seconds.*
- *Drink two glasses of water 20 minutes BEFORE meals, not during.*
- *Have a protein-rich snack in between meals – this will help you control your appetite.*
- *Dish out protein and carb portions the size of your palm.*

## MY FAVOURITE AFTERNOON SNACK IDEAS

*Go for a wholesome, satiating and protein-rich snack when the afternoon munchies hit.*

- *JSHealth Protein Smoothie without the fruit (see page 147).*
- *250 ml Greek yoghurt sweetened with ground cinnamon and stevia – add 1 tablespoon protein powder if you wish.*
- *4 tablespoons raw nuts and sliced carrot.*
- *Veggie sticks with 2 tablespoons hummus/tahini.*
- *A boiled egg.*
- *JSHealth sugar-free protein balls (see page 269).*
- *Celery filled with almond butter.*
- *Sweet cottage cheese – mix 3–4 tablespoons cottage cheese with stevia, ground cinnamon and vanilla powder.*

# MY DAILY EATING GUIDE

## Breakfast: 7.30–9 am

*It's like they always say: breakfast is the most important meal of the day. It kickstarts your digestion and metabolism and feeds your body with the vitamins and minerals it needs to perform. Try to eat within one hour of waking, and always include protein and fat. Have your one coffee around this time too.*

## Snack: 11 am

*Have your green juice and a small snack around mid-morning. Snacks must contain a protein component. This snack is optional as some people simply are not hungry at this stage. Tune in to your appetite.*

## Lunch: 12.30–1 pm

*For lunch, combine dark leafy greens with one or two servings of protein, one unit of good fat and one unit of starch – your choice of starchy veggies, gluten-free grains or legumes. Chances are you'll feel fuller when you add a portion of fat. Lunch will ensure your body slowly releases energy over the rest of the day so you don't experience the dreaded afternoon slump.*

## Snack: 4–5 pm

*Choose a protein-rich snack to keep your blood sugar stable until dinner. Avoid coffee and fruit in the afternoon – they won't do your cravings, stress or blood-sugar levels any favours.*

## Dinner: 7 pm

*Dinner should be your lightest meal of the day. A protein with non-starchy veggies, including lots of greens, or a small portion of starchy carbs (like sweet potato, pumpkin, quinoa or brown rice) is a good choice.*

## Supper

*I'm a big believer in moderation, so I encourage you to treat yourself to a sweet treat once or twice a week after dinner (see pages 249–86).*

# A WEEK OF NUTRITIOUS EATING

Here's an example of how my meals tend to look. On the weekends I enjoy a spelt scone from my local organic bakery and in the evening I'll have a glass or two of organic red wine with dinner and some dark chocolate or a scoop of gelato without the guilt. Yum. Remember, you can tailor your plan too!

|  | DAY 1 | DAY 2 | DAY 3 |
|---|---|---|---|
| **BREAKFAST** | JSHealth Protein Smoothie (see page 147) topped with crushed nuts/seeds/homemade paleo granola (see page 141) – it's the best! | 1–2 poached or scrambled eggs and sautéed greens and ¼ avocado and 1 slice of gluten-free bread. | 8 tablespoons cooked oats topped with ½ banana sliced, a handful of blueberries and 2 tablespoons vanilla pea protein powder or 2 tablespoons LSA mix (linseed, sunflower and almond meal) for the protein boost. |
| **SNACK** | Green apple with a sprinkle of ground cinnamon and a handful of raw almonds. Or this may be a good time to have a green juice or coffee. | Carrot sticks with 1–2 tablespoons hummus or tahini. | 2 JSHealth Sugar-free Protein Balls (see page 269). Or a handful of raw almonds. |
| **LUNCH** | Large green salad with grated carrot, ¼ avocado, tomato, cucumber, onion, 75 g cooked sweet potato and 100–150 g chicken or turkey breast. Use the JSHealth Clean Life Dressing (see page 297). | Large tuna salad with cucumber, onion, tomato and a sprinkle of cooked quinoa. Use the JSHealth Clean Life Dressing (see page 297). | Brown rice salad (70 g cooked brown rice) with 150 g grilled chicken, salmon or 1 boiled egg, with steamed broccoli florets and a drizzle of tahini and lemon. |
| **SNACK** | 150–200 g Greek yoghurt/coconut milk yoghurt mixed with ground cinnamon and stevia powder. | JSHealth Protein Smoothie (see page 147) without the fruit. Or 2 brown rice cakes with a smear of almond butter and a sprinkle of cinnamon. | Carrot sticks with 1–2 tablespoons hummus or tahini. |
| **DINNER** | Grilled Cajun salmon fillet with sautéed garlic broccoli/broccoli mash and a green salad. | Garlic and ginger chicken/salmon stir-fry with broccoli, green beans, mushrooms and pak choi. (Use sesame oil/olive oil and tamari when stir-frying.) | San Choy Bau (see page 224). Fill lettuce cups with protein of choice and diced tomato, cucumber and avocado and 4 tablespoons cooked quinoa (optional). |
| **SUPPER** | Decaf chai tea with almond milk and ground cinnamon (optional – add stevia/raw honey to sweeten) And 1 bliss ball (see pages 268–9). | Decaf chai tea with almond milk and ground cinnamon. If I'm still hungry or craving something sweet, I'll have 125 ml Greek yoghurt with ground cinnamon and a handful of blueberries. | Decaf chai tea with almond milk and ground cinnamon. And 1–2 pieces of 70–80 % dark/raw cacao chocolate. |

| DAY 4 | DAY 5 | DAY 6 | DAY 7 |
|---|---|---|---|
| JSHealth Protein Smoothie (see page 147) topped crushed nuts/seeds/ homemade paleo granola (see page 141). | 8 tablespoons cooked oats topped with ½ banana sliced, a handful of blueberries and 2 tablespoons vanilla pea protein powder or 2 tablespoons. LSA mix for the protein boost. | 1–2 poached or boiled eggs served with ¼ avocado and sautéed greens and 2 slices of gluten-free toast or 2 brown rice cakes. | 2-egg omelette. (Whisk eggs with a dash of almond milk, salt and pepper then add sautéed spinach, tomato, mushrooms to the middle and flip over into an omelette.) Serve with ¼ avocado, and 1 slice of gluten-free toast or 2 brown rice cakes if you're hungry. |
| Carrot sticks with 1–2 tablespoons hummus or tahini. | 2 JSHealth Sugar-free Protein Balls (see page 269). Or 250 ml Greek yoghurt with ground cinnamon and stevia. | Green apple with a sprinkle of ground cinnamon. | 2 JSHealth Sugar-free Protein Balls (see page 269). Or a handful of raw almonds and carrot sticks. |
| Big chopped salad with grilled chicken/turkey breast/salmon fillet/boiled egg and diced tomatoes, cucumber, onion, lettuce, broccoli and carrots. Top with protein. Use the JSHealth Clean Life Dressing (see page 297). | Brown rice bowl with grilled salmon/can of tuna/lentils and sautéed greens of choice. Drizzle with tahini, olive oil and lemon juice. | Chicken/tuna lettuce wrap filled with avocado and veggies of choice. | Brown rice sushi (salmon/ tuna/chicken/tempeh). Or a chicken and quinoa mixed green salad. |
| 2 JSHealth Sugar-free Protein Balls (see page 269). Or 3 tablespoons cottage cheese mixed with ground cinnamon. | JSHealth Protein Smoothie (see page 147) without the fruit. | Carrot and celery sticks with 1–2 tablespoons hummus or tahini. | 250 ml Greek yoghurt sweetened with ground cinnamon or stevia. Or one of my favourite froyo recipes (see page 262). |
| Grilled fish fillet with sautéed garlic spinach/kale. Drizzle with lemon juice. | Grilled fillet steak with roasted cauliflower or cauliflower mash and a green salad. | Grilled salmon served with a tomato, onion and avocado salsa and 70 g brown rice. | Grilled Moroccan spiced chicken breast served with roasted sweet potato/sweet potato mash and a mixed green salad with a drizzle of olive oil and balsamic. |
| Decaf chai tea with almond milk and ground cinnamon. | Decaf chai tea with almond milk and ground cinnamon (add stevia or raw honey to sweeten if you like). | Decaf chai tea with almond milk and ground cinnamon. | Decaf chai tea with almond milk and ground cinnamon. |

# EATING OUT

When trying to stick to the healthy life, eating out or going to dinner parties can be tricky!

Whilst I would suggest only eating out once or twice a week, it is also important to say yes to socialising, indulge moderately without the guilt and to enjoy life! Next time you're heading out, don't stress. Just do the best you can to make the healthiest choices possible.

Here are my top tips for healthy dining in a restaurant setting.

- *Enjoy a protein-rich snack and drink two glasses of water before you go out. This will curb your hunger, and stop you from overeating.*

- *Always consider the salad options. If salads are limited, check out the 'sides' – often you will find a garden salad, or steamed greens. These are perfect options for before, or during, your main meal. I always start my meal with a green salad.*

- *Choose food that is grilled, steamed or roasted rather than deep fried.*

- *Hold off on rice, bread and potatoes.*

- *Keep dressings and sauces on the side.*

- *Don't avoid eating that day. Eat balanced meals as usual or you will likely overeat.*

- *Choose your protein wisely. Try grilled fish, chicken or lean meat.*

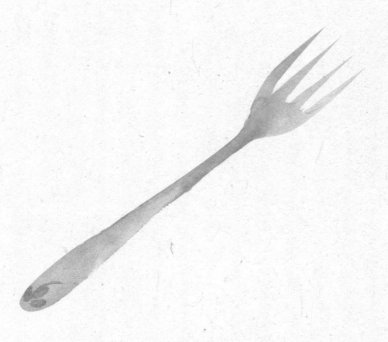

# Takeaway options

Be careful when ordering takeaway. Limit it to once or twice a week, and follow this guide for different cuisines.

| | BETTER CHOICES | AVOID |
|---|---|---|
| GLOBAL | Lean protein (grilled, steamed or barbecued)<br>Green veggies or salad<br>Optional: Small serve of brown rice or quinoa on the side<br>I usually go straight for the sides: roasted brussels sprouts, sweet potato chips, steamed greens with lemon juice and olive oil.<br>Perfect! Ask for salad dressings on the side | Fried foods and creamy dressings |
| CHINESE | Lean protein (chicken or seafood) stir-fry<br>Colourful veggies (steamed or stir-fried)<br>Poached, grilled or steamed options that use simple flavours like chilli, garlic and ginger<br>Boiled rice | Dumplings<br>Spring rolls<br>Fried meats<br>Fried rice |
| THAI | Lean protein<br>Asian veggies (e.g. pak choi and Chinese broccoli)<br>Steamed fish with ginger<br>Stir-fries made with lime, lemongrass, ginger, basil, chilli or garlic (sauce on the side)<br>Tom yum soup<br>Thai beef salad | Spring rolls<br>Chicken wings<br>Moneybags<br>Pad Thai<br>Satay sauce |
| INDIAN | Chicken tikka/tandoori chicken (oven-baked or grilled)<br>Veggies<br>Brown, jasmine or basmati rice<br>Roti | Creamy curries<br>Fried foods<br>Gravies |
| VIETNAMESE | Vermicelli salad with lean beef/chicken<br>Soup with rice noodles and protein<br>Steamed or poached seafood or meat with fresh herbs<br>Rice paper rolls with dipping sauces that are light and thin<br>Vietnamese-style salad | Fried foods<br>Creamy sauces<br>Dumplings |
| JAPANESE | Miso soup<br>Edamame<br>Sashimi (white fish is best)<br>One fish/chicken sushi roll with brown rice<br>Chicken/beef teriyaki with Asian veggies (ask for sauce on the side as they are high in sugar)<br>Sashimi salad with seaweed and avocado | Tempura dishes<br>Mayo and heavy sauces |
| ITALIAN | Grilled chicken/veal/steak/fish<br>Steamed or grilled veggies<br>Italian garden salad<br>Choose thin, gluten-free pizza bases topped with loads of veggies like tomato, peppers, onion and mushroom, and ask for no cheese | Creamy pasta dishes<br>Processed meats<br>Thick pizza bases with lots of cheese |

# ALCOHOL

I believe alcohol can be part of a healthy lifestyle – as long as it's consumed responsibly and moderately. My personal rule is no more than one or two drinks in one sitting – and even then, I only drink on weekends or special occasions. I consider it a treat.

As for healthy drink options, gin, vodka and whisky with mineral water or water are best. Using cordials, juices or soft drinks as mixers is disastrous. Red wine is a better choice than white for its antioxidant value. I go for organic and biodynamic red wine.

Always eat something small and protein-rich before drinking.

Also, though alcohol can promote relaxation, it's when we rely on it to de-stress that it becomes a major problem. If you 'need' a bottle of wine after work to wind down, there's a bigger issue at play here. Chat to a health professional about why you need that kind of release and find healthier ways to deal with stress.

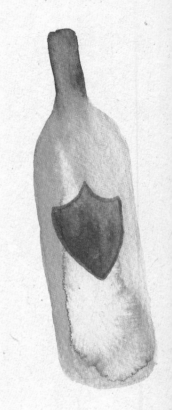

# COFFEE

In my opinion, the issue with coffee is not coffee itself. The additions of sugar, milk, cream and sweeteners are what make that innocent cup of coffee not so innocent! In fact, they may be the reason behind many of your health issues.

Caffeine can cause a rise in cortisol and adrenaline, so be careful if you're stressed and drinking coffee. Too much coffee also has a major impact on liver and digestive function which affects sleep and blood sugar. Say 'yes, please!' to one cup a day and leave it at that. The following are all good options:

- *A long black – a black coffee with an optional dash of good-quality organic cow's milk or almond milk (if you prefer to go dairy-free).*

- *A piccolo – one shot of espresso with only a small amount of milk added. This is what I have. When I'm cleansing, I enjoy it with almond milk instead of cow's milk.*

- *A macchiato or Americano – mostly coffee with a tiny dash of milk.*

- *A ½ latte/flat white – one shot of espresso with about 125 ml milk.*

- *A small ¾ latte/flat white – one shot of espresso with about 75 ml milk and no added sugar or sweetener.*

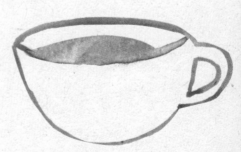

## NEED TO CUT BACK ON YOUR CAFFEINE?

One cup of coffee a day can be healthy but I suspect most people actually drink about three to six cups! If this sounds like you, please consider reducing your intake. The problem with too much caffeine goes beyond the jitters – it can cause anxiety, sleep issues and serious hormonal imbalances. I know this habit isn't an easy one to break, so these are my top tips for cutting down on caffeine.

- *Start your day with warm lemon water before you have any coffee.*
- *Drink your coffee before noon on a full stomach. I try to drink mine around 9 am.*
- *Skip the afternoon coffee because caffeine can stay in your system for hours and make it difficult to fall asleep.*
- *When the craving for your second or third cup comes, opt for a chai tea with hot almond milk and ground cinnamon, a dandy coffee, green juice or homemade Healthy Chai Latte (see page 308).*
- *If you're craving the pick-me-up you get from coffee, try having something nutritious but sweet, like my Cacao Sea Salt Truffles – it will lift you right up! (See page 268.)*
- *Ensure you're eating enough protein and good fats at each meal to keep your blood sugar balanced. When you don't eat these macronutrients, you'll crave things like caffeine.*
- *Make sleep a priority. For most people, that means a solid eight hours a night. When you're well rested, I bet you won't even miss those extra morning coffees.*

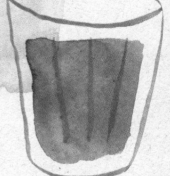

I see many vegans and vegetarians in my clinic and I'm passionate about helping them to eat a balanced diet.

It can be challenging to consume all the right nutrients when certain food groups are missing. Some vegans find they feel fatigued a lot of the time, which often means there is a nutrient deficiency in their diet. It's important to tune in to your body, recognise your symptoms and alter your diet if you're not feeling your best.

* *Always carry healthy snacks with you in your bag – e.g. nuts, seeds, fruit or vegan bars.*

* *Eat lots of greens. Cook some veggies in a pan with a little water and tamari, and add lots of baby spinach. This is a fab nutrient-dense side.*

* *Don't be scared of carbs – sweet potatoes, brown rice and quinoa are great options.*

* *Increase your B12 vitamin intake with the help of lentils, beans and leafy greens like broccoli, spinach and kale.*

* *Boost your zinc by eating nuts, dark leafy greens, beans, grains, pumpkin seeds and sunflower seeds. Sprinkle seeds onto your oatmeal and salads.*

* *Up your iron levels with dark leafy greens like spinach, plus lentils, tahini, nuts, and blackstrap molasses.*

* *Ensure you're getting enough protein on a daily basis. Nuts, seeds, legumes, beans,*

quinoa, tempeh, broccoli, avocado and rice/pea protein powder are all good sources.

* *Incorporate smoothies and juices into your diet for an extra protein and nutrient hit.*

* *Find a good-quality vegan protein powder and throw it into your smoothies.*

* *Use spices instead of sauces to add flavour to your food. Many sauces contain gelatin and other animal-derived thickeners and flavourings.*

* *Drizzle flaxseed oil onto your salads for its essential fatty acids.*

* *Watch your oil intake and choose healthy oils. Rather than cooking all your veggies in oil, steam them and add spices for flavour.*

* *Avoid the refined starches: white bread, white rice, bagels, cereals and pasta. Just because you are more limited doesn't mean you can only eat these! It's easy to fall into the trap of eating bread at every meal. Choose gluten-free grains instead.*

* *Be careful not to have too much soy, as it's in a lot of vegan replacements. If you're a coffee drinker, coconut milk is a great alternative for soya milk.*

* *Eat six small meals throughout the day to stabilise your blood sugar.*

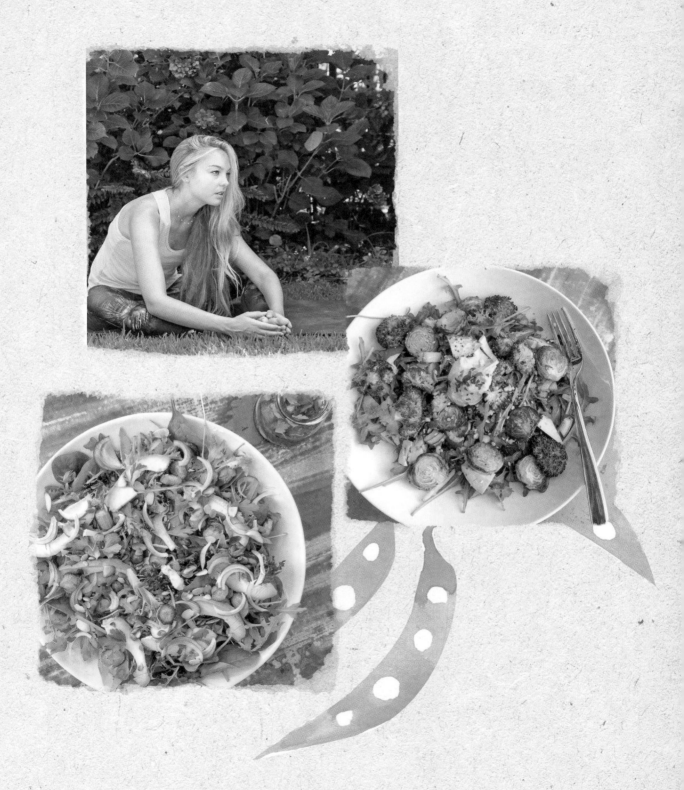

# VEGAN/VEGETARIAN MEAL PLAN

| | MONDAY | TUESDAY | WEDNESDAY |
|---|---|---|---|
| **EXERCISE** | Listen to your body. See page 80 for tips on working out. | Listen to your body. See page 80 for tips on working out. | Listen to your body. See page 80 for tips on working out. |
| **BREAKFAST** Pre-breakfast: enjoy warm lemon water. | Vanilla, Flaxseed, Chia & Banana Parfait (see page 168). | Oatmeal (see page 152) and a serve of pea or rice protein powder. | Mum's Coconut & Mango Chia Overnight Oats (see page 153). |
| **MID-MORNING SNACK** Enjoy your one daily coffee or a green juice. | Green apple with a smear of almond or peanut butter and a sprinkle of cinnamon. | Carrot and celery sticks with 2 tablespoons tahini or hummus. | Breakfast bar (see pages 164–7). |
| **LUNCH** | Brown rice pasta with pesto and pumpkin seeds, topped with cashew cheese, if desired. | Cumin-spiced Lentils with Shaved Brussels Sprouts (see page 202). | Roasted sweet potato filled with ¼–⅓ avocado, beans, rocket leaves and a sprinkle of roasted pumpkin seeds. |
| **MID-AFTERNOON SNACK** | Carrot and celery sticks with 2 tablespoons tahini or hummus. | 2 brown rice cakes topped with almond butter, cinnamon and banana (optional). | 2 Tahini Balls (see page 269). |
| **DINNER** | Comforting Veggie Curry (see page 218) with lentils. | Courgette Mushroom Alfredo (see page 215) with brown rice pasta or mung bean pasta. | Mushroom, leek and tempeh stir-fry. |
| **SUPPER** Try to stick to herbal tea, but feel free to treat yourself after dinner 2–3 times a week. | Caffeine-free herbal tea of your choice. | Caffeine-free herbal tea of your choice. A vegan sweet treat (see pages 248–87) or 2 pieces of raw cacao chocolate. | Caffeine-free herbal tea of your choice. |
| **SYMPTOMS / EMOTIONS** Are you a more mindful eater? | | | |

*Tahini Balls (see page 269)*

*Healing Aubergine Bruschetta (see page 244)*

| THURSDAY | FRIDAY | SATURDAY | SUNDAY |
|---|---|---|---|
| Listen to your body. See page 80 for tips on working out. | Listen to your body. See page 80 for tips on working out. | Listen to your body. See page 80 for tips on working out. | Listen to your body. See page 80 for tips on working out. |
| Papaya with cinnamon, 2 tablespoons coconut milk yoghurt, chopped almonds or granola, and a drizzle of lime juice. | Paleo Coconut, Date & Almond Cereal (see page 136). | Vegan Breakfast Salad (see page 177). | Thick & Creamy Peanut Butter Acai Bowl (see page 136). |
| 125 g of berries sprinkled with desiccated coconut. | Carrot and celery sticks with 2 tablespoons tahini or hummus. | Breakfast bar (see pages 164–7). | Green apple with a smear of almond or peanut butter and a sprinkle of cinnamon. |
| Energy Chop Chop Salad (see page 185) with beans or lentils and a drizzle of JSHealth Clean Life Dressing (see page 297). | Roasted or steamed broccoli with brown rice, ¼–⅓ avocado and a sprinkle of sesame seeds. | Energy Chop Chop Salad (see page 185) with a mix of beans and lentils. | Courgette Mushroom Alfredo (see page 215) with brown rice pasta or mung bean pasta. |
| Carrot and celery sticks with 2 tablespoons tahini or hummus. | Flaxseed crackers served with ¼–⅓ avocado or 2 tablespoons hummus. | 2 brown rice cakes topped with almond butter or tahini and a sprinkle of cinnamon. | 2 brown rice cakes topped with almond butter, cinnamon and banana (optional). |
| Comforting Veggie Curry (see page 218) with quinoa. | Healing Aubergine Bruschetta (see page 244) with cashew cheese. | Courgette Mushroom Alfredo (see page 215) with lentils. | Garlic & Mushroom San Choy Bau (see page 224) with quinoa. |
| Caffeine-free herbal tea of your choice. | Caffeine-free herbal tea of your choice. | Caffeine-free herbal tea of your choice. Fig & Pistachio Chocolate Bark (see page 276). | Caffeine-free herbal tea of your choice. |

*Thick & Creamy Peanut Butter Acai Bowl (see page 136)*

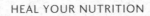

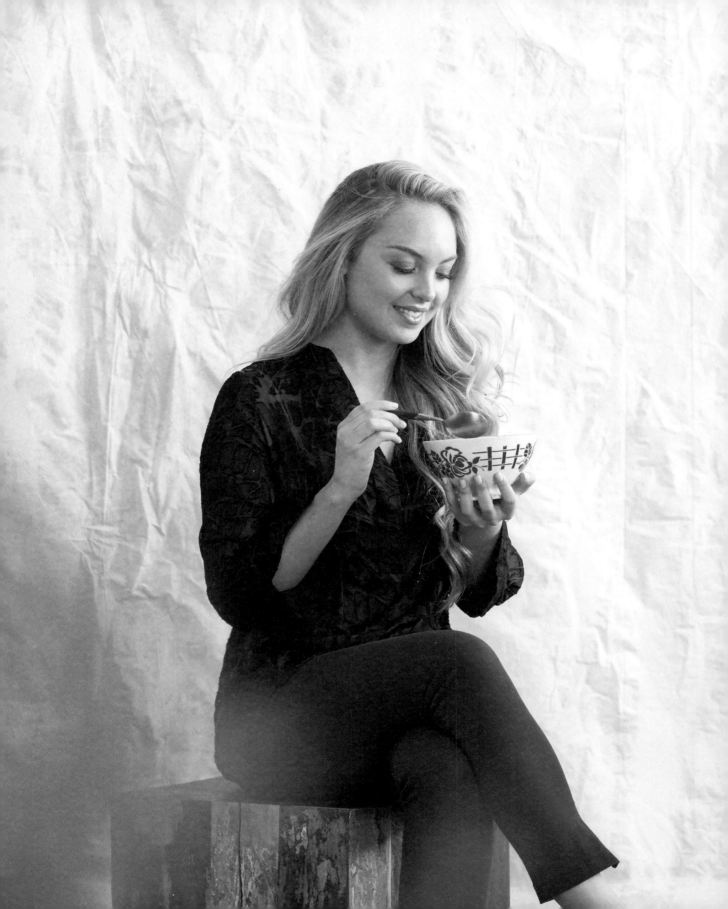

# THE 8-WEEK ACTION PLAN

*I know the information in this book can feel a little overwhelming. So I've created an 8-week action plan to help you on your journey to living a healthier life. It will give you a holistic guide to the most important principles you need to heal your relationship with food, your body, your life and your nutrition. I've also created an 8-week online program on jessicasepel.com that specialises in helping you combat disordered eating and give up fad-dieting forever. Vow to give up dieting and turn to a balanced, wholefood way of eating today. Remember to share your journey with me at #jshealth because I'm so excited to see you living the healthy life. Start by signing the commitment contract.*

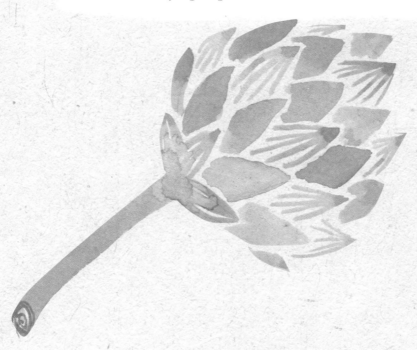

# COMMITMENT CONTRACT

I, _____ , promise to give up dieting for

GOOD. I commit to becoming a mindful eater, someone who eats with

joy and pleasure. I will respect my body and give it the fuel it needs to

thrive. From this point on, I will let go of the guilt, anxiety and panic

about food. I will be health-conscious, not weight-conscious. I choose to

be healthy and glowing, not depleted and deprived. I vow to give thanks

for my meals, and remind myself that food is abundant. I will tune in to

my hunger and satiety signals and respond to them accordingly. I will

keep tabs on my emotions and if/how they're affecting my eating. I will

remember that I am enough, and food does not have power over me.


SIGNED _____


DATE _____

# WEEK ONE

*Healing your relationship with food won't happen overnight, but Week One is the perfect time to start. This week, I want you to concentrate on removing the negative emotions surrounding food and concentrate on building a more positive mindset towards eating. I'm with you!*

## FOOD

Work on reducing stress with eating – tune in to mindful eating, put down your phone when you eat, look at your food, chew it, enjoy it and deal with guilty thoughts.

## BODY

Throw away the scales for three months for now and see how much less anxiety you feel.

Delete apps that make you count your food/calories as it causes your body stress and anxiety.

Stress is the root of so many of our health problems. This week, dig down to the root of the issue and combat your stress with this stress-busting action plan (see page 30). Most importantly, enter the JSHealth SFZ daily for 10–20 minutes per day. Include the SFZ in your calendar to ensure you make the time – this is the best thing you can do for your body.

## LIFESTYLE

Make a mental note to avoid rushing – try and take things slower this week. When you catch yourself running, say to yourself, 'I have all the time I need'.

Switch off your phone at 8 pm to help with sleep and stress. Take any tech gadgets out of your bedroom. Remind yourself that you've had the whole day to work hard and you'll have the whole day tomorrow too.

## RITUALS

Do 20 deep belly breaths or alternate nostril breathing every night before bed (see page 34).

Put your legs up against a wall for 10 minutes every day (see page 34).

Try some stress-reducing vitamins. Take some magnesium dyglicinate in powder form before bed. Invest in a good-quality adrenal formula, recommended by a practitioner, and trial it for six weeks.

SAY THESE AFFIRMATIONS EVERY DAY:

*'I love and approve of myself.'*
*'I am safe and loved.'*
*'I have a fulfilling life.'*
*'I am blessed.'*
*'I celebrate the uniqueness of my body.'*

*If your mindset hasn't
started to change yet,
never fear, it will get easier.
Stop being so hard on yourself.
Remember, you're doing your best
and you're about to enter Week Two
and I'm with you all the way.*

## FOOD

Practise mindful eating (see page 21).

Enjoy a protein-rich dinner every night to help induce a good night's sleep and balance your blood-sugar levels. See the recipe section for delicious protein-rich meals.

Stop drinking caffeine after midday. Stick to one per day, every day. (See page 114 for more.)

Avoid alcohol this week and see if your sleep improves.

Fill up half your plate with greens at each meal.

## BODY

Swap two of your high-intensity workout sessions – e.g. boot camp, spinning, crazy gym workout – to a yoga class or a brisk walk or a rest day – just for this week. And notice if you feel calmer, sleep better and feel more energetic.

## LIFESTYLE

Prioritise sleep: A good night's sleep will do you the world of good. This week, prioritise sleep and reap the benefits.

Head to your local farmers markets this weekend instead of the supermarket to buy your veggies and fruit for the week. Use this opportunity to clear your head and enjoy your weekend away from work.

Make a shopping list and plan your meals for the week ahead to save time and money.

## RITUALS

Before bed, enjoy a couple of extra special sleep-inducing moments to yourself.

- *A hot bath with Epsom salts or shower with lavender oil.*
- *After your bath, put your legs up against the wall for 10 minutes and breathe deeply.*
- *Jump into bed and enjoy decaf chai tea with cinnamon and warm coconut or almond milk or chamomile tea in bed with a book.*

Say affirmations while you eat. Repeat after me: 'This food is nourishing for me!'

Practise gratitude. (See page 28.)

## FOOD

What does your body need? Note how you feel after each meal. To boost energy, eat:

- *Greens – lots of them!*
- *Iron-rich foods: meat, legumes and beans, spinach and other dark leafy greens, nuts and seeds.*
- *Fruit: banana, berries, mango, green apples and citrus fruits.*
- *Gluten-free wholegrains: brown rice, quinoa, oats.*
- *White and oily fish (like salmon).*
- *Virgin organic coconut oil and avocado.*
- *Organic sources of dairy.*
- *And, of course, drink 2 litres of water a day!*

Avoid: gluten, refined carbs (such as cereal, white bread, white pasta), sugar and processed foods.

## LIFESTYLE

When I hit the gym once or twice a week, I do a quick 30-minute workout. Give it a go! For a cardio workout, I do interval training on the treadmill for 20 minutes. This involves jogging for one minute, then sprinting for 30 seconds.

For a strength workout, I do tricep dips, sit-ups, one-minute plank hold and 15–20 weighted squats (I hold a five kilo weight in each hand). I repeat this circuit three times.

## BODY

Listen to your hunger or fullness signals, and respond accordingly. You'll feel so much better.

Find a unique plan that works for you. Design your own lifestyle and experiment until you find what works for your body. How often do you need to eat? When are your energy levels highest? Adjust your eating and exercise habits accordingly.

## RITUALS

Think about establishing healing routines. Sit down to eat your meals – no phones, no TV and no distractions. Just you and your delicious plate of food.

Carve out some time for a morning routine, even if it's just 15 minutes. Try to include exercise, lemon water/tea, meditation or breathing exercises, yoga and a commitment to no phones/emails.

Set yourself up a relaxing night routine. Try to include cooking a delicious nourishing dinner, spending time with your loved ones, switching your phone/emails off by 8 pm, drinking herbal tea and taking some time to just relax and enjoy doing nothing. The body is meant to rest and restore itself at night. Give it time to do so.

# WEEK FOUR

*This week, I want you to give yourself a break. A break from the guilt you may be feeling around food, exercise, friends, family, work and anything else that may be bothering you. This week, I want you to choose self-love and acceptance over guilt.*

## FOOD

At dinnertime, eat more cooked meals as opposed to raw foods. Enjoy soups/slow cooked meats/sautéed veggies in virgin organic coconut oil – they are so nourishing for the nervous system.

When it's your turn to cook, treat your friends and family to a fabulous healthy meal. Celebrate the wonderful people in your life and enjoy their company.

## BODY

Let go of guilt. Every time a guilty feeling pops up, jot it down, take a deep breath and say, 'I let go'. Then breathe out.

If you don't eat as well as you could, let it go and breathe out.

If you don't exercise every day, let it go and breathe out.

When you feel guilt around food, practise my guilt-free tips (see page 13).

## LIFESTYLE

Take some time to consider if you have a negative relationship with yourself. What is the source of this? Talk it through with a counsellor, family member or trusted friend.

Stop apologising for yourself! You are amazing just as you are.

Build up your confidence. (See page 28.)

## RITUALS

Even if you don't feel thankful for your body right now, you need to fake it till you make it. Make the JSHealth Body Love Scan a part of your daily routine and know that the gratitude for your body will start to feel real soon. Here's how it works:

* *Close your eyes and think about being loved and accepted.*

* *Breathe deeply and visualise love pouring into your head, onto your face. Thank those body parts for working hard for you and bestow health on them.*

* *Move down to your mouth, thyroid and chest area, and visualise the same. Thank those parts of your body.*

* *Keep moving down your body, visualising love and giving thanks for everything those parts do. For example, I say, 'Thank you for my healed digestive system', 'Thank you for my healing thyroid', 'Thank you for my clean liver', and 'Thank you for my strong legs that help to carry me around'.*

# WEEK FIVE

*When you've got lots of energy,
the world is your oyster so in
Week Five we'll focus on stoking that
internal fire and getting your buzz back!*

## FOOD

Practise indulgence with moderation in mind. Treat yourself today, and enjoy it with gratitude and zero guilt.

Give up refined sugar. Flick to page 105 to find ways to reduce your sugar cravings. Then, go to Sweet Treats & Healthy Snacks on pages 249–86 to see just how deliciously sweet wholefoods can be *without* the help of refined sugar.

See page 15 to help you decrease binge eating and emotional eating – the first step is to remove diets from your vocabulary or mentality. Dieting + restriction + deprivation results in overeating and bingeing. Commit to eating wholefoods for life – this is the only way that works long term.

## LIFESTYLE

Make stillness part of your life. Take the time out for yourself. Focus on resting and restoring, not pounding the gym. This week, have more rest days and on the days you do exercise, work out *smarter*, not harder.

Identify anyone who seems to be draining you – they may be calling/texting/nagging you all the time – and put up some boundaries with them.

Commit to getting eight hours of quality sleep every night.

Time for technology boundaries! Take some time off from social media and emails – perhaps one day a week to start. Unfollow people on Instagram who cause even one per cent anxiety for you.

## BODY

If you are still struggling with fatigue – get your iron and thyroid tested with your doctor this week. Start by taking care of your gut and liver for more energy – see Heal Your Thyroid on page 36.

## RITUALS

Enjoy a YOU day this week. Just be on your own for a day or even half a day and treat yourself to a rejuvenating activity: whatever you like best.

* *Have a bath with a scented candle and magazine.*

* *Take a 20-minute nap in the afternoon.*

* *Listen to relaxing music or read.*

* *Dance in your room.*

* *Enjoy a Thai massage or acupuncture session.*

* *Watch a movie in bed with a cup of tea.*

*There's nothing like a good cleanse to make you feel whole and well again.*

## FOOD

Focus on eating cleansing foods like:

- *Dark leafy greens (like spinach)*
- *Lean protein: fish, chicken, beans, legumes etc.*
- *All herbs and spices, especially garlic, parsley, coriander, ginger and turmeric*
- *Grated carrot with lemon juice*
- *Apple cider vinegar*
- *Dandelion root tea*
- *Citrus fruits, particularly lemon*
- *All berries.*

Trial cutting alcohol out during the week and keep it to weekends – no more than two glasses. Want to take it a step further? Challenge yourself to one month without alcohol to clean up your gut and liver.

If you suffer from anxiety, avoid or cut back on caffeine, refined sugar and alcohol. They affect energy levels and sleep, and a lack of sleep inevitably worsens anxiety.

## LIFESTYLE

This is a good time to make the 3-day liver reboot a part of your monthly schedule – put it into your calendar, starting on Monday next week.

Try and cut back your coffee to one cup a day. Trial this for one week and you will notice you need less. Swap the other cups with chai tea.

This week, focus on embracing the people who bring you joy and distancing yourself from those who bring you down. Give yourself permission to say no to social arrangements where you are extra stressed or your energy is low. Start creating boundaries with the people in your life who seem to drain you. Spend time with them when you have the energy. Put yourself first.

## RITUALS

Enjoy an Epsom salt bath two to three times this week – so cleansing.

Practise grounding affirmations in moments of anxiety. Use affirmations that work for you.

## BODY

Listen to your food voice. (See page 13.)

# WEEK SEVEN

*This week isn't about eradicating the 'last' or 'extra' two kilos you've been obsessing about. It's about arriving at a balanced, natural weight that your body can sustain.*

## FOOD

By now, you would have tried different aspects of living a healthy life. Let's start bringing it all together; the food lists in the nutrition chapter are designed to achieve a balanced, sustainable weight and ensure you nourish your body with wholesome foods.

❧ *Eat protein at every meal.*

❧ *Cut all refined carbs and switch to gluten-free grains this week.*

❧ *Give up sugar, for life.*

❧ *Add 1 tablespoon apple cider vinegar to a small glass of water and drink before meals – great for digestion and blood-sugar balance.*

❧ *Limit dairy to two portions per day – organic versions only.*

❧ *Add 1–2 tablespoons chia seeds or psyllium husk to your breakfast daily for extra fibre.*

## BODY

Take care of your stress levels (see page 30). Then the next step will be taking care of your gut and liver for a healthy weight (see page 58). Make sure you are eating to balance your blood-sugar levels (see page 105).

## LIFESTYLE

Make eating out a treat, not the norm. Try not to eat out more than once or twice per week.

Plan your exercise routine to maximise healing and strengthening. See page 80 for my thoughts on working out. Ensure you get one to two rest days too, please.

Lower the pressure on yourself and try some new strategies for combating anxiety. Remember to be kind to yourself. Perhaps this is a good time to find a good therapist to help support you.

## RITUALS

Reinforce your affirmations and give thanks for the wonderful, strong, powerful body you have. Feel grateful for your body and it will make you feel physically lighter.

Follow these steps to make peace with your body:

❧ *Forgive yourself for the past, surrender to what is and just do your best to make the best choices in this moment. Focus on your bright future ahead.*

❧ *When you wake up, picture the best version of yourself. Imagine looking and feeling your best and then feel excited that you are becoming that person.*

❧ *From now on you aren't allowed to leave a mirror without paying yourself a compliment! No more criticism allowed!*

# WEEK EIGHT

*It's the last week, but certainly not the least important. It's time to focus on taking care of your hormones.*

## FOOD

Find hormone-balancing foods on page 70. Identify and remove any food intolerances that can trigger an autoimmune response. For those with Hashimoto's, I recommend going gluten-free.

Be mindful of foods that can interfere with thyroid function, such as soybeans, peanuts, millet, strawberries, turnips, watercress and raw veggies in the brassica family (such as broccoli and kale). (See page 41.)

Eat more iodine – add seaweed and dulse flakes to your soups and salads.

## LIFESTYLE

Take care of your adrenals by prioritising rest and solitude daily. Breathe deeply. High cortisol levels are directly linked to lower thyroid function, so it's important to de-stress. Re-read Heal Your Stress on page 30.

Detox your environment. (See page 76.)

## RITUALS

Catch up with a friend/family member. Spend time with people who make you feel good.

Create a vision board for your life after the 8-week plan. (See page 83.)

I say my affirmations every morning as I wake up. Create five affirmations for yourself. Make sure they're in the present tense to keep that good energy pulsating. For instance, instead of saying 'I want a fulfilling career,' say, 'Thank you for my fulfilling career'.

## BODY

Choose two thyroid-healing exercises on page 42 and commit to doing them. Your overall health will thank you for it!

Incorporate rest periods into your day. All you need is 10–20 minutes each day.

Get your thyroid levels checked (TSH, T4, T3 and thyroid antibodies).

Healthy thyroid function depends on healthy gut bacteria. (See page 52 for more on gut health and cleansing functions.)

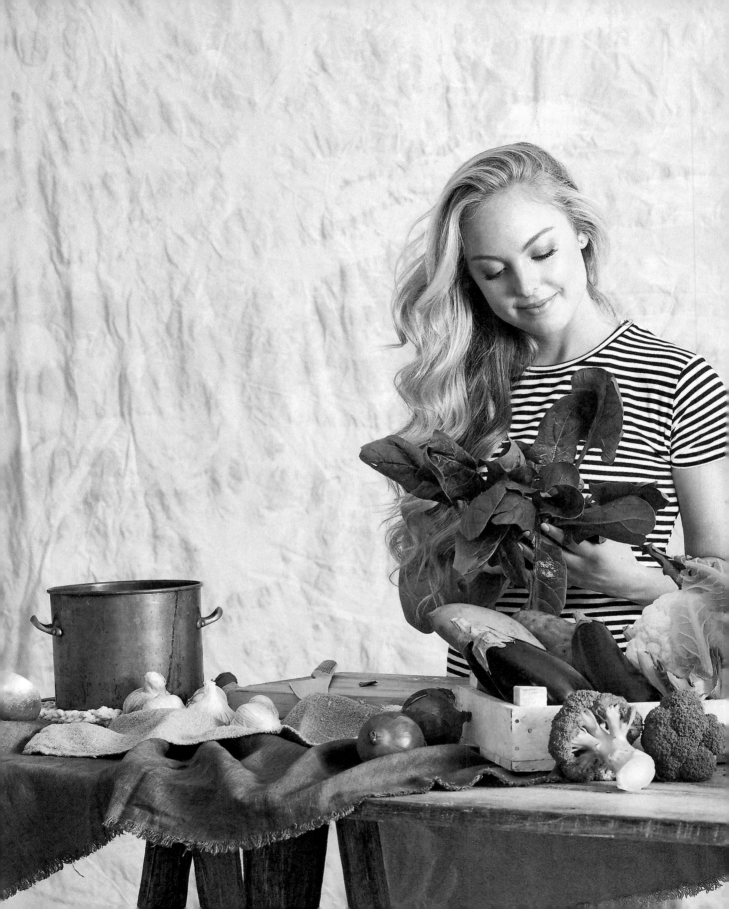

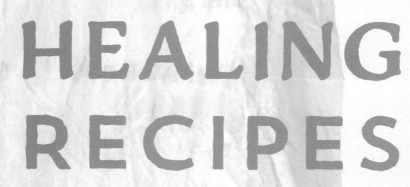

# HEALING
# RECIPES

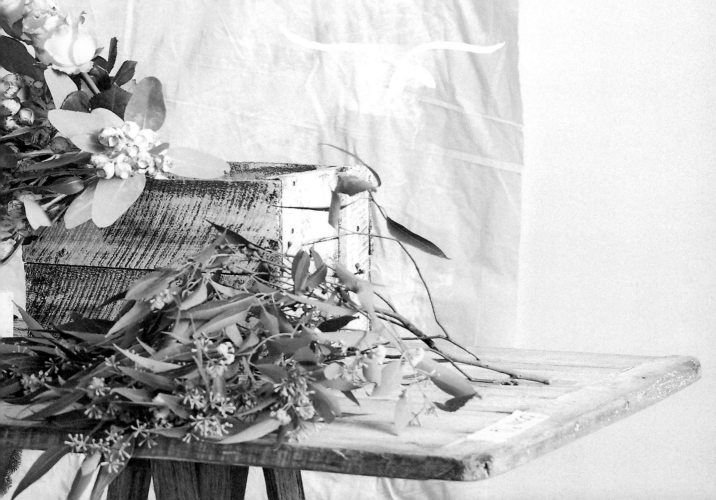

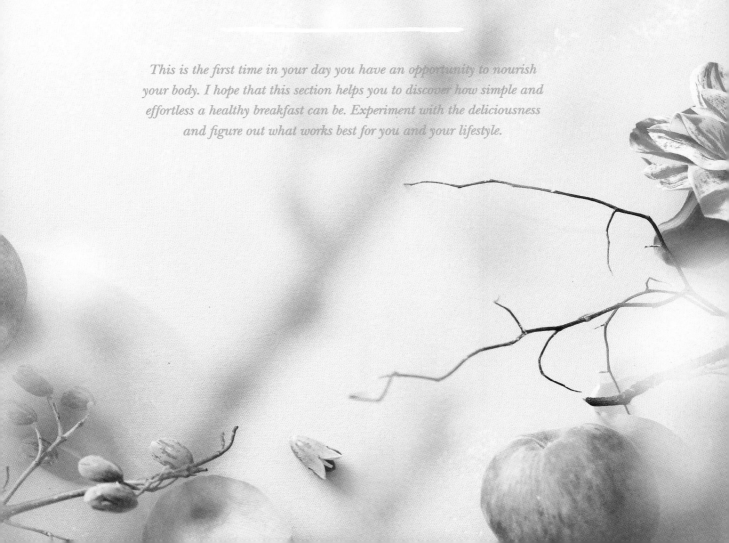

# BREAKFASTS

This is the first time in your day you have an opportunity to nourish
your body. I hope that this section helps you to discover how simple and
effortless a healthy breakfast can be. Experiment with the deliciousness
and figure out what works best for you and your lifestyle.

# PALEO COCONUT, DATE & ALMOND CEREAL

*This vegan, refined sugar-free, no-grain breakfast cereal is so nourishing, and far healthier than any store-bought cereal. Once you're hooked, you can increase the quantities to make a big batch and store in an airtight container for the week.*

SERVES 1
PREP TIME: 10 minutes

2–3 heaped tablespoons flaked almonds, almond meal or crushed raw almonds
1–2 tablespoons ground flaxseed
2 tablespoons desiccated coconut or coconut flakes
2 medjool dates, pitted and sliced
a handful of pumpkin or sunflower seeds
1–2 tablespoons pea protein powder (optional, for an extra protein hit)
250 ml coconut milk
½ banana, sliced
a handful of fresh or frozen blueberries
¼ teaspoon ground cinnamon
raw honey, for drizzling (optional)
a handful of raw almonds or hazelnuts, to serve (optional)

Combine the almonds, flaxseed, coconut, dates, seeds and protein powder (if using) in a breakfast bowl or mason jar.

Alternatively, whiz the ingredients in a blender or food processor for a finer texture.

Top the cereal with the coconut milk, banana slices, berries and cinnamon, and a drizzle of honey, if you like. If you're in need of extra sustenance, finish with a handful of raw almonds or hazelnuts.

# THICK & CREAMY PEANUT BUTTER ACAI BOWL

*I am all about healthy low-sugar versions of acai bowls – without fruit juice and too much sweetener. This recipe is so nutritionally balanced.*

SERVES 1
PREP TIME: 5 minutes

100 g unsweetened acai, frozen and chopped
1 frozen banana, chopped
75 g frozen berries
½ teaspoon ground cinnamon
a pinch of Celtic sea salt
1 heaped tablespoon 100% peanut butter
1½ teaspoons stevia granules or raw honey
125 ml coconut milk
1 serve vegan or whey protein powder (optional)
extra berries, banana slices, shredded coconut or homemade granola (see pages 140–1), to serve (optional)

Place the acai, banana, berries, cinnamon, salt, peanut butter, stevia or honey, coconut milk and protein powder (if using) in a blender and blend until the mixture is thick but smooth.

Pour the mixture into a bowl and top with berries, banana, shredded coconut and/or granola.

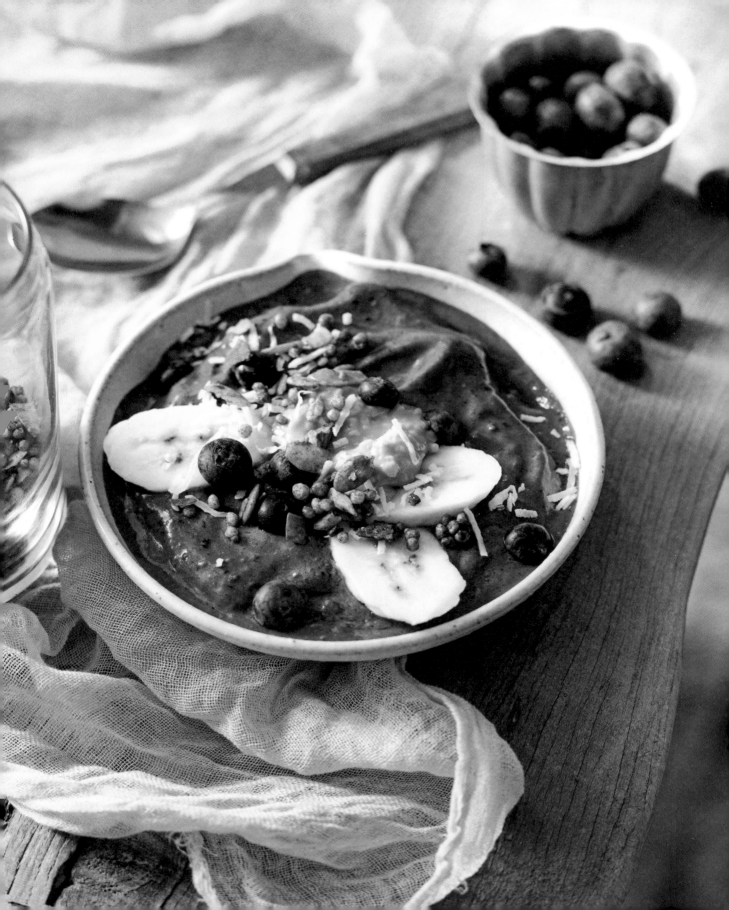

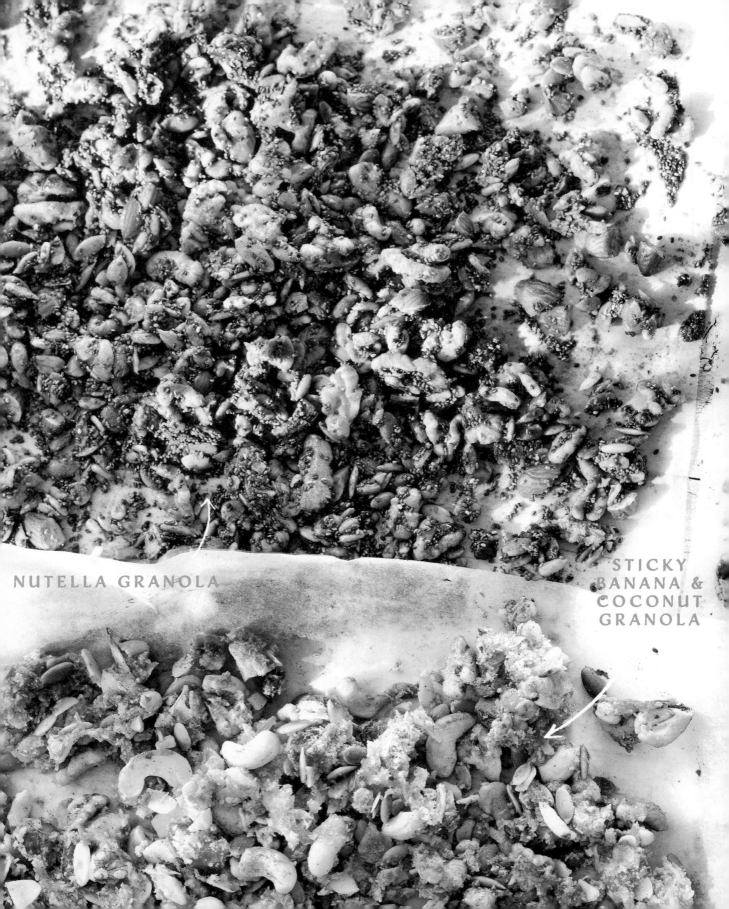

NUTELLA GRANOLA

STICKY
BANANA &
COCONUT
GRANOLA

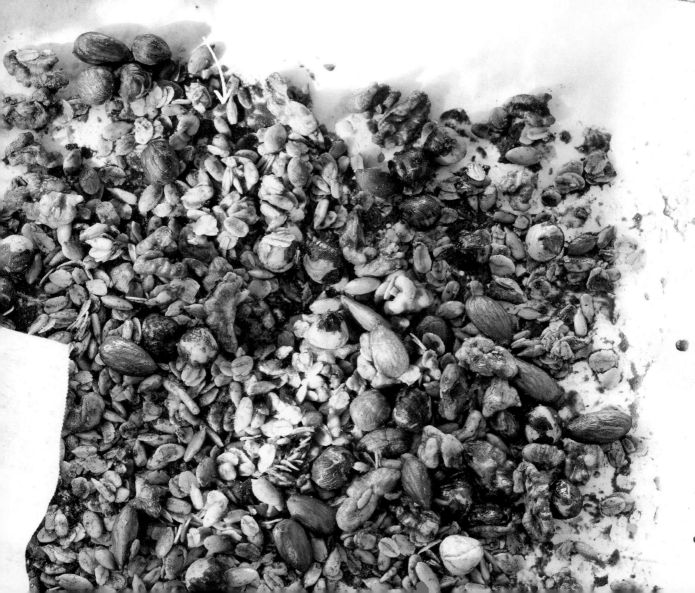

# WAYS WITH GRANOLA

*Granola is an easy prep-ahead breakfast that you can make your own with all of your favourite nuts, seeds and fruits. I love coming up with new combinations of flavours! Recipes overleaf.*

**CHAI-SPICED PALEO GRANOLA**

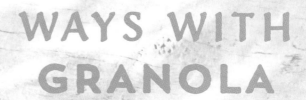

## 'NO RECIPE GRANOLA'

*It is so easy to make homemade granola, and it's cheaper than buying it ready-made too!*

BASE
2 x 250 ml cups mixed nuts, seeds, coconut flakes, buckinis (you can use any of these – sometimes I just use mixed nuts and seeds to keep it simple)
50 g optional grains (organic or gluten-free oats or quinoa flakes) – omit for a grain-free paleo version
ground cinnamon or cardamom or grated nutmeg, to taste
a pinch or two of Celtic sea salt
70 g virgin organic coconut oil, melted
2 tablespoons sweetener (maple syrup, rice malt syrup, raw honey or mashed banana)
thick Greek-style yoghurt, or almond or coconut milk, to serve

Preheat the oven to 180°C (160°C fan/gas 4) and line a baking tray with baking paper.

Pick and mix 2 x 250 ml cups of your base ingredients and an optional grain (if using), and place in a bowl. Sprinkle with your choice of spices and a pinch or two of sea salt.

Pour the melted coconut oil over the mixture, then drizzle over the sweetener and mix well.

Bake for 10 minutes. Take out and stir the mixture, then bake for another 5–10 minutes or until golden.

Remove from the oven and allow the granola to cool for at least 10 minutes. Serve with yoghurt or your choice of milk.

## STICKY BANANA & COCONUT GRANOLA

*I made this one fine morning when living in LA. It kind of happened accidentally and it was a massive hit – my husband couldn't get over the way the granola transformed into caramel-like pieces. This pairs so well with some fresh banana slices and a sprinkle of crushed walnuts.*

MAKES about 3½ cups (850 ml)
PREP TIME: 40 minutes, including cooking and cooling

2 x 250 ml cups mixed seeds and nuts (pumpkin seeds, cashews, walnuts and flaked almonds)
30 g coconut flakes
1 teaspoon ground cinnamon
2 pinches of Celtic sea salt
4 medjool dates, pitted and finely chopped (optional)
70 g virgin organic coconut oil, melted
2 tablespoons raw honey or maple syrup (optional)
½ banana, mashed
1 tablespoon coconut flour
thick Greek-style yoghurt, or almond or coconut milk, to serve

Preheat the oven to 180°C (160°C fan/gas 4) and line a baking tray with baking paper.

Place the mixed seeds and nuts in a bowl. Stir in the coconut flakes, cinnamon, salt and dates (if using).

Pour the coconut oil over the mixture, then drizzle over the raw honey or maple syrup (if using). Stir until well combined. Add the banana and mix with your hands so it coats the granola. Spread out evenly on the prepared tray and sprinkle the coconut flour over the top. Bake for 10 minutes. Take out and stir the mixture, then bake for another 5–10 minutes or until golden.

Remove from the oven and allow the granola to cool for at least 10 minutes. Serve with yoghurt or your choice of milk.

# NUTELLA GRANOLA

*Chocolate and hazelnut goodness that goes so deliciously with thick and creamy coconut milk yoghurt.*

MAKES about 4 cups (1 litre)
PREP TIME: 40 minutes, including cooking and cooling

2 x 250 ml cups mixed seeds and nuts (such as pumpkin and sunflower seeds, almonds, hazelnuts and walnuts)
70 g hazelnuts, whole or halved, extra
100 g organic or gluten-free oats (optional)
2 tablespoons raw cacao powder
1 teaspoon ground cinnamon
70 g virgin organic coconut oil, melted
2–3 tablespoons maple syrup (omit for a sugar-free version)
thick Greek-style yoghurt, or almond or coconut milk, to serve

Preheat the oven to 180°C (160°C fan/gas 4) and line a baking tray with baking paper.

Place the mixed seeds and nuts, extra hazelnuts and oats (if using) in a bowl. Stir in the cacao powder and cinnamon.

Pour the coconut oil over the mixture, then drizzle over the maple syrup (if using). Stir until well combined.

Spread out evenly on the prepared tray and bake for 10 minutes. Take out and stir the mixture, then bake for another 5–10 minutes or until golden.

Remove from the oven and allow the granola to cool for at least 10 minutes. Serve with yoghurt or your choice of milk.

# CHAI-SPICED PALEO GRANOLA

*The delicious smell that comes out of the oven while this is baking makes this recipe a household must. It is so nourishing and goes beautifully with thick and creamy Greek-style yoghurt. It's perfect for people on a low- or no-gluten diet.*

MAKES about 2½ cups (600 ml)
PREP TIME: 40 minutes, including cooking and cooling

2 x 250 ml cups mixed seeds and nuts (such as pumpkin, sunflower and chia seeds, almonds and walnuts)
1 teaspoon chai spice blend
1 teaspoon ground cinnamon
1 teaspoon vanilla powder
70 g virgin organic coconut oil, melted
2 tablespoons maple syrup
thick Greek-style yoghurt, or almond or coconut milk, to serve

Preheat the oven to 180°C (160°C fan/gas 4) and line a baking tray with baking paper.

Place the mixed seeds and nuts in a bowl. Stir in the chai spice, cinnamon and vanilla powder.

Pour the coconut oil over the mixture, then drizzle over the maple syrup. Stir until well combined.

Spread out evenly on the prepared tray and bake for 10 minutes. Take out and stir the mixture, then bake for another 5–10 minutes or until golden.

Remove from the oven and allow the granola to cool for at least 10 minutes. Serve with yoghurt or your choice of milk.

## TIP

*Make a big batch of any of these granolas and store in an airtight container for up to a week.*

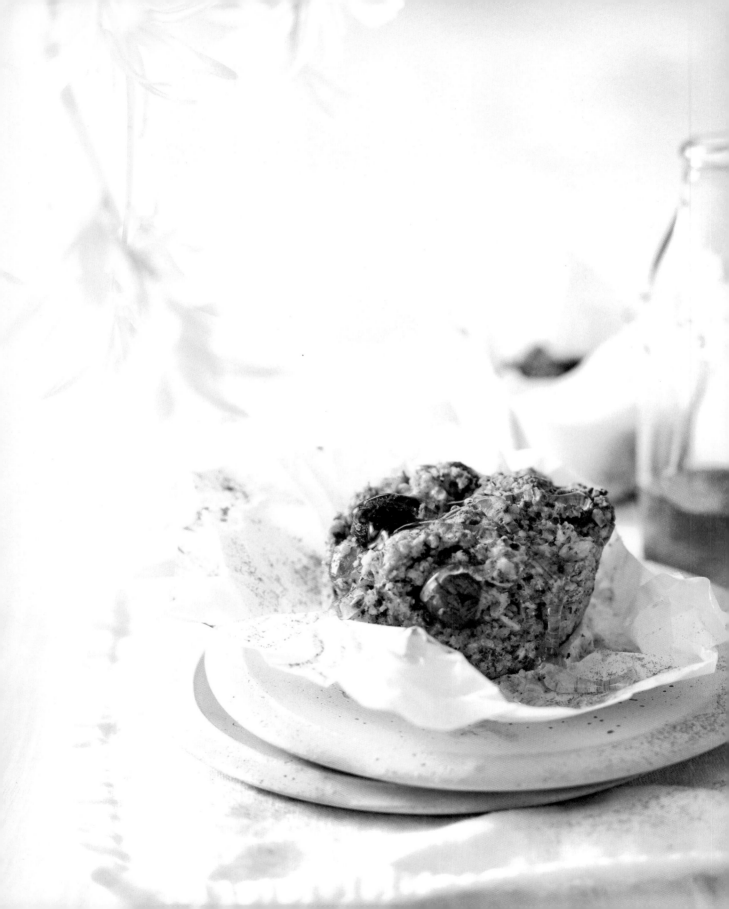

# CHIA, BLUEBERRY & BANANA BREAKFAST MUFFINS

**MAKES 10**
**PREP TIME:** 50 minutes, including cooking

200 g hazelnut meal
  or almond meal
75 g organic or gluten-free
  oats
2 tablespoons chia seeds
2 teaspoons baking powder
½ teaspoon ground
  cinnamon, plus extra for
  sprinkling (optional)
½ teaspoon ground ginger
a pinch of Celtic sea salt
3 eggs, lightly beaten
3 tablespoons virgin organic
  coconut oil, melted
90 g medjool dates, pitted
  and roughly chopped
2 large ripe bananas,
  mashed with a fork
2 tablespoons natural
  yoghurt or coconut
  milk yoghurt
75 g blueberries
2 tablespoons raw honey
  or maple syrup

*Muffins are my favourite indulgence. I love these in particular as they don't leave you feeling heavy and bloated.*

Preheat the oven to 180°C (160°C fan/gas 4). Line 10 standard muffin-tin holes with baking paper or paper cases.

In a large bowl, combine the hazelnut or almond meal, oats, chia seeds, baking powder, cinnamon, ginger and salt.

Whisk together the eggs, coconut oil, dates, bananas and yoghurt in a large jug. Add to the dry ingredients and mix well, then fold through the blueberries.

Divide the mixture evenly among the muffin holes.

Bake for 30–35 minutes or until the muffins are golden brown. Remove from the oven and cool slightly in the tin. These can be served warm or at room temperature.

Drizzle with honey or maple syrup just before serving and finish with a sprinkle of cinnamon, if desired.

# WAYS WITH SMOOTHIES

*These nutritionally balanced smoothies are the ultimate meal-on-the-go, and so easy and quick to make. Buy the best quality blender you can – they're a great investment! Recipes overleaf.*

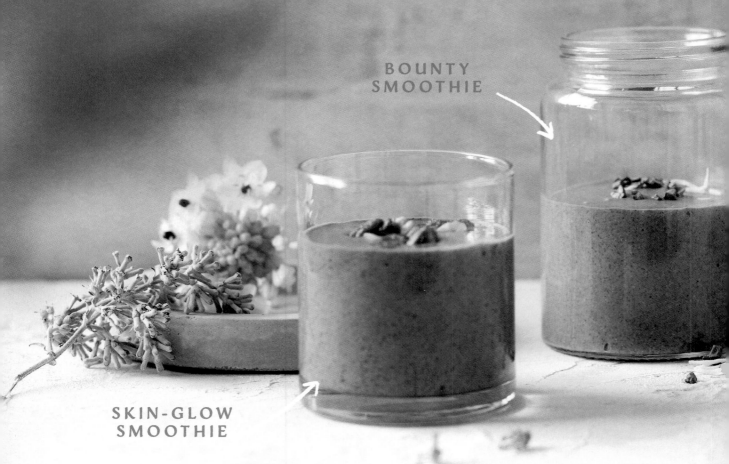

BOUNTY
SMOOTHIE

SKIN-GLOW
SMOOTHIE

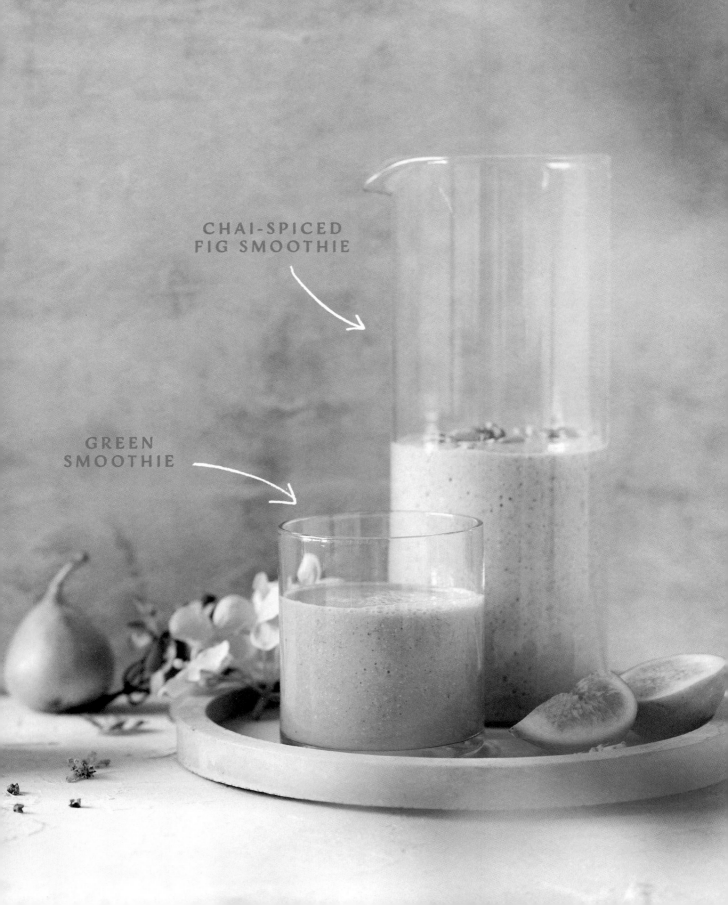

CHAI-SPICED
FIG SMOOTHIE

GREEN
SMOOTHIE

## SKIN-GLOW SMOOTHIE

SERVES 1

*Chia seeds and flaxseed provide essential fatty acids that will make your skin glow, and berries and pumpkin seeds help with skin cell repair and growth.*

½–1 frozen banana, chopped
50–100 g blueberries and/or
   strawberries, fresh or frozen
250 ml coconut milk
1 teaspoon ground cinnamon
2 tablespoons goji berries
1 tablespoon chia seeds
1 tablespoon ground flaxseed
250 ml ice cubes
1 tablespoon coconut butter
   (optional)
walnuts, pumpkin seeds and
   extra goji berries, to serve

Place the banana, berries, coconut milk, cinnamon, goji berries, chia seeds, flaxseed, ice cubes and coconut butter (if using) in a blender and blend until smooth.

Pour into a glass and top with walnuts, pumpkin seeds and extra goji berries.

## BOUNTY SMOOTHIE

SERVES 1

*Because I love Bounty bars and wanted a healthy version!*

2 tablespoons raw cacao
   powder
½–1 frozen banana, chopped
3 tablespoons desiccated
   coconut
2 medjool dates, pitted and
   chopped
1 teaspoon chia seeds
125 ml coconut or almond
   milk
1 tablespoon almond butter or
   coconut butter
4 ice cubes
¼ teaspoon xanthan gum,
   to thicken (optional)
1–2 teaspoons stevia granules
   (optional)
raw cacao nibs and extra
   desiccated coconut, to serve

Place the cacao powder, banana, coconut, dates, chia seeds, milk, butter, ice cubes, xanthan gum and stevia (if using) in a blender and blend until smooth.

Pour into a glass and top with cacao nibs and an extra sprinkle of desiccated coconut.

## GREEN SMOOTHIE

SERVES 1

*I created this smoothie to soothe all tummy troubles – mint, ginger and chia are incredibly good for the digestive system. Plus rocket, lime and cucumber are excellent detoxifiers and absolutely full of nutrients. So next time you're feeling bloated, weighed down or just a bit under the weather, give it a try.*

½ frozen banana, chopped
250 ml coconut water
a handful of baby spinach
   or rocket leaves
juice of ½ lime
½ Lebanese or ridge cucumber
1 teaspoon chia seeds
3–4 mint leaves
½ teaspoon grated ginger
4–5 ice cubes

Place all the ingredients in a blender and blend until smooth.

Pour into a glass and enjoy!

## CHAI-SPICED FIG SMOOTHIE

SERVES 1

*I'm in love with anything chai and anything fig so this combo is divine.*

½–1 frozen banana, chopped
1 serve vanilla protein powder
1–2 tablespoons organic or
 gluten-free oats
2 dried or fresh figs, sliced
1 tablespoon hulled tahini
1 teaspoon ground cinnamon
1 teaspoon stevia granules or
 raw honey
½ teaspoon chai spice blend
a pinch of grated nutmeg and/
 or ground cardamom
250 ml ice cubes
250 ml almond milk
crushed walnuts, mixed seeds
 and extra sliced fresh fig and
 ground cinnamon, to serve

Place the banana, protein powder, oats, figs, tahini, cinnamon, stevia or honey, chai spice blend, nutmeg and/ or cardamom, ice cubes and almond milk in a blender and blend until smooth.

Pour into a glass and top with crushed walnuts, mixed seeds and extra fig and cinnamon.

## SALTED CARAMEL SMOOTHIE

SERVES 1

*Salty and sweet is my absolute favourite combo. This divine smoothie tastes like a salted caramel ice-cream.*

250 ml almond milk
1 frozen banana, chopped
2 medjool dates, pitted and
 chopped
1 teaspoon Celtic sea salt
1 tablespoon hulled tahini
 or almond butter
1 teaspoon vanilla powder
3 ice cubes
homemade granola
 (see pages 140–1) and extra
 Celtic sea salt, to serve

Place the almond milk, banana, dates, salt, tahini or almond butter, vanilla powder and ice cubes in a blender and blend until smooth.

Pour into a glass and top with granola and extra salt.

## JSHEALTH PROTEIN SMOOTHIE

SERVES 1

*My signature smoothie which is too popular not to include! I start my days with this one; it's very nutritionally balanced.*

1 serve protein powder
1 teaspoon chia seeds or
 psyllium husk
60 g frozen berries
25 g baby spinach leaves
 (optional)
1 teaspoon vanilla powder
½ teaspoon ground cinnamon
4–5 ice cubes
250 ml almond milk
1 teaspoon stevia granules
½ frozen banana (optional)

Place the protein powder, chia seeds, berries, baby spinach leaves, vanilla powder, cinnamon, ice cubes, almond milk, stevia and banana (if using) in a blender and blend until smooth.

Pour into a glass and enjoy!

### TIP

*You can make all these smoothies 'blood-sugar friendly' by replacing the banana and dates with berries or stevia granules and cinnamon.*

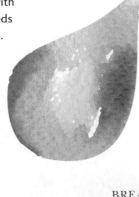

# BAKED BANANA WITH TAHINI CARAMEL SAUCE

*Enjoy these bananas just as they are, or add yoghurt or oats if you like. Not just for breakfast, this is a great pick-me-up snack to avoid that afternoon slump. It knocks over my sweet tooth when I have it with Greek-style yoghurt.*

SERVES 1
PREP TIME: 15 minutes, including cooking

1 banana, halved lengthways
1 teaspoon virgin organic coconut oil (or use coconut oil spray)
ground cinnamon, for dusting
3 tablespoons walnuts, crushed
Greek-style yoghurt or coconut milk yoghurt, to serve (optional)

TAHINI CARAMEL SAUCE:
2 tablespoons hulled tahini
2 tablespoons maple syrup
1 teaspoon ground cinnamon, or to taste
3 tablespoons filtered water

Preheat the oven to 180°C (160°C fan/gas 4) and line a baking tray with baking paper.

Place the banana halves on the prepared tray, cut side up. Drizzle or spray with coconut oil and dust with cinnamon.

Top the banana halves with the crushed walnuts and bake for 7–10 minutes or until golden.

Meanwhile, to make the caramel sauce, combine all the ingredients in a small bowl.

Top the banana halves with the caramel sauce and serve warm with Greek-style yoghurt or coconut milk yoghurt, if liked.

# CINNAMON, CARDAMOM & ORANGE ZEST BIRCHER MUESLI

*For those who prefer to eat gluten-free, you are welcome to use quinoa flakes, gluten-free oats or a combo of chia seeds and flaxseed instead of the oats.*

SERVES 2
PREP TIME: 10 minutes + overnight soaking

100 g organic or gluten-free oats
250 ml milk of choice or filtered water
1 tablespoon finely grated orange zest
1 tablespoon freshly squeezed orange juice
70 g raw almonds, roughly chopped
1 tablespoon shredded coconut
1 small pear, grated
2 tablespoons Greek-style yoghurt
1 teaspoon ground cinnamon, plus extra to serve (optional)
½ teaspoon ground cardamom
maple syrup or raw honey, fresh full-fat ricotta, blueberries or dates, to serve

Soak the oats in the water or milk overnight. Make sure they are completely covered.

In a bowl, combine the oats with the orange zest, juice, almonds, coconut, pear, yoghurt, cinnamon and cardamom – the texture should be thick but smooth.

To serve, drizzle with maple syrup or honey and top with ricotta, blueberries or torn fresh dates. Sprinkle with a little extra cinnamon, if desired.

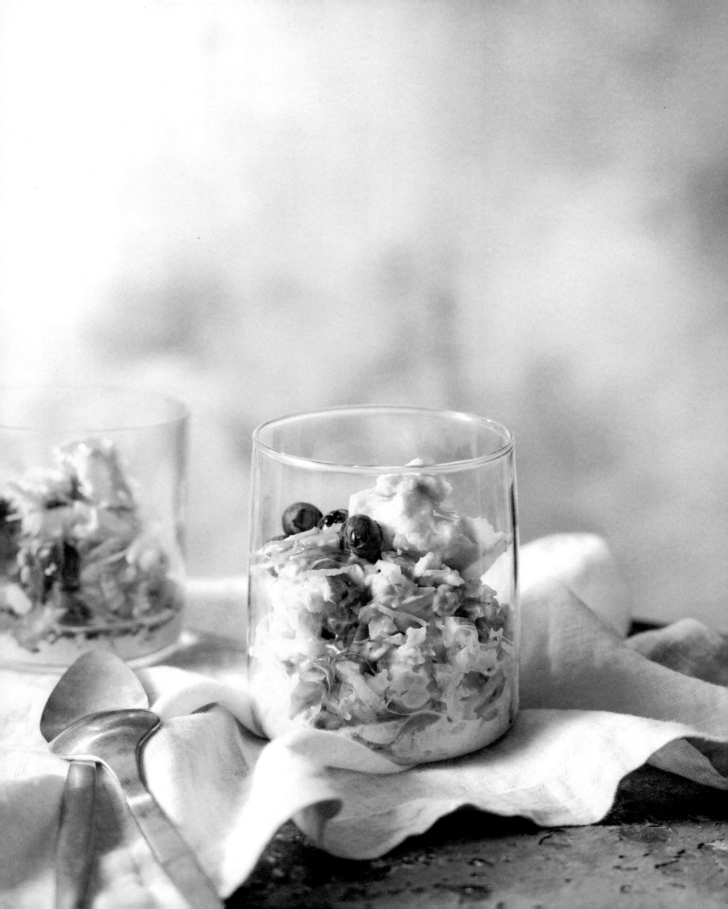

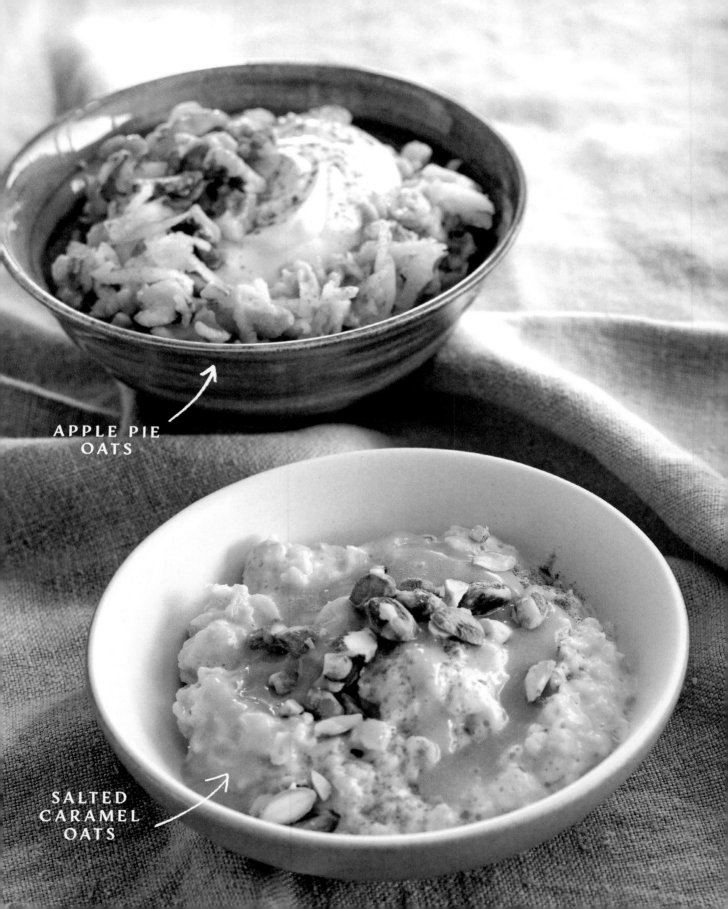

APPLE PIE
OATS

SALTED
CARAMEL
OATS

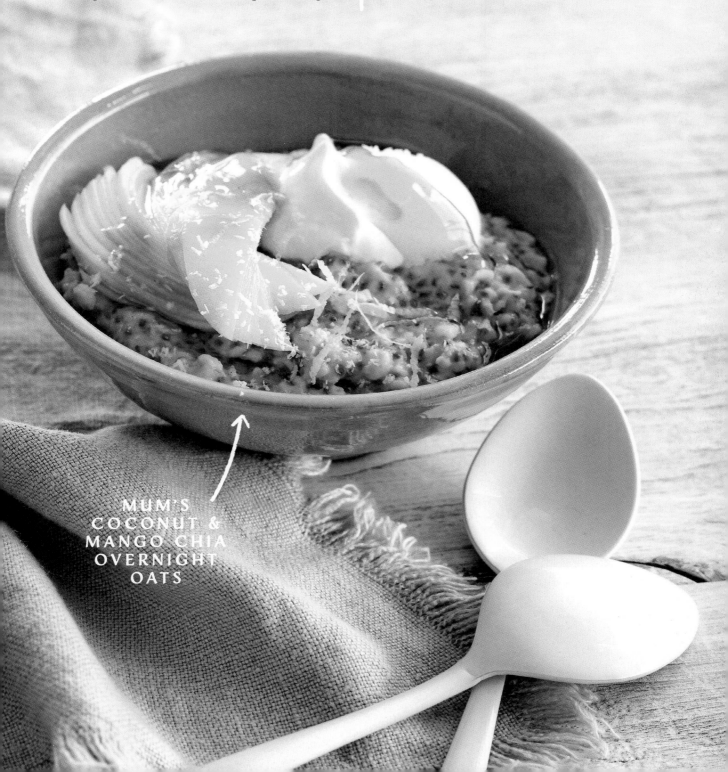

A bag of oats goes a long way! Oats are versatile, inexpensive and very nourishing – they are high in fibre and B vitamins. Eating oats for breakfast will keep you nice and full until lunchtime. Recipes overleaf.

# WAYS WITH OATS

MUM'S COCONUT & MANGO CHIA OVERNIGHT OATS

## OATMEAL

*If you are gluten-intolerant or suffer from coeliac disease, swap your oats for quinoa flakes in any of these recipes. Gluten-free oats are now available too.*

SERVES 1
PREP TIME: 15 minutes, including cooking

50 g organic or gluten-free oats
125 ml milk of choice (almond, coconut,
    cow's milk etc.)
125 ml filtered water

Combine the oats, milk and water in a saucepan and bring to the boil over high heat.

Reduce the heat to medium and simmer, covered, for 10–12 minutes or until the oats are soft.

Choose one of the delicious toppings from the recipes that follow and enjoy.

## TIP

---

*Add grated apple to your morning oats and finish with toasted almonds and Greek-style yoghurt! Heavenly. A personal fave of mine.*

---

## APPLE PIE OATS

*Do you love the taste and smell of apple pie and ice-cream? Then make this nutritious version – you won't be sorry.*

SERVES 1
PREP TIME: 15 minutes, including cooking

50 g organic or gluten-free oats
250 ml almond milk, coconut milk or
    filtered water
1 teaspoon ground cinnamon
½ teaspoon grated nutmeg
¼ teaspoon ground ginger and/or cardamom
a squeeze of lemon juice
a pinch of Celtic sea salt

TOPPING:
2 tablespoons walnuts, crushed
½ green apple, grated
1 tablespoon maple syrup
2 heaped tablespoons Greek-style yoghurt
    or coconut milk yoghurt (optional)
ground cinnamon, extra, to serve

Combine the oats and milk or water in a saucepan and bring to the boil over high heat.

Reduce the heat to medium and simmer, covered, for 10–12 minutes or until the oats are soft.

Still over medium heat, stir the cinnamon, nutmeg, ginger and/or cardamom, lemon juice and salt into the oats.

Spoon the oats into a bowl and top with the crushed walnuts, apple, maple syrup, yoghurt (if using) and finish with a dusting of cinnamon.

# SALTED CARAMEL OATS

*This combination happened accidentally, but now you need to make it ASAP!*

SERVES 1
PREP TIME: 15 minutes, including cooking

50 g organic or gluten-free oats
250 ml almond milk, coconut milk or filtered
  water
a handful of pistachio kernels
ground cinnamon, to serve

CARAMEL SAUCE:
1 heaped tablespoon hulled tahini
a pinch of Celtic sea salt
1 tablespoon maple syrup
a few drops of hot water

Combine the oats and milk or water in a saucepan
and bring to the boil over high heat.

Reduce the heat to medium and simmer, covered,
for 10–12 minutes or until the oats are soft.

Meanwhile, to make the caramel sauce, mix together
all the ingredients until smooth and well combined.

Spoon the oats into a bowl and top with the caramel
sauce, pistachios and a dusting of cinnamon.

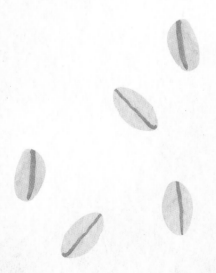

# MUM'S COCONUT & MANGO CHIA OVERNIGHT OATS

*My mum has been making this version of oats
recently for breakfast and it is absolutely divine.
It tastes of summer!*

SERVES 1
PREP TIME: 15 minutes, including cooking +
overnight soaking

50 g organic or gluten-free oats
1 tablespoon chia seeds
250 ml almond milk, coconut milk or filtered
  water, plus extra milk if needed
½ teaspoon ground cinnamon
a pinch of Celtic sea salt

TOPPING:
½ mango, sliced
1 tablespoon desiccated coconut
1 tablespoon maple syrup
1 tablespoon finely grated lemon zest
2 heaped tablespoons Greek-style yoghurt or
  coconut milk yoghurt
ground cinnamon and flaked almonds
  (optional), to serve

Combine the oats and chia seeds in a bowl, pour
in enough water to cover and soak overnight.

The next morning, combine the oat mixture and milk
or water in a saucepan and bring to the boil over
high heat.

Reduce the heat to medium and simmer, covered,
for 10–12 minutes or until the oats are soft.

Stir in the cinnamon and salt and perhaps a little
more milk, if liked.

Spoon the oats into a bowl and top with the mango,
coconut, maple syrup, lemon zest and yoghurt.
Finish with a dusting of cinnamon and, if liked,
a handful of flaked almonds.

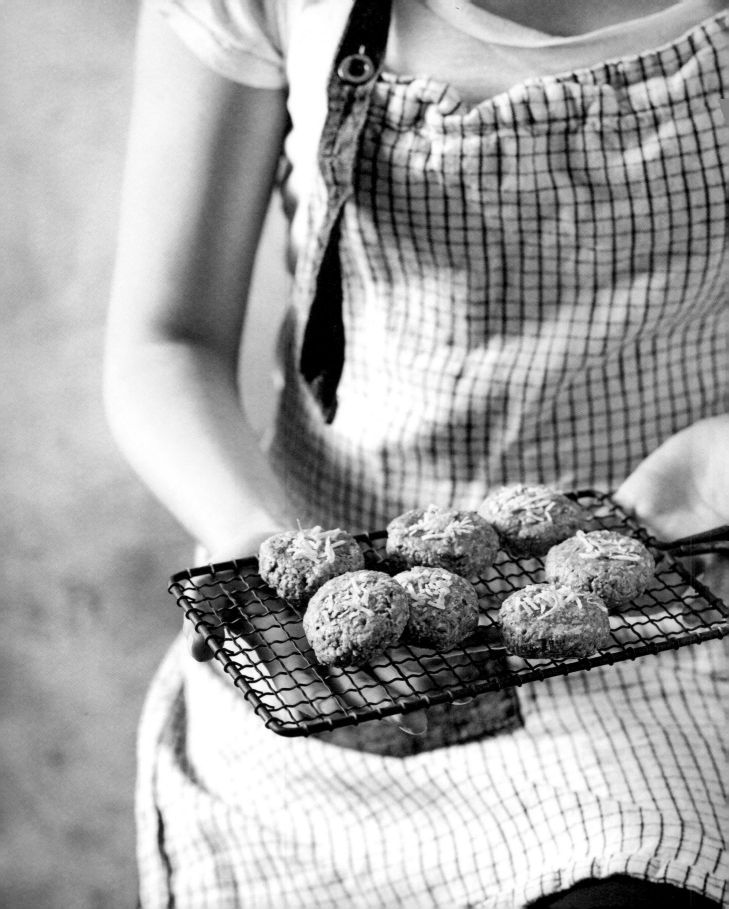

# BREAKFAST CINNAMON OAT COOKIES

MAKES 10
PREP TIME: 30 minutes, including cooking

70 g organic or gluten-free oats

3 tablespoons almond butter

2 tablespoons sunflower seeds

2 tablespoons pumpkin seeds

1 tablespoon sesame seeds

2 tablespoons vanilla protein powder or 1 teaspoon vanilla extract

2 teaspoons ground cinnamon

a pinch of Celtic sea salt

1½ tablespoons maple syrup or raw honey

2–3 tablespoons filtered water

1 tablespoon shredded coconut

*Who loves dunking cookies in tea? I do. These are so clean and wholesome and can be a great addition to breakfast picnics. The kiddies will love them too.*

Preheat the oven to 160°C (140°C fan/gas 3) and line a baking tray with baking paper.

Blend the oats, butter, seeds, vanilla, cinnamon, salt, maple syrup or honey and water in a food processor until well combined.

Using damp hands, roll heaped tablespoons of the mixture into balls. Flatten the balls onto the prepared tray and sprinkle the tops with the coconut. Bake for 12–15 minutes or until golden and cooked through. Remove and cool on a wire rack. Store in an airtight container for up to 5 days.

For a raw version, roll the mixture into balls, sprinkle with the coconut and place in the freezer for 30 minutes. Refrigerate in an airtight container for up to 5 days.

# GLUTEN-FREE GREEN BREAD

MAKES 1 loaf
PREP TIME: 1 hour,
including cooking

200 g almond meal, plus
  extra for coating
50 g LSA or ground
  flaxseed
75 g chia seeds
4 tablespoons crushed raw
  almonds
4 tablespoons psyllium
  husk
1½ teaspoons baking
  powder
1 teaspoon Himalayan pink
  rock salt
handful of kale, stalk
  removed and leaf finely
  chopped
2 handfuls of baby spinach
  leaves, finely chopped
2 tablespoons finely
  chopped flat-leaf parsley
1 tablespoon finely
  chopped thyme
3 eggs
2 tablespoons virgin
  organic coconut oil
75 ml milk of choice
  (I usually use almond
  milk), plus extra if
  needed
coconut oil spray
1 tablespoon flaked
  almonds
olive oil, to serve (optional)

*I make this loaf every week and keep it in the fridge. It goes with everything and is completely unprocessed, unlike most breads you buy. In addition, it's gluten-free, very high in fibre and a great way to get in the greens. I'll have a slice with eggs for breakfast most mornings – it's hard to resist!*

Preheat the oven to 180°C (160°C fan/gas 4).

Combine the almond meal, LSA or flaxseed, chia seeds, almonds, psyllium husk, baking powder and salt in a large mixing bowl. Add the kale, spinach, parsley and thyme and stir well.

Whisk together the eggs, coconut oil and milk in a measuring jug.

Slowly pour the wet ingredients into the bowl, stirring until everything is well combined. If the batter is too wet, add extra almond meal; if it is too dry, add more milk.

Lightly oil a standard loaf tin (approximately 21 cm x 11 cm) with coconut oil spray, then coat liberally with extra almond meal to prevent the bread from sticking. Spoon the batter into the tin and scatter over the flaked almonds.

Bake for 35–45 minutes. To check if it's cooked, insert a skewer into the middle of the loaf – if it comes out dry, it's done. If the top is starting to brown, cover with foil and continue baking until cooked through. It will feel more solid than regular bread.

Remove the loaf from the oven and cool completely in the tin. Cut into slices and serve with olive oil, if liked, or use to make sandwiches.

Keep covered in the fridge for up to 1 week. It also freezes well.

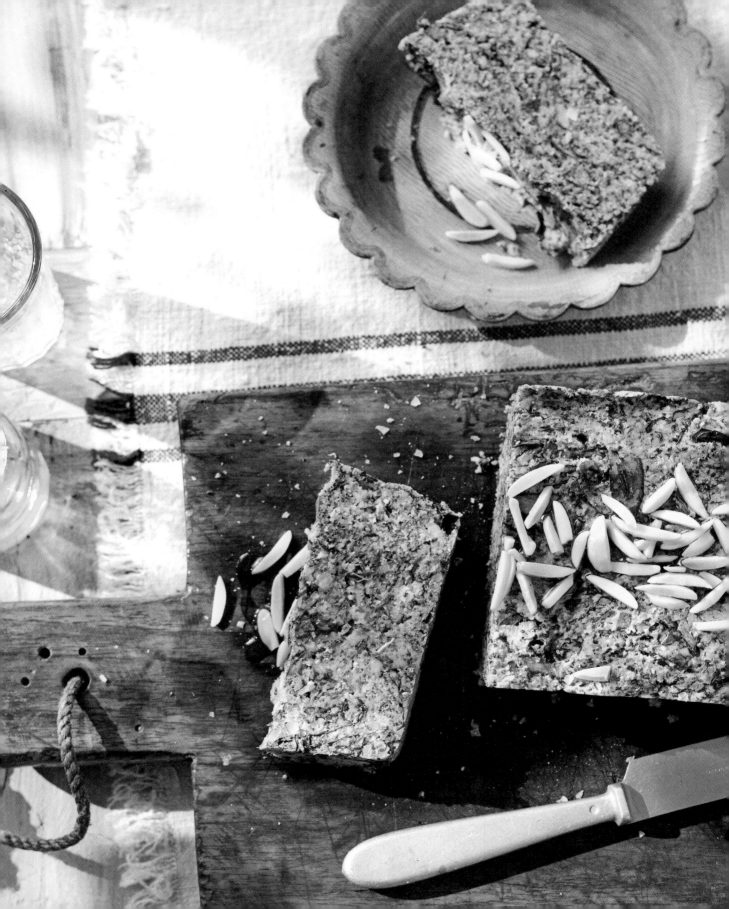

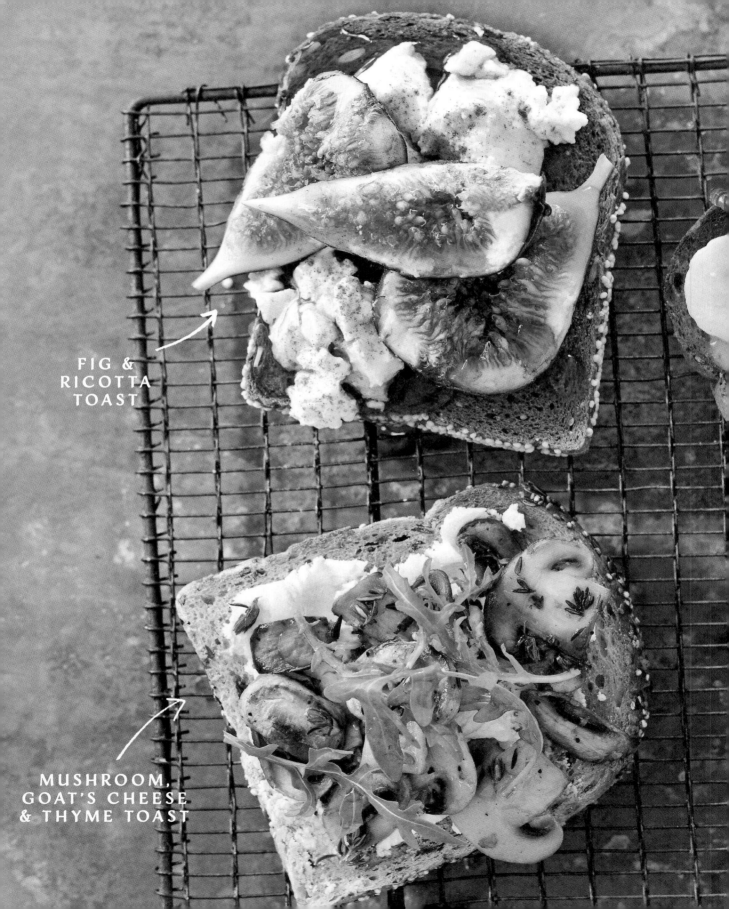

FIG &
RICOTTA
TOAST

MUSHROOM,
GOAT'S CHEESE
& THYME TOAST

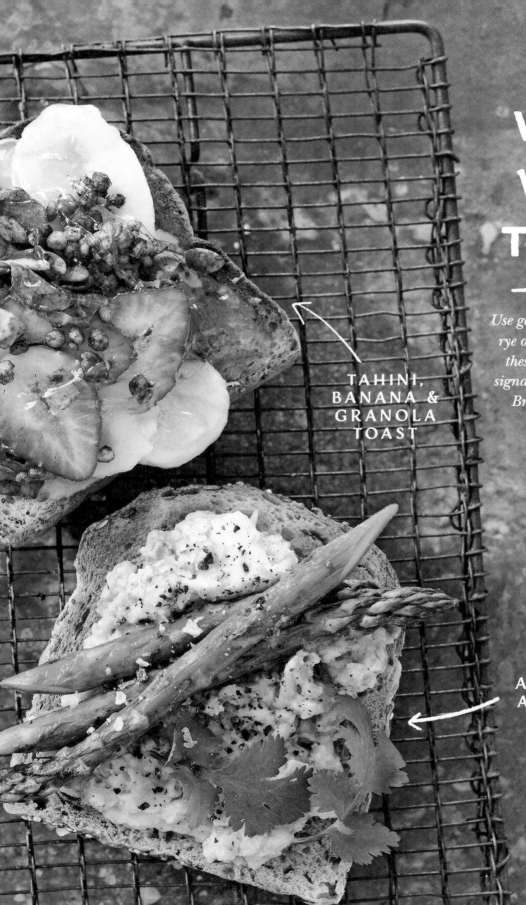

# WAYS WITH TOAST

*Use good-quality sourdough, rye or gluten-free bread for these toasts, or make my signature Gluten-free Green Bread (see page 156). Recipes overleaf.*

TAHINI, BANANA & GRANOLA TOAST

AVOCADO & ASPARAGUS TOAST

## FIG & RICOTTA TOAST

### SERVES 1

Spread fresh full-fat ricotta on your toast, then layer on 1 sliced fresh fig. Sprinkle with ground cinnamon and drizzle with maple syrup. Finish with fresh mint leaves, if you like.

## TAHINI, BANANA & GRANOLA TOAST

### SERVES 1

Spread 1 tablespoon hulled tahini on your toast, then layer on 1 sliced banana. Drizzle with raw honey and sprinkle with ground cinnamon. Sprinkle with homemade granola (see pages 140–1) and, if you like, crushed nuts and seeds, toasted coconut flakes or strawberry slices.

## MUSHROOM, GOAT'S CHEESE & THYME TOAST

### SERVES 1

Heat a little olive oil in a frying pan over medium heat and cook 1 crushed garlic clove until softened. Add 75 g sliced button mushrooms, a handful of thyme sprigs, Celtic sea salt and ground pepper and sauté until the mushrooms are cooked. Spread 1 tablespoon goat's cheese or hummus on your toast, then top with the mushroom mixture and some baby rocket leaves. (Alternatively, roughly crumble the cheese and scatter it over the mushrooms.)

## AVOCADO & ASPARAGUS TOAST

### SERVES 1

Mash ½ avocado with Celtic sea salt, ground pepper and a drizzle of olive oil and spread on your toast. Pan-fry 2–3 asparagus spears in a little virgin organic coconut oil and crushed garlic and season with salt and pepper (or any spices of choice). Top the avocado toast with the asparagus and some fresh flat-leaf parsley.

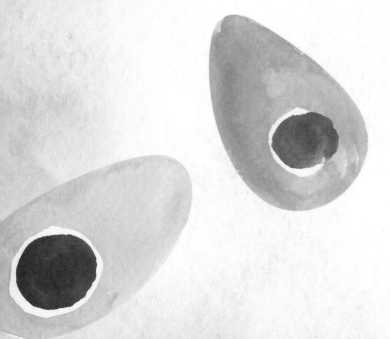

# IS TOAST YOUR COMFORT FOOD?

When I'm having a 'low day', I don't turn to pizza or burgers any more. I try to choose foods that will nourish my body instead, like toast made from good quality bread, oats, almond butter, banana, avocado, coconut or thick, creamy Greek-style yoghurt. And the best part?? I feel GOOD after eating them. When we turn to junk foods we feel even worse about ourselves. Tuning into your body and your mind (and choosing real food) will help heal your body and your relationship with food. Here are the foods I turn to when I need extra self-loving and healing.

- Almond butter smeared on delicious gluten-free toast with banana slices and ground cinnamon – my ultimate comfort meal
- Avocado smashed with Himalayan pink rock salt and olive oil on good-quality sourdough/rye or gluten-free toast
- Warm porridge cooked in almond or coconut milk and ground cinnamon, topped with almond butter
- Black tea with coconut milk, honey and ground cinnamon
- Delicious homemade Healthy Chai Latte (see page 308)
- Fresh dates filled with nut butter or hulled tahini and ground cinnamon
- Brown rice bowl with chicken or salmon and sautéed greens
- 1–2 teaspoons almond butter – out of the jar!

- Hulled tahini or drizzled on anything
- Homemade granola (see pages 140–1) served with warm almond milk
- Organic eggs served with avocado and stir-fried greens in coconut oil
- Quinoa bowl with scrambled eggs and avocado, topped with pesto (see page 292)
- Organic egg omelettes
- Brown rice cakes smeared with tahini and ground cinnamon
- Chia, Blueberry & Banana Breakfast Muffins (see page 143)
- Avocado sushi
- Homemade Banana Hazelnut Chocolate Bread (see page 265) with a smear of almond butter
- Homemade Nice-cream (see page 260)

# BREAKFAST BROWNIES

*These prove just how delicious and indulgent healthy living can be. They are high in fibre and good fats and will keep you full. Double the recipe and make a big batch to share.*

MAKES 8 large brownies
PREP TIME: 45 minutes, including freezing

115 g walnuts
2 heaped tablespoons raw cacao powder
175 g medjool dates, pitted and chopped
a pinch of Celtic sea salt
½ teaspoon ground cinnamon
15 g rice puffs or quinoa puffs
1 tablespoon virgin organic coconut oil
2 tablespoons ground flaxseed
3–4 tablespoons filtered water

TOPPING (OPTIONAL):
2 tablespoons almond butter
1 tablespoon raw cacao powder
ground cinnamon, for dusting

Place the walnuts, cacao powder, dates, salt, cinnamon, rice or quinoa puffs, coconut oil and flaxseed in a food processor. Add 3 tablespoons of the water and blend until the mixture is moist and chunky, but not runny. Add more water if needed.

Line a 20 cm square baking tin with baking paper, then press the mixture firmly and evenly into the tin.

If you are adding the topping, spread the almond butter over the brownie mixture and sprinkle with the cacao powder and cinnamon.

Cover and refrigerate for at least 30 minutes. Remove from the fridge and cut the brownie into eight even bars.

# HEALTHY COCO POPS

*Your kiddies will truly fall in love with this recipe. A must for all healthy mums, bubs and teenagers.*

MAKES about 200 g
PREP TIME: 50 minutes, including cooking and cooling time

90 g rice puffs
100 g flaked almonds
2 tablespoons virgin organic coconut oil, melted
2 tablespoons rice malt syrup or maple syrup
2 tablespoons raw cacao powder
1 teaspoon ground cinnamon
almond milk, coconut milk or yoghurt, to serve
fresh berries, banana slices and/or chia seeds,
  to garnish (optional)

Preheat the oven to 180°C (160°C fan/gas 4) and line a large baking tray with baking paper.

Place the rice puffs and almonds in a bowl.

Drizzle the coconut oil and syrup over the rice puffs and almonds, and sprinkle with the cacao powder and cinnamon.

Use your hands to mix it all together – make sure you do this gently as you don't want to squash the rice puffs.

Spread out evenly on the prepared tray and bake for 15–20 minutes, stirring halfway – take care not to overcook it as the mixture can burn easily.

Remove from the oven and set aside to cool completely.

Serve with almond milk, coconut milk or yoghurt. If you like, top with berries, banana slices and/or chia seeds.

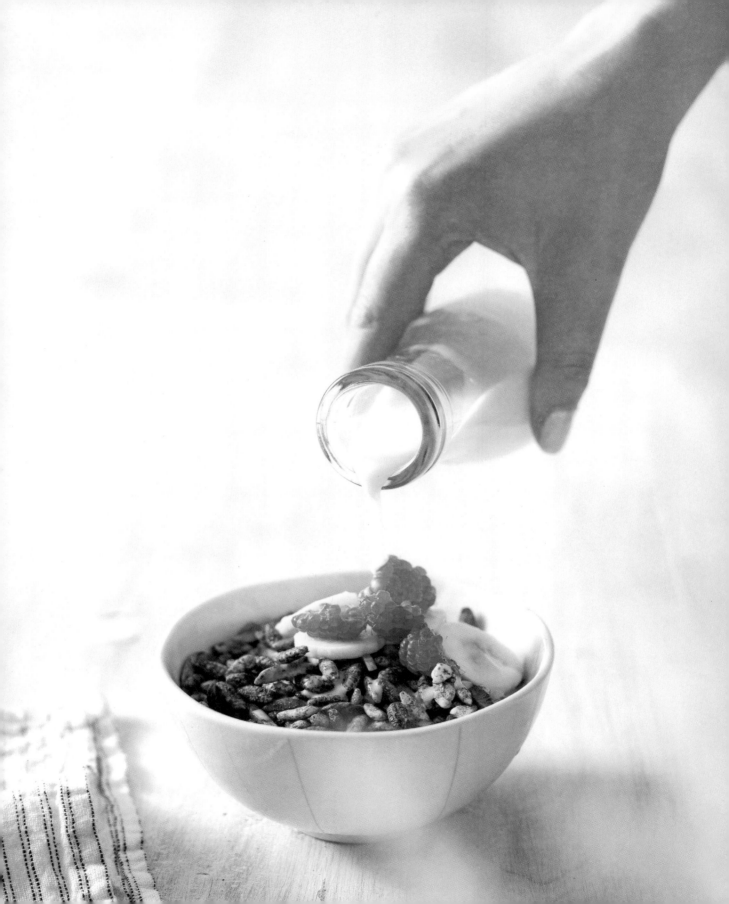

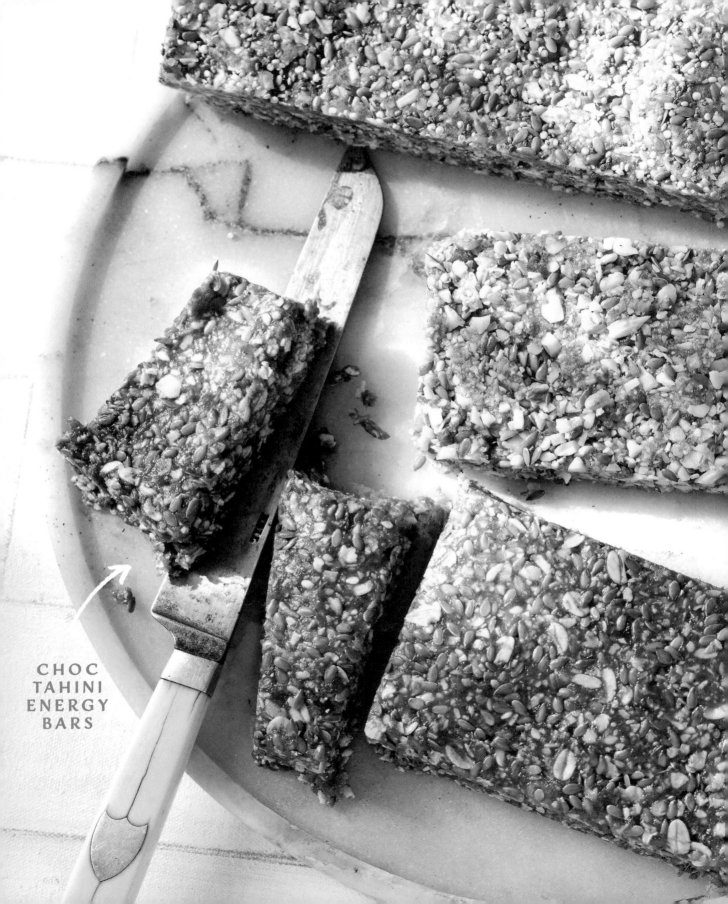

CHOC
TAHINI
ENERGY
BARS

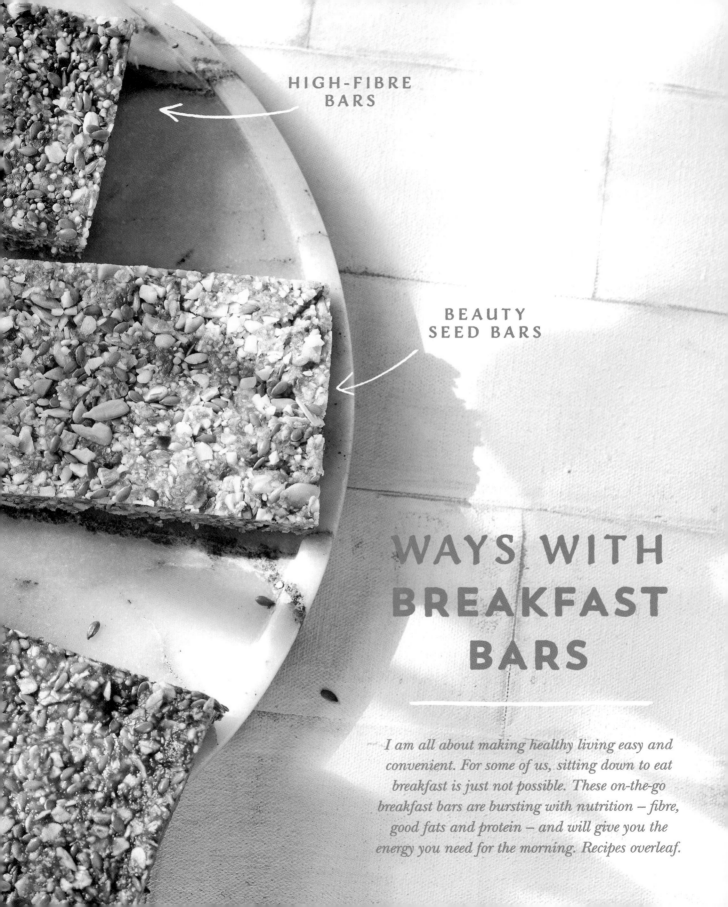

HIGH-FIBRE
BARS

BEAUTY
SEED BARS

# WAYS WITH BREAKFAST BARS

*I am all about making healthy living easy and convenient. For some of us, sitting down to eat breakfast is just not possible. These on-the-go breakfast bars are bursting with nutrition — fibre, good fats and protein — and will give you the energy you need for the morning. Recipes overleaf.*

## CHOC TAHINI ENERGY BARS

*This combination of nutritious ingredients and amazing flavours will lift you right up.*

MAKES 10
PREP TIME: 55 minutes, including freezing

10 medjool dates, pitted and chopped
125 g organic or gluten-free oats or quinoa
55 g flaxseed
2 tablespoons sesame seeds
3 tablespoons raw cacao powder
¼ teaspoon Celtic sea salt
50 g hulled tahini
70 g virgin organic coconut oil, melted
2 tablespoons coconut nectar, raw honey
  or maple syrup

Place all the ingredients in a food processor and pulse until well combined – the mixture should be firm but soft.

Grease and line a 20 cm square baking tin and press the mixture in evenly with the back of a spoon.

Cover and freeze for 30–40 minutes or until firm.

Remove from the freezer and cut into 10 bars. Store in an airtight container in the fridge for up to a week.

## BEAUTY SEED BARS

*Packed with good fats and antioxidants for glowing skin and hair.*

MAKES 8
PREP TIME: 55 minutes, including freezing

10 medjool dates, pitted and chopped
70 g sunflower seeds
70 g pumpkin seeds
70 g raw almonds
50 g organic or gluten-free oats or quinoa
3 tablespoons flaxseed
2 tablespoons sesame seeds
2 tablespoons goji berries
3 tablespoons almond butter
2 tablespoons virgin organic coconut oil, melted
2 tablespoons coconut nectar, raw honey
  or maple syrup

Place all the ingredients in a food processor and pulse until well combined – the mixture should be firm but soft.

Grease and line a 20 cm square baking tin and press the mixture in evenly with the back of a spoon.

Cover and freeze for 30–40 minutes or until firm.

Remove from the freezer and cut into eight bars. Store in an airtight container in the fridge for up to a week.

## HIGH-FIBRE BARS

*Very satiating – the fibre and good fats will keep you full all morning.*

MAKES 8
PREP TIME: 55 minutes, including freezing

10 medjool dates, pitted and chopped
3 tablespoons chia seeds
55 g white quinoa
3 tablespoons flaxseed
2 tablespoons LSA or ground flaxseed
2 tablespoons psyllium husk
125 g organic or gluten-free oats
¼ teaspoon Celtic sea salt
3 tablespoons almond butter
2 tablespoons virgin organic coconut oil, melted
2 teaspoons coconut nectar, raw honey
  or maple syrup

Place all the ingredients in a food processor and pulse until well combined – the mixture should be firm but soft.

Grease and line a 20 cm square baking tin and press the mixture in evenly with the back of a spoon.

Cover and freeze for 30–40 minutes or until firm.

Remove from the freezer and cut into eight bars. Store in an airtight container in the fridge for up to a week.

## LUNCHBOX FILLERS

*Choc Tahini Energy Bars are the perfect lunchbox nut-free snack. Here are some more nutritious and nut-free snacks that your kids will love.*

- Rice paper rolls
- Chia pudding
- Frittata or chicken kebabs with salad
- Air-popped popcorn with organic butter and Celtic sea salt
- Homemade nut-free cookies
- Fresh dates filled with tahini
- Lentil and bean salad
- Cut-up veggies (carrots, cucumber, celery) with boiled eggs, hummus or tahini
- Mountain bread wraps with egg or tuna and salad
- Fresh berries with Greek-style yoghurt, a sprinkle of ground cinnamon and shredded coconut
- Lettuce wraps filled with your choice of protein and quinoa
- Quinoa tabbouleh salad, without the nuts!
- Sliced green apple with cinnamon
- Bliss balls (see pages 268–9)
- Nut- and sugar-free granola with Greek-style yoghurt
- Brown rice cakes with avocado or tahini and cinnamon spread
- Homemade nut-free trail mix (sunflower, pumpkin seeds, goji berries, cranberries)
- Homemade quinoa/brown rice sushi

# HERB, ONION & CAULIFLOWER SHAKSHUKA

*I adore this savoury breakfast. It's a favourite on a Sunday morning, enjoyed with a creamy coffee that my hubby has brought home for me. Plain passata is delicious but you could also sauté a plum tomato in olive oil with a clove of crushed garlic. I love to add leftover roasted veggies to this dish, especially Crispy Brussels by Cayley (see page 238).*

SERVES 1
PREP TIME: 25 minutes, including cooking

1 tablespoon olive oil
1 garlic clove
½ red onion, roughly chopped
175 g cauliflower florets
125 ml organic tomato passata
2 eggs
a handful of flat-leaf parsley leaves
2 tablespoons goat's cheese (optional)
1 teaspoon za'atar
Celtic salt flakes and ground pepper

Heat the olive oil in a small frying pan over medium heat, add the garlic and onion and sauté until softened. Then add the cauliflower and cook for 1–2 minutes or until slightly heated.

Stir in the tomato passata.

Make two wells in the middle and crack the eggs into the wells.

Cover with a lid and cook until the egg whites are just set but the yolks are still runny.

Scatter over the parsley, goat's cheese and za'atar, season with salt and pepper and serve.

# VANILLA, FLAXSEED, CHIA & BANANA PARFAIT

*I love this delicious but oh-so-easy breakfast dish. It's full of fibre too, making it the perfect cleansing option for breakfast. In addition, this recipe is gluten-free and vegan.*

SERVES 1
PREP TIME: 10 minutes

1–2 tablespoons ground flaxseed
50 g chia seeds
250 ml vanilla almond or coconut milk, plus extra if needed
1 teaspoon virgin organic coconut oil, melted
1 medjool date, pitted and chopped
½ teaspoon vanilla powder
½ teaspoon ground cinnamon
½ banana, mashed
a handful of walnuts
a pinch of Celtic sea salt
banana slices, homemade granola (see pages 140–1) and extra crushed walnuts, to serve

In a blender or food processor, blend the flaxseed, chia seeds, milk, coconut oil, chopped date, vanilla, cinnamon, banana, walnuts and salt. You may need to add a little more milk, depending on the consistency – it should have a pudding-like texture.

Transfer to a jar or bowl to eat straight away or soak in the fridge overnight.

Serve topped with banana slices, granola and crushed walnuts.

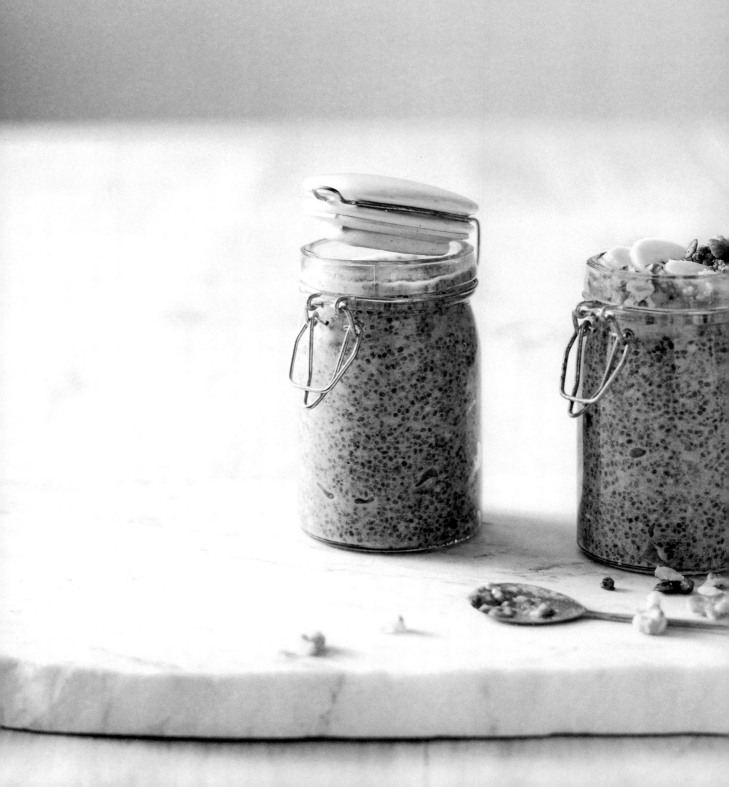

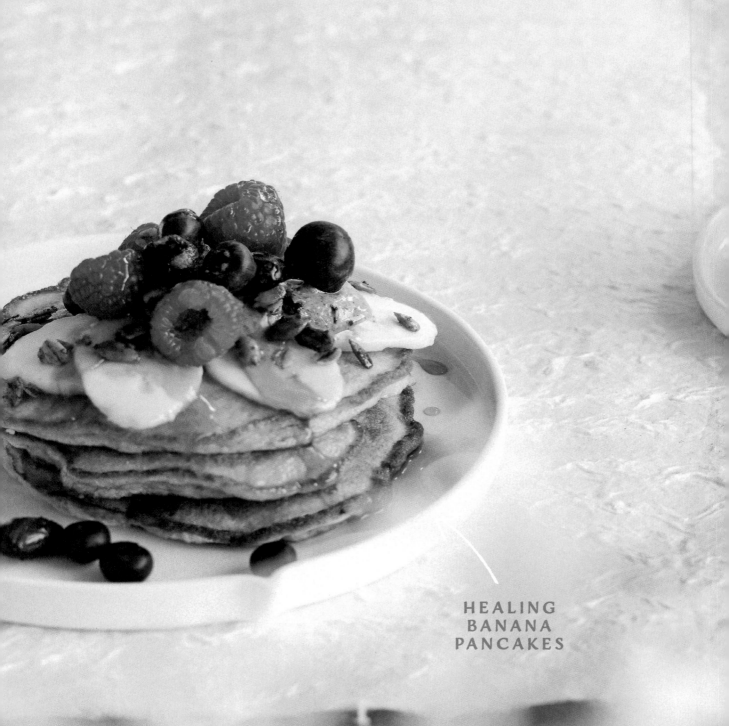

HEALING
BANANA
PANCAKES

# WAYS WITH PANCAKES

*There is something so relaxing about enjoying a sunny morning in the kitchen whipping up breakfast for your loved ones. Seeing the delight on their faces when everyone digs into their stack of pancakes is made even better when you know there is nothing naughty about them!*
*Recipes overleaf.*

APPLE CRUMBLE
PANCAKES

BANANA & CHOC
COCONUT CREPES

## HEALING BANANA PANCAKES

*These simple gluten-free pancakes are a lovely breakfast to enjoy on a weekend morning or when you want to impress the kids. It's a great way of showing them how delicious healthy living is.*

SERVES 1
PREP TIME: 10 minutes, including cooking

2 eggs, beaten
1 banana, mashed
2 heaped tablespoons coconut flour
a pinch of ground cinnamon
2 tablespoons almond or coconut milk
1 teaspoon virgin organic coconut oil
your choice of homemade granola (see
   pages 140–1), Greek-style yoghurt, sliced
   banana, almond butter or fresh berries, to serve

Place the egg, mashed banana, coconut flour, cinnamon and milk in a bowl and mix well.

Melt the coconut oil in a non-stick frying pan over medium heat. Add 3 tablespoons of batter for each pancake and cook for 2 minutes and then flip and cook the other side for another 2 minutes.

Plate up and finish with your choice of topping.

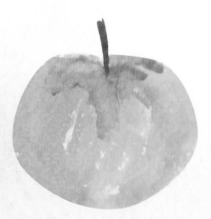

## APPLE CRUMBLE PANCAKES

*Apple crumble is my favourite treat so it's only fair to share these decadent pancakes with you.*

SERVES 2
PREP TIME: 20 minutes, including cooking

4 tablespoons coconut flour
½ teaspoon baking powder
1 teaspoon ground cinnamon
a pinch of grated nutmeg
a pinch of Celtic sea salt
2 eggs, beaten
75 ml coconut milk
½ teaspoon vanilla extract
1–2 tablespoons maple syrup, raw honey
   or stevia granules
1 teaspoon virgin organic coconut oil
Greek-style yoghurt or coconut milk yoghurt,
   to serve

APPLE CRUMBLE TOPPING:
1 teaspoon virgin organic coconut oil
½ green apple, cut into chunks
a handful of walnuts
a pinch each of ground cinnamon,
   cardamom and ginger
maple syrup, for drizzling

Place the coconut flour, baking powder, cinnamon, nutmeg, salt, egg, milk, vanilla and maple syrup, honey or stevia in a bowl and mix well.

Melt the coconut oil in a non-stick frying pan over medium heat. Add 3 tablespoons of batter for each pancake and cook for 2 minutes, then flip and cook the other side for another 2 minutes.

Meanwhile, to make the apple crumble topping, melt the coconut oil in a small frying pan over medium–high heat. Add the apple, walnuts and spices and a drizzle of maple syrup and sauté for 4–5 minutes only or until golden. Sprinkle the apple topping over the pancakes and serve with a dollop of yoghurt.

# BANANA & CHOC COCONUT CREPES

*Who doesn't like crepes? And who said you can't enjoy them if you are health conscious? These are the healthiest crepes you will ever have – and so delicious. Also high in protein so they keep you really full until your next meal.*

SERVES 2
PREP TIME: 15 minutes, including cooking

6 egg whites
2 tablespoons almond milk

¼ banana, mashed

1 heaped tablespoon raw cacao powder
3 tablespoons desiccated coconut

1 tablespoon psyllium husk

2 tablespoons LSA or ground flaxseed
2 tablespoons Greek-style yoghurt

1–2 teaspoons stevia granules, 4 drops vanilla
   stevia or 1 tablespoon maple syrup
1 tablespoon ground cinnamon

1 tablespoon virgin organic coconut oil
coconut flakes, raw cacao powder and finely
   grated orange zest, to serve

PROTEIN YOGHURT FILLING:

2 tablespoons Greek-style yoghurt

1 tablespoon maple syrup

1 tablespoon pea, whey, rice or vanilla
   protein powder

1 tablespoon almond or coconut milk

Place the egg whites, almond milk, banana, cacao powder, coconut, psyllium husk, LSA or flaxseed, yoghurt, stevia or maple syrup and cinnamon in a bowl and mix well.

Melt the coconut oil in a non-stick frying pan over medium heat. Pour half the batter into the pan and cook for 2 minutes, then flip and cook the other side for another 2 minutes. Remove and repeat with the remaining batter to make a second crepe.

Meanwhile, to make the yoghurt filling, mix all the ingredients together in a bowl until creamy and well combined.

Lay the crepes out flat on plates and divide the filling between them, spooning it evenly over one half. Flip the other half over the filling to make crepe sandwiches.

Sprinkle with coconut flakes, cacao powder and orange zest and serve.

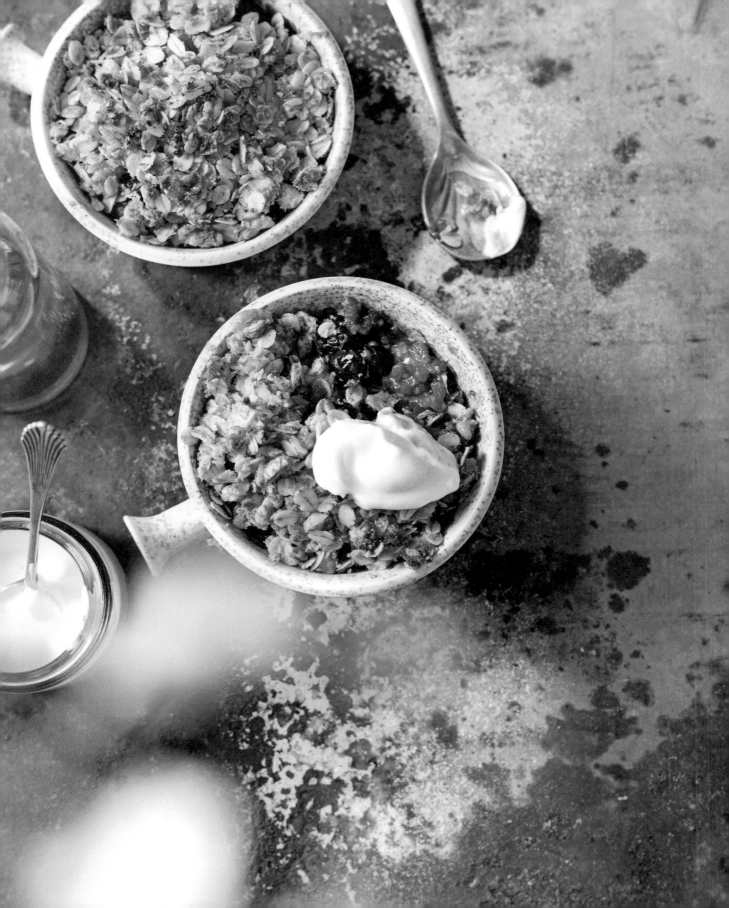

# BERRY BREAKFAST CRUMBLE

SERVES 2
PREP TIME: 25 minutes,
including cooking

225 g mixed berries,
   fresh or frozen
1 teaspoon ground
   cinnamon
Greek-style yoghurt or
   coconut milk yoghurt,
   to serve

CRUMBLE:
3 tablespoons organic
   or gluten-free oats
1 tablespoon crushed
   walnuts
1 tablespoon desiccated
   coconut
1 tablespoon virgin organic
   coconut oil, melted
1 teaspoon raw honey
   or maple syrup
½ teaspoon ground
   cinnamon
a pinch of grated nutmeg
   (optional)

*This warm nourishing crumble is like eating dessert for breakfast.
Enjoy it with a nice cup of chai.*

Preheat the oven to 200°C (180°C fan/gas 6).

Combine the berries and cinnamon in a small baking dish or two ramekins.

To make the crumble topping, combine all the ingredients in a bowl.
Sprinkle the crumble evenly over the berries.

Bake the breakfast crumble for 10–15 minutes or until golden.

Serve with a generous dollop of Greek-style yoghurt or coconut milk yoghurt.

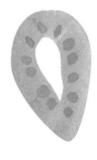
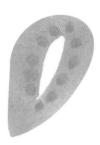
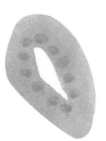

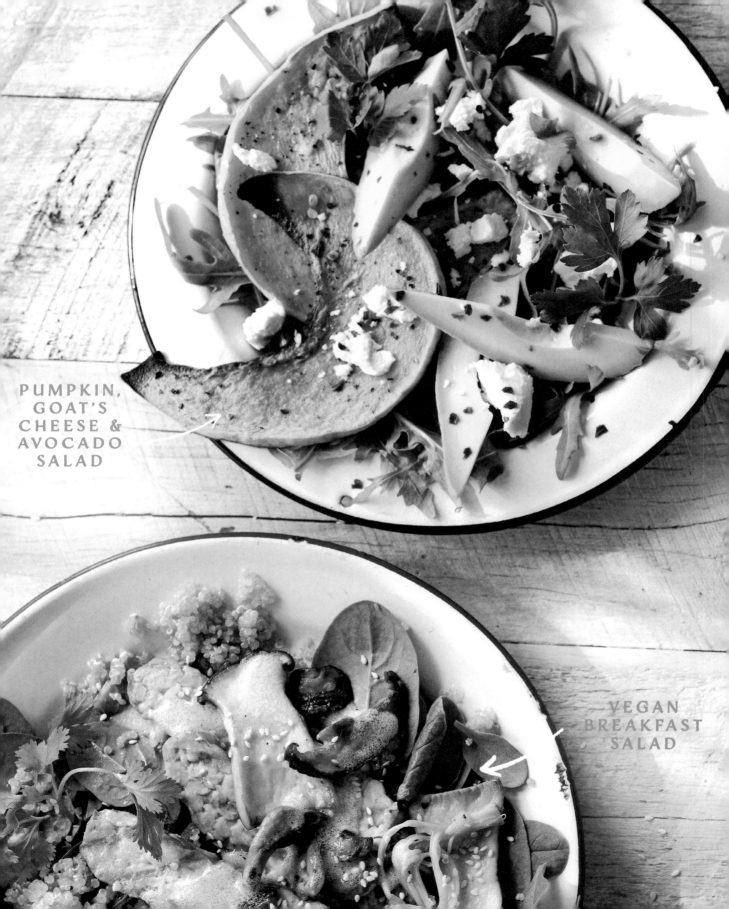

PUMPKIN,
GOAT'S
CHEESE &
AVOCADO
SALAD

VEGAN
BREAKFAST
SALAD

# VEGAN BREAKFAST SALAD

*Who says you can't have salad for breakfast? Both these salads are delicious and a great way to fuel your body for the busy day ahead. The basic building blocks of a nourishing, satisfying salad are fresh greens, veggies sautéed in coconut oil, your chosen protein and 100 g cooked grains. Have a play with your favourite flavours and you'll be a salad-for-breakfast convert in no time!*

SERVES 2
PREP TIME: 10 minutes

1 tablespoon virgin organic coconut oil
200 g mushrooms
100 g tempeh
200 g steamed quinoa
2 handfuls of baby spinach leaves
Lemony Tahini Dressing (see page 297)

Heat the oil in a large non-stick frying pan over medium–high heat. Add the mushroom and sauté for 4–5 minutes.

Meanwhile, place the tempeh under a hot grill and grill for 2–3 minutes.

Combine the sautéed mushrooms, grilled tempeh, quinoa and baby spinach leaves in a bowl. Serve with Lemony Tahini Dressing.

# PUMPKIN, GOAT'S CHEESE AND AVOCADO SALAD

SERVES 2
PREP TIME: 40 minutes

1 tablespoon virgin organic coconut oil
½ small pumpkin, peeled and cut into wedges
40 g goat's cheese, crumbled
1 avocado, sliced
2 handfuls of rocket leaves
boiled or poached egg (optional)
flat-leaf parsley, to serve
chilli flakes, to serve (optional)

Preheat the oven to 200°C (180°C fan/gas 6).

Melt the oil in a roasting tin, add the pumpkin and roast for 25–30 minutes or until golden and tender.

Place the roasted pumpkin, crumbled goat's cheese and avocado slices on a pile of fresh rocket leaves. Add a boiled or poached egg if you like.

Serve scattered with flat-leaf parsley and chilli flakes.

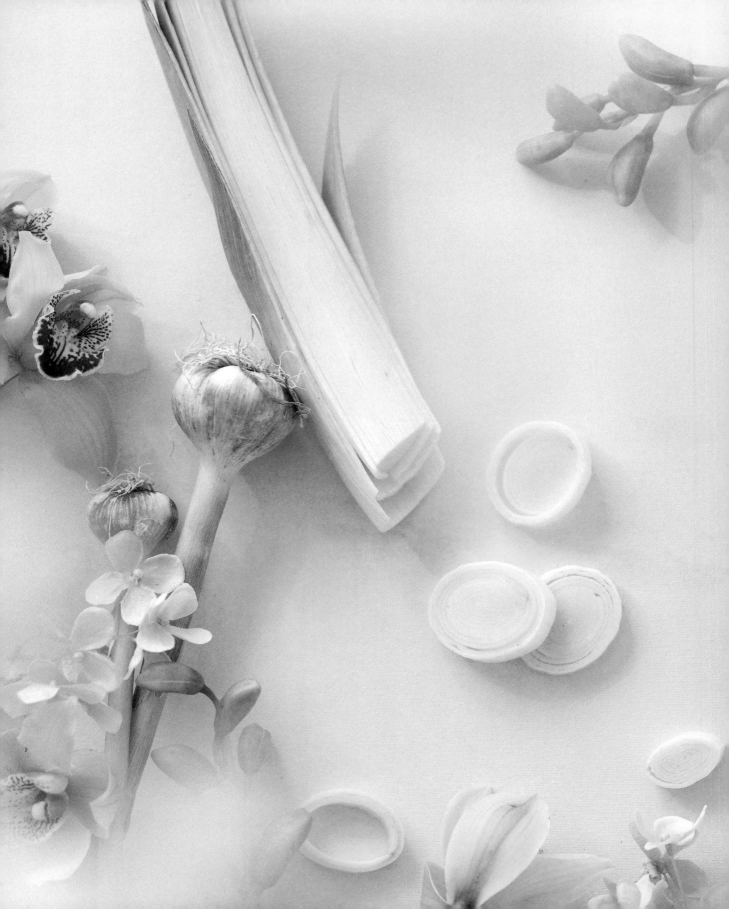

# SALADS & SOUPS

When you embrace a healthy life, salads make your life so much easier, and tastier! They also require very little fuss – it's all about throwing your favourite veggies into a bowl and pairing them with a clean protein and a delicious dressing. Salads are great for lunch, and can also be served with your choice of protein for dinner.

Similarly, the nourishing soups included here are designed to help you during busier times in your life – you can freeze them and enjoy when you just don't have the time to cook.

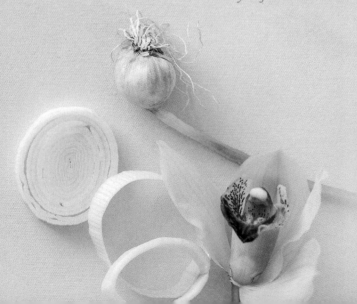

# ICEBERG LETTUCE WEDGE SALAD

*If you love Japanese flavours as much as I do, you must make this salad. The sesame dressing brings everything together. It's so simple to prepare.*

SERVES 2 for lunch, 4 as a side
PREP TIME: 15 minutes

1 iceberg lettuce
1 avocado, cut into cubes
1 tablespoon white sesame seeds
1 tablespoon black sesame seeds
2 spring onions, thinly sliced on the diagonal

HEALING SESAME DRESSING:
125 ml tamari
3 tablespoons white balsamic vinegar
2 tablespoons organic Dijon mustard
2 tablespoons sesame oil
1 tablespoon raw honey
a handful of sesame seeds
a small handful of chopped spring onion

Cut the lettuce in half lengthways, then cut it again into small wedges.

Place the wedges on a platter.

Top each wedge with avocado chunks, and sprinkle with the sesame seeds and spring onion.

To make the Healing Sesame Dressing, place ingredients in a bowl and whisk until combined. Drizzle the dressing over the salad and serve.

# CAULIFLOWER, LABNEH & HARISSA SALAD

SERVES 4
PREP TIME: 40 minutes, including cooking

1 large head cauliflower, cut into florets
2 tablespoons harissa paste
4 tablespoons olive oil
Celtic sea salt and ground pepper
250 g cherry tomatoes, halved
1 x 400 g tin chickpeas, drained and rinsed
50 g rocket leaves
80 g labneh
Lemony Tahini Dressing (see page 297), for drizzling
a small handful of mint leaves (optional)

Preheat the oven to 180°C (160°C fan/gas 4) and line a baking tray with baking paper.

Place the cauliflower, harissa and 3 tablespoons of the olive oil in a bowl. Season with salt and pepper and mix so the cauliflower is well coated in the harissa and oil.

Spread out the cauliflower on the prepared tray and roast for 25–30 minutes or until tender.

Meanwhile, line a second baking tray. Scatter the tomatoes and chickpeas over the tray, drizzle over the remaining olive oil and season with a good pinch of salt.

Transfer to the oven and cook for 10–15 minutes or until lightly roasted.

Put the rocket leaves in a salad bowl or scatter over a platter and top with the roasted chickpeas, tomatoes and cauliflower. Scatter over some clumps of labneh (this is so delicious!).

Drizzle over the dressing and garnish with a handful of mint leaves, if you like.

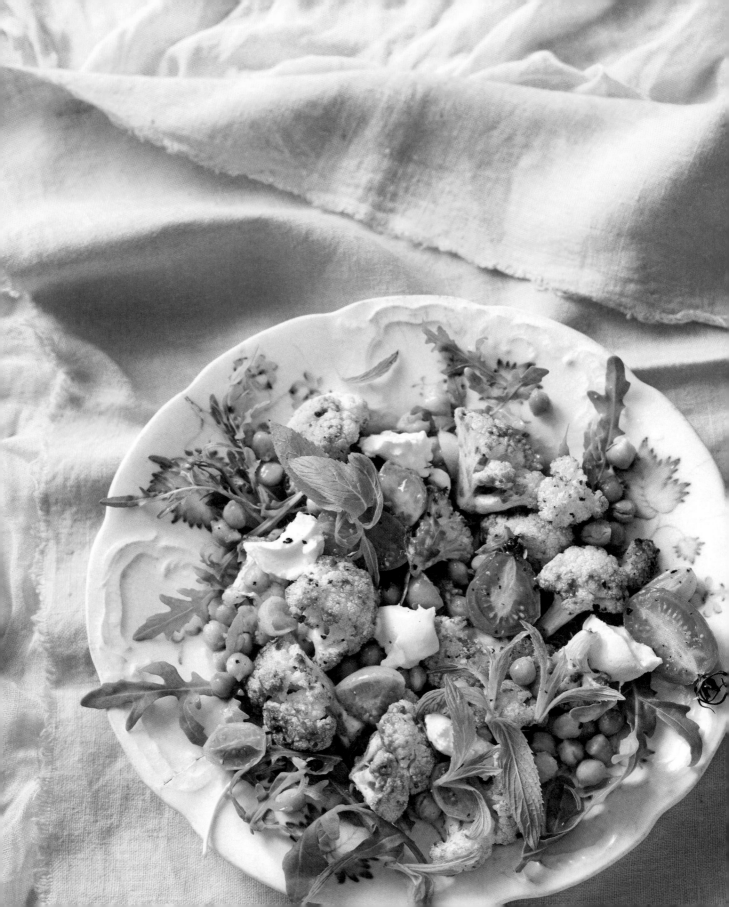

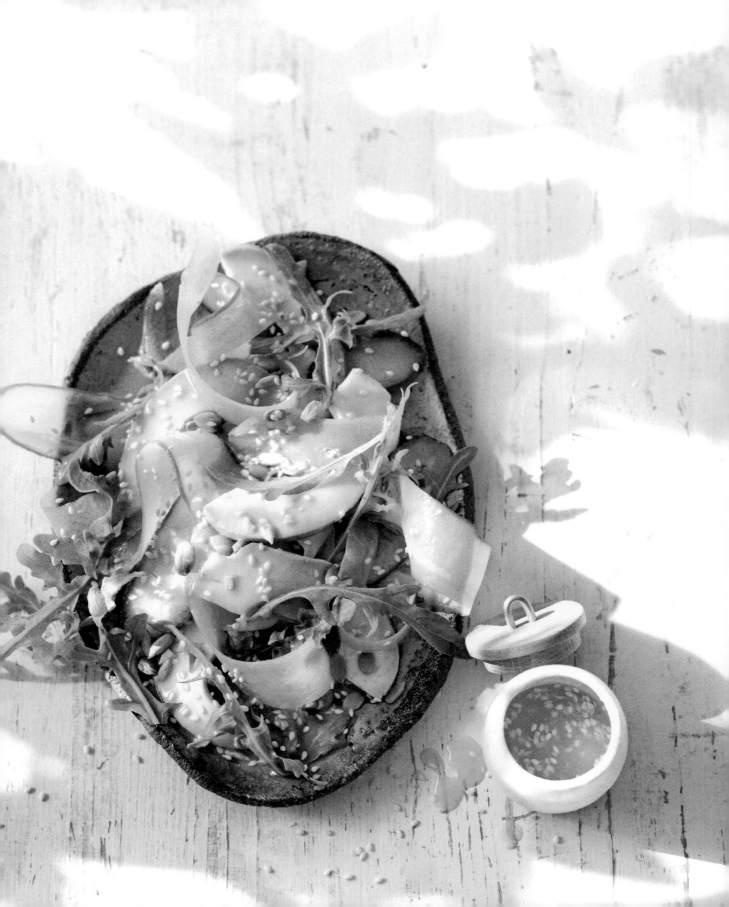

# CUCUMBER & CARROT SALAD WITH CRUNCHY SEEDS

*I love the crunch factor in my salads! You too? It works really well with grilled fish and the miso dressing makes it divine!*

SERVES 4
PREP TIME: 15 minutes, including cooking

100–150 g rocket leaves
4 carrots
4 Lebanese or ridge cucumbers
1 avocado, sliced
4 tablespoons sunflower seeds
4 tablespoons pumpkin seeds
2 tablespoons sesame seeds
olive oil, for drizzling
Himalayan pink rock salt
Miso Salad Dressing (see page 297), for drizzling

Place the rocket leaves in a large salad bowl.

Using a vegetable peeler or mandolin, peel the carrots and cucumbers lengthways to create ribbons.

Scatter the carrot, cucumber and avocado over the rocket in the bowl.

Lightly roast all the seeds in a dry frying pan over medium–low heat for 3 minutes or until just lightly golden. Drizzle over a little olive oil and toss some salt through the seeds, then continue to dry-fry until crunchy and golden. Transfer to a bowl and set aside to cool.

Sprinkle the cooled seeds over the salad, then drizzle over the miso dressing and serve.

# WARM MUSHROOM & RICOTTA SALAD

*Warm ricotta and mushrooms – what a divine combination. I use full-fat ricotta fresh from the deli as it's the 'whole' food version and of course it tastes better.*

SERVES 2
PREP TIME: 20 minutes, including cooking

3–4 tablespoons olive oil
1 garlic clove, crushed
150 g mixed mushrooms, sliced if large
a handful of thyme leaves
1–2 teaspoons Himalayan pink rock salt
125 g mixed salad leaves or rocket leaves
4 tablespoons fresh full-fat ricotta

Heat 2 tablespoons of the olive oil in a frying pan over medium heat, add the garlic and cook until softened.

Add the mushrooms and thyme to the pan, then drizzle over the remaining olive oil and season with the salt, to taste. Sauté the mushrooms until cooked and smelling amazing.

Put the salad or rocket leaves in a large salad bowl. Add the warm mushrooms and dollops of fresh ricotta.

Mix all the ingredients well until the ricotta, warmed and softened by the mushrooms, has spread nicely through the salad.

*Lunchbowls are nutritious bowls of goodness that you can eat at home or on-the-go, for lunch or dinner. I like to use wholesome brown rice as a base. Try these three delicious versions, then make up your own! All these lunchbowls serve one person.*

## PESTO CHICKEN BOWL WITH BROCCOLI & PUMPKIN SEEDS

Marinate a chicken breast in pesto (see page 292), then grill or bake it until cooked through. Meanwhile, sauté broccoli florets in garlic and olive oil. Combine in a bowl with the shredded or sliced chicken, chopped avocado, pumpkin seeds and a good handful of rocket leaves.

## BROWN RICE BOWL WITH SMOKED TROUT AND AVOCADO

Sauté 3 large torn kale leaves in olive oil and garlic until wilted. Tip 70 g cooked brown rice into a bowl and add 150–200 g smoked trout, flaked into pieces. Add ½ chopped avocado and the kale, then sprinkle with sesame seeds and dulse flakes to taste and drizzle with Miso Salad Dressing (see page 297).

## BROWN RICE BOWL WITH SESAME SALMON, AUBERGINE & TAHINI

Remove the skin and bones from a salmon fillet, then coat in tamari and sesame seeds and place on a greased baking tray. Add 1 sliced aubergine to a second baking tray, then salt the slices and drizzle with olive oil. Bake with the salmon in a preheated 200°C (180°C fan/gas 6) oven until tender. Combine the salmon, aubergine and 70 g cooked brown rice in a bowl and drizzle with Healing Peanut Sesame Dressing (see page 297).

## HEALTHY PACKED LUNCHES

I like to eat home-cooked lunches most days. You feel so much better when you eat out less and of course you save money too. I often make extra of these lunchbowls for dinner so I can have the leftovers for lunch the next day. I pack them up in mason jars or glass storage containers as plastic ones can leach chemicals.

# ENERGY CHOP CHOP SALAD

*This is my daily go-to salad to make at home. I sometimes add goat's cheese, or you can add any protein of your choice to make it more substantial. I was living in LA for a few months last year and wherever you go you can have a chopped salad. It was a happy discovery for me as chopped veggies burst with flavour, as you will see. To save yourself some elbow grease you can shred and slice the vegetables in a food processor, if preferred.*

SERVES 2
PREP TIME: 15 minutes

2 carrots, grated
a handful of flat-leaf parsley or basil leaves,
  chopped
¼–½ iceberg lettuce, shredded
½ red cabbage, thinly sliced
½ white cabbage, thinly sliced
½ avocado, diced
3 tablespoons pumpkin seeds, roasted if liked
Celtic sea salt and ground pepper
Miso Salad Dressing or JSHealth Clean Life
  Dressing (see page 297), for drizzling

Combine the carrot, parsley or basil, lettuce, cabbage, avocado and pumpkin seeds in a bowl. Season with salt and pepper and gently toss.

Drizzle on the dressing and toss again, then serve.

# CHOP CHOP TUNA SALAD

*This is a great everyday salad. As much as I love it with tuna my advice would be to only eat tuna twice a week at the most to avoid mercury overload.*

SERVES 2
PREP TIME: 15 minutes

1 iceberg lettuce, shredded
1 x 185 g tin Italian tuna in olive oil, drained and
  flaked
1 plum tomato, diced
½ red onion, diced
2 tablespoons tinned cannellini beans or
  chickpeas
1–2 tablespoons goat's cheese (optional)
Celtic sea salt and ground pepper
JSHealth Clean Life Dressing or Lemony Tahini
  Dressing (see page 297), for drizzling

Combine the lettuce, tuna, tomato, onion, beans or chickpeas and goat's cheese (if using) in a bowl.

Season with salt and pepper to taste and drizzle over your choice of dressing. Toss gently to combine and serve.

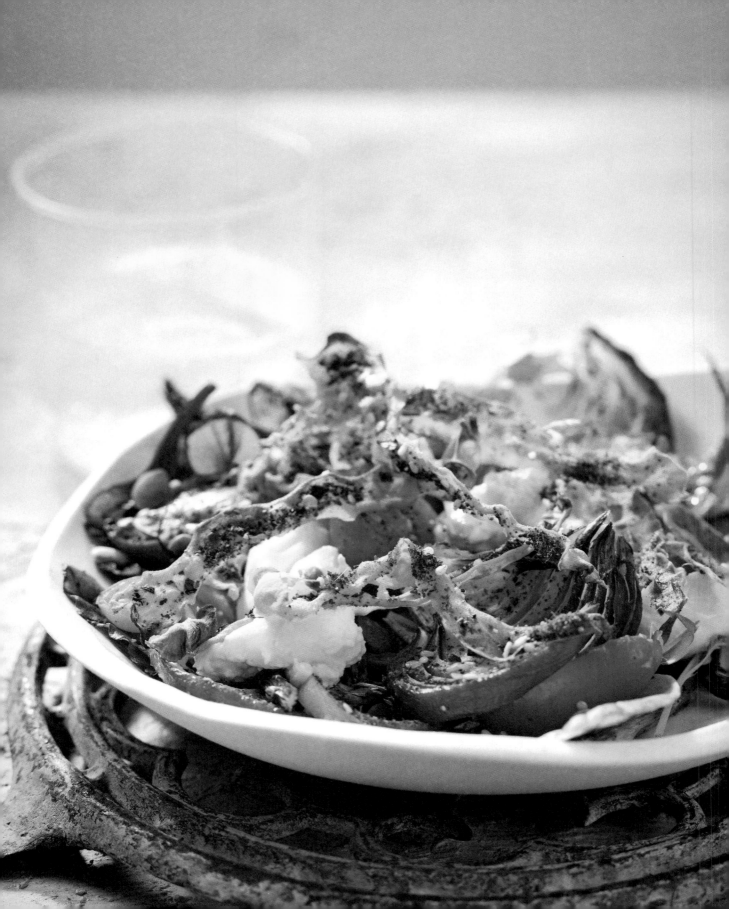

# ZA'ATAR CARROT CHIP SALAD WITH CINNAMON SEEDS

**SERVES 4**
**PREP TIME:** 35 minutes, including cooking

3 large carrots, cut into long strips with a vegetable peeler or mandolin
250 g cherry tomatoes, halved
1 bunch asparagus, trimmed and cut into short lengths
1 red onion, thinly sliced (optional)
olive oil or coconut oil spray
½ teaspoon chilli flakes
1 teaspoon za'atar
Celtic sea salt and ground pepper
4 tablespoons mixed seeds (such as sesame, sunflower and pumpkin seeds)
1 teaspoon ground cinnamon
100–150 g rocket leaves or mixed lettuce leaves
2 tablespoons labneh

*I adore za'atar – a delicious Middle Eastern spice blend that is full of flavour with a crunchy texture. It goes really well with carrots and chicken.*

Preheat the oven to 180°C (160°C fan/gas 4) and line two large baking trays with baking paper.

Divide the carrot, tomato halves, asparagus and onion (if using) between the prepared trays.

Spray with oil, then sprinkle over the chilli flakes, za'atar and some salt and pepper.

Bake for 15–20 minutes.

Meanwhile, roast the seeds and cinnamon in a dry frying pan over medium–low heat until golden and wonderfully fragrant.

Transfer the roasted vegetables to a large bowl and combine with the salad leaves. Top with the labneh and cinnamon seeds.

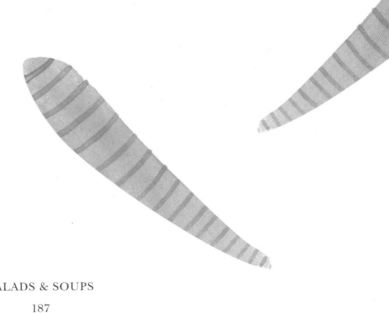

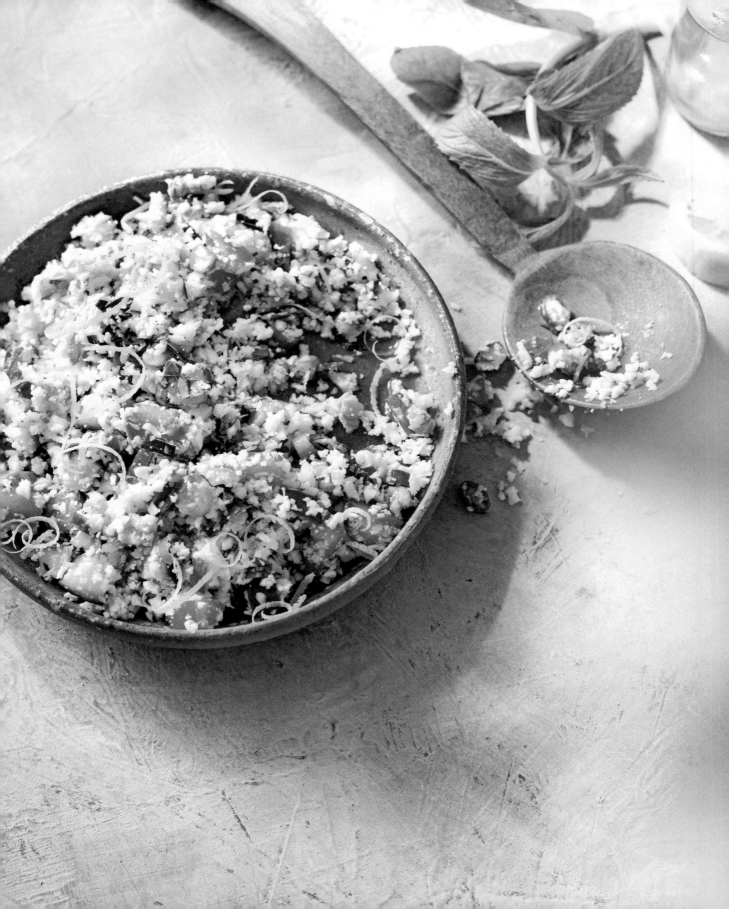

# CAULIFLOWER & WALNUT TABBOULEH

*A gluten-free, grain-free alternative to your traditional couscous tabbouleh. It is incredibly fresh and light to enjoy with your protein of choice.*

SERVES 2 as a main, 4 as a side
PREP TIME: 20 minutes

1 small head cauliflower, cut into florets
2 plum tomatoes, diced
1 Lebanese or ridge cucumber, diced
2 spring onions, thinly sliced
50 g flat-leaf parsley leaves, chopped
4 tablespoons chopped mint
115 g walnuts, chopped
Celtic sea salt and ground pepper

DRESSING:
4 tablespoons olive oil
finely grated zest and juice of 1 lemon
Celtic sea salt

Steam the cauliflower florets for 10 minutes or until tender but still a little crisp. Cool the cauliflower completely. Pulse the cauliflower in a food processor to the consistency of fine breadcrumbs.

Tip the cauliflower into a mixing bowl.

Add the tomato, cucumber, spring onion, parsley, mint and walnuts. Season with salt and pepper to taste.

To make the dressing, whisk together all the ingredients in a small bowl.

Add the dressing to the tabbouleh and gently toss to coat.

# ASPARAGUS, AVOCADO & ALMOND SALAD

*This delicious summer salad makes a beautiful light meal in its own right, perhaps topped with a poached or soft-boiled egg, but it is just as welcome as a side for a lazy weekend lunch.*

SERVES 4
PREP TIME: 20 minutes, including cooking

4 bunches asparagus, trimmed
100 g flaked almonds
115 g sliced spring onion
2 avocados, cut into cubes
Celtic sea salt, ground pepper and chilli flakes (optional)

DRESSING:
2 tablespoons organic Dijon mustard
2 tablespoons olive oil
125 ml white balsamic vinegar
juice of ½ lemon
1 tablespoon raw honey
Celtic sea salt and ground pepper

Steam the asparagus for 5–10 minutes or until tender but still a little crisp.

Meanwhile, roast the flaked almonds in a dry frying pan over medium–low heat until lightly golden.

To make the dressing, whisk together all the ingredients in a small bowl.

Combine the asparagus, almonds, spring onion and avocado in a bowl, add the dressing and toss to coat. Season with salt, pepper and chilli flakes, if you like.

# BRUSSELS SPROUT & CARAMELISED ONION SALAD

*I absolutely adore this salad. I made it for a family Sunday lunch and everyone loved it so much they keep asking me to make it again!*

SERVES 4-6
PREP TIME: 20 minutes, including cooking

750 g brussels sprouts, trimmed and thinly
   sliced or shredded
1 tablespoon virgin organic coconut oil
2 red onions, thinly sliced
70 g raw almonds
1 tablespoon olive oil
1 teaspoon Celtic sea salt
1 teaspoon chilli flakes, or to taste
finely grated zest of 1 lemon

Steam the brussels sprouts for 7–10 minutes or until just tender.

Meanwhile, melt the coconut oil in a large frying pan over high heat and fry the onion for 5–10 minutes or until softened and golden.

Blitz the almonds in a food processor so they are crushed, but stop before they form a paste.

Combine the sprouts and onion in a bowl and mix through the olive oil, salt, chilli and lemon zest. Top with crushed almonds and serve.

# SHAVED BRUSSELS SPROUTS WITH POMEGRANATE

*Inspired by a beautiful salad on the Green Kitchen Stories blog, this salad is a total crowd-pleaser as part of a brunch spread.*

SERVES 2 as a main, 4 as a side
PREP TIME: 25 minutes, including cooking

300 g brussels sprouts, trimmed and shredded
340 g frozen broad beans
125 g hazelnuts  or walnuts (or a mixture of both)
seeds from 1 pomegranate
40 g goat's cheese, crumbled (optional)
mint sprigs, to garnish

DRESSING:
2–3 tablespoons olive oil
2 tablespoons hulled tahini
1 tablespoon raw honey
1 tablespoon organic Dijon mustard
2 teaspoons lemon juice
½ teaspoon Celtic sea salt

To make the dressing, whisk together all the ingredients in a small bowl.

Steam the shredded sprouts for 7–10 minutes or until tender. Meanwhile, cook the broad beans in a saucepan of salted boiling water until tender, then drain and peel. Combine the sprouts and beans in a large bowl. Drizzle with the dressing and toss well to coat.

Roast the nuts in a dry frying pan over medium heat until golden – watch them carefully as they burn easily. Set aside to cool, then add to the bowl with the pomegranate and combine.

Scatter over the goat's cheese (if using) and garnish with mint. It's ready to eat now, but it's also lovely if you let it sit for an hour or so before serving.

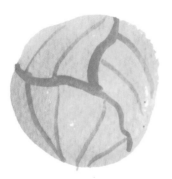

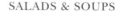

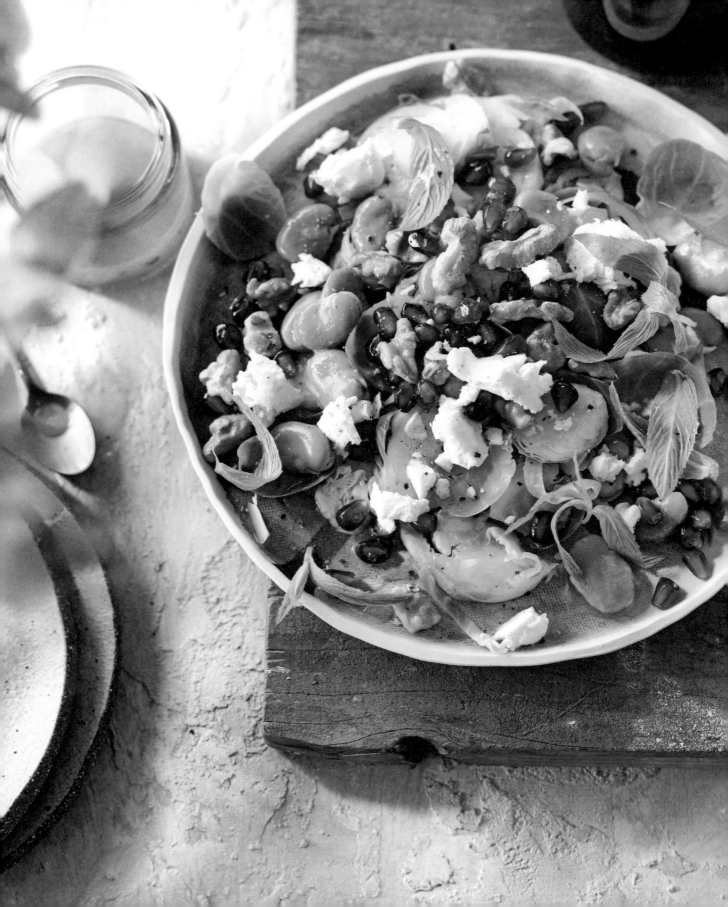

# CAULIFLOWER & BRAZIL NUT SOUP

SERVES 4
PREP TIME: 50 minutes,
including cooking

2 tablespoons virgin
 organic coconut oil
1 leek, pale part only,
 trimmed and thinly sliced
Himalayan pink rock salt
 and ground pepper
1.25 litres vegetable stock
1 large head cauliflower,
 cut into florets
150 g Brazil nuts, roughly
 chopped

NUT TOPPING:
1 tablespoon virgin organic
 coconut oil
75 g Brazil nuts, chopped
 and lightly roasted
flat-leaf parsley leaves,
 to serve

*Cauliflower is wonderful in soups because it's so creamy. Brazil nuts are high in selenium which supports your thyroid. What a combo!*

Melt the coconut oil in a large saucepan over medium heat. Add the leek and a pinch of salt and cook gently for 10 minutes or until softened and golden.

Add the stock and most of the cauliflower florets (reserve a large handful of small florets for garnish).

Bring to the boil, then reduce the heat and simmer, covered, for 20 minutes or until the cauliflower is tender.

Add the Brazil nuts, then blend with a stick blender until smooth and creamy. Season to taste with salt and pepper.

To make the topping, melt the coconut oil in a frying pan over medium–high heat. Chop the reserved cauliflower florets into a rough crumb, add to the pan and cook until just crunchy.

Top each bowl of soup with the crunchy cauliflower, chopped Brazil nuts and parsley.

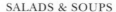

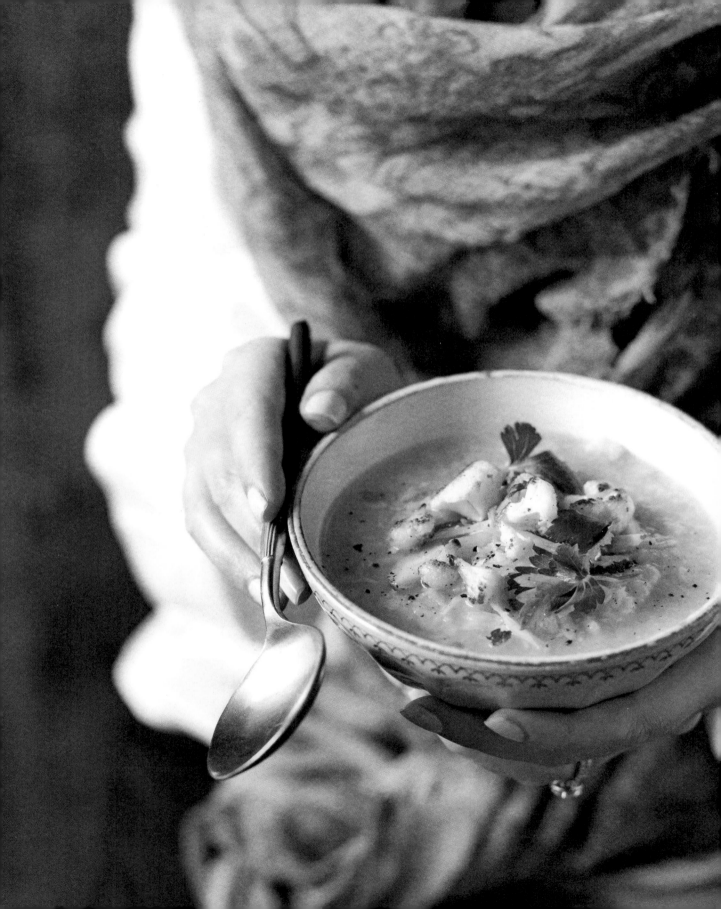

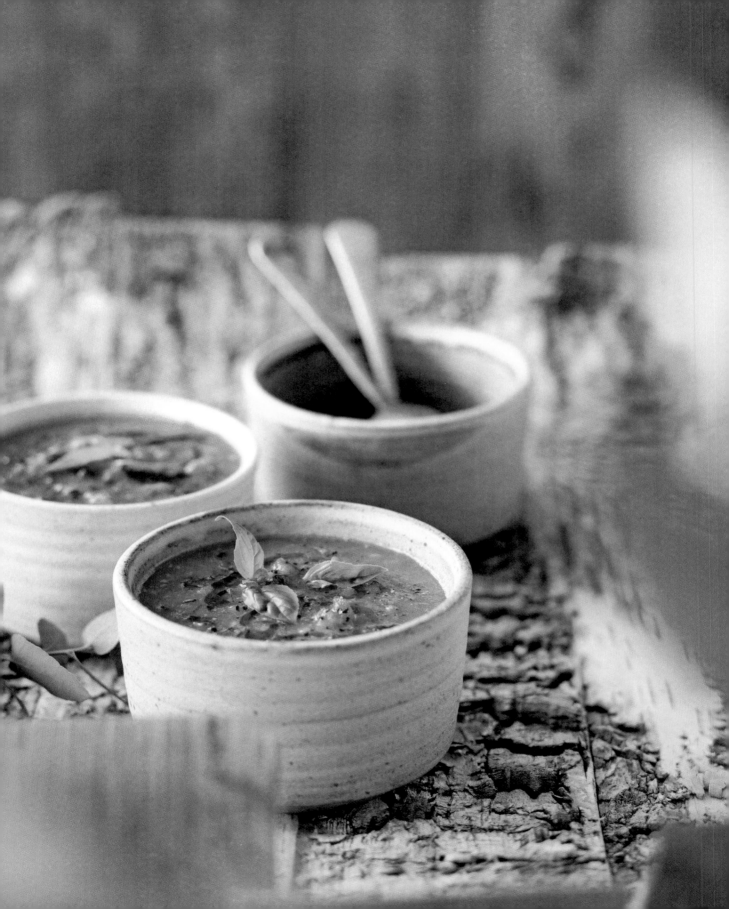

# TOMATO & RED PEPPER SOUP

SERVES 4
PREP TIME: 1 hour 35
minutes, including cooking

3 large red peppers
3 tablespoons olive oil
6 plum tomatoes
1 red onion, finely chopped
1 garlic clove, crushed
2 teaspoons smoked
  paprika
a pinch of chilli flakes
Celtic sea salt and ground
  pepper
1 bunch basil, chopped,
  reserving a few small
  leaves for garnish
750 ml vegetable stock

*My wonderful mum, Nicky Sepel, has been making this soup for years and we all beg her to make it every Friday night – it's that good!*

Preheat the oven to 200°C (180°C fan/gas 6) and line two baking trays with baking paper.

Cut the peppers into quarters and remove the seeds and membranes. Arrange on one of the prepared trays and drizzle over 1 tablespoon of the olive oil.

Cut the tomatoes into quarters and arrange on the second tray, cut side up. Drizzle over 1 tablespoon of the olive oil.

Place the trays in the oven and roast the vegetables for 30 minutes.

Meanwhile, heat the remaining olive oil in a large heavy-based saucepan over medium heat, add the onion and garlic and cook until softened.

Add the paprika and chilli and season to taste with salt and pepper.

Add the roasted pepper and tomato, then stir in the chopped basil and sauté for 20 minutes or until softened and collapsed.

Pour in the stock and bring to the boil, then reduce the heat to medium–low and simmer for a further 20 minutes.

Blend the soup with a stick blender until smooth and creamy.

Taste and adjust the seasoning if necessary, then serve garnished with the reserved basil leaves.

# GREEN DETOX SOUP

SERVES 4
PREP TIME: 45 minutes,
including cooking

1 tablespoon olive oil
1 large onion, roughly
  chopped
2 garlic cloves, crushed
1 leek, pale part only,
  trimmed and thinly sliced
2 large courgettes, cut into
  1 cm pieces
1 large head broccoli,
  cut into florets, stems
  chopped
1 bulb fennel, trimmed and
  cut into 1 cm pieces
1.25 litres vegetable stock,
  plus extra if needed
1 teaspoon ground
  coriander
1 teaspoon ground cumin
½ teaspoon chilli flakes
Celtic sea salt and ground
  pepper
½ bunch kale, stalks
  removed and leaves torn
100 g baby spinach leaves
25 g mixed herbs (such
  as coriander, mint and
  flat-leaf parsley), roughly
  chopped
coriander or mint sprigs,
  lemon wedges and
  Rosemary Chilli Crackers
  (see page 251) to serve
  (optional)

*This soup proves the powerful healing nature of food. It is loaded with enzymes and nutrients that will really support your body's own cleansing functions. If you are feeling run down or your immune system is weaker than usual, make a pot of this and feel better for it. As a delightful bonus, it will also give your skin a natural glow.*

Heat the olive oil in a large saucepan over medium heat, add the onion, garlic and leek and cook for 5 minutes or until softened. Add the courgette, broccoli and fennel and cook for 2–3 minutes.

Pour in the stock, then stir in the ground coriander, cumin and chilli flakes and season to taste with pepper.

Bring to the boil, then reduce the heat and simmer for 10 minutes.

Add the kale and simmer for 5 minutes or until the vegetables are tender, adding a little water or extra stock if necessary.

Add the spinach and simmer for 1 minute. Remove from the heat.

Using either a stick blender or food processor, blend the soup until smooth. Stir through the mixed herbs and season to taste with salt and pepper.

Ladle the soup into bowls and garnish with coriander or mint sprigs.
Serve with lemon wedges and Rosemary Chilli Crackers, if desired.

## TIP

*My favourite thing is to roast almonds with rosemary and sea salt and scatter them over my soup. So delicious, and it also adds a fantastic crunch factor.*

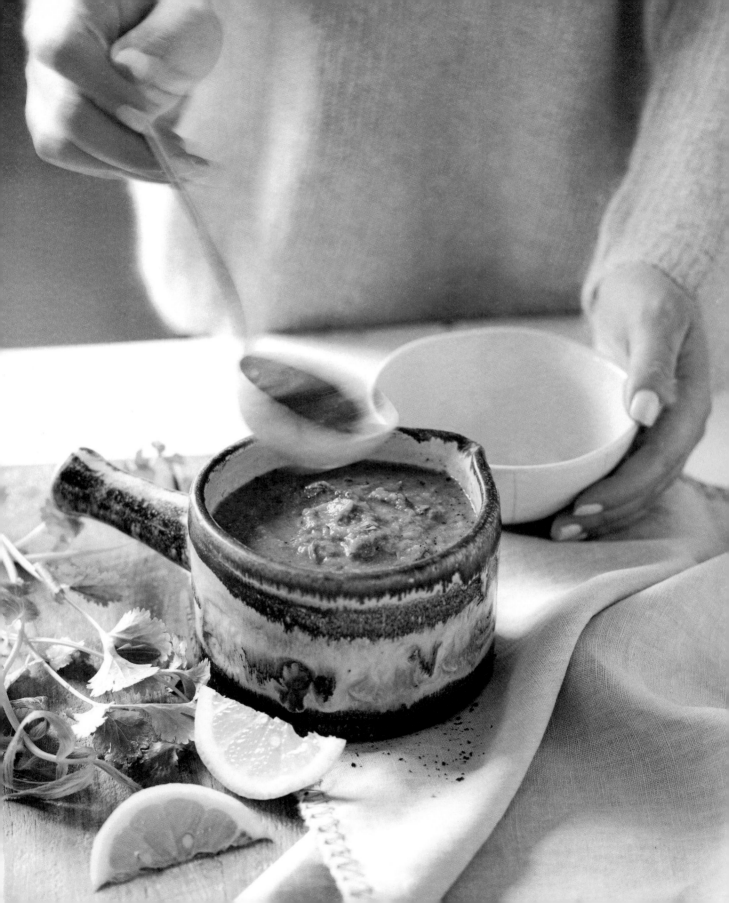

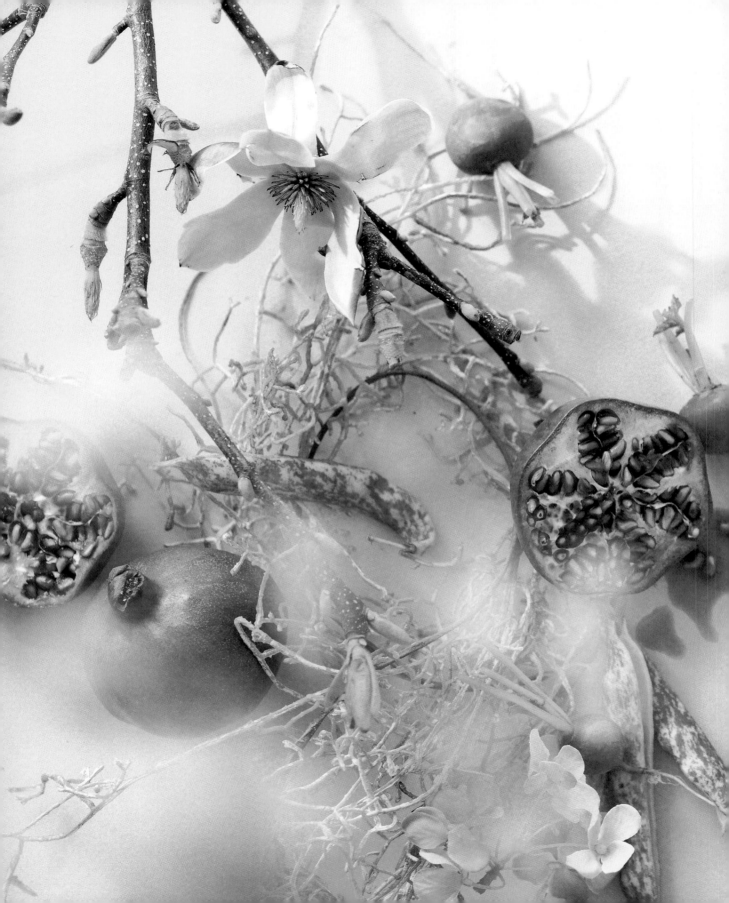

# MAINS

*I'm more of a savoury than a sweet kind of gal. The recipes in this chapter are my go-to dishes – simple, wholesome meals that prove how easy it is to make healthy food for you and your loved ones. Being time-poor means I need to create quick and easy meals that are also nourishing and delicious. I hope you like the results!*

*One strategy that helps me is to double or triple the quantities every time I cook so we always have leftovers the next day, or that can be stored in the freezer for another night when I'm not in the mood to cook. I encourage you to do the same with the recipes in this chapter.*

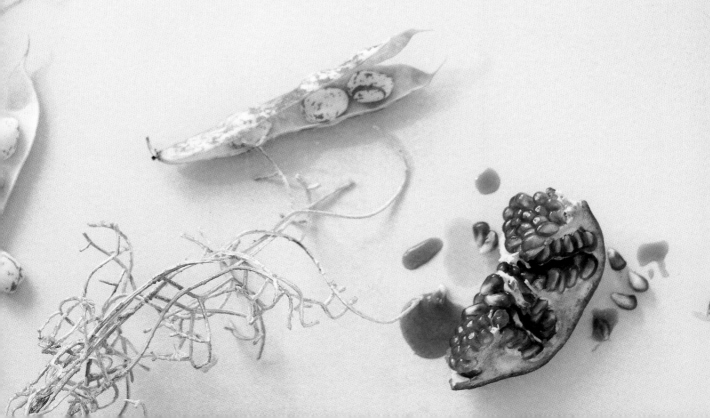

## BUILDING BLOCKS TO CREATING A WHOLESOME AND HEALING MAIN MEAL

- Choose a protein to grill, roast or steam.

- Choose your herbs, spices and condiments to flavour your protein: such as chilli, ginger, cumin, rosemary, basil, lemon juice, organic Dijon mustard, tamari and olive oil.

- Choose a Veggie Side (see pages 231–47).

- Always serve with some fresh mixed greens.

- KEEP IT SIMPLE! THIS IS MY GOLDEN RULE.

## A MATTER OF TASTE

When it comes to seasoning your food it's obviously a matter of personal taste. We all enjoy things differently. I love a lot of chilli, for example, but I know many people who don't. Because I develop recipes to suit my tastes some of you may find there is too much heat in certain dishes, so I'd advise you to tune in to your own taste buds. The same goes for salt and pepper: taste the food as you go and make it work for you.

## MY FAVOURITE WEEKDAY MEALS

During the week I make dinner for Dean and myself most nights. Here are some quick and easy dinners that we both love.

- Teriyaki Salmon Bowl (see page 206) served on Thai-style Fried 'Rice' (see page 247) or Truffle Cauliflower Purée (see page 242)

- Chilli & Rosemary Steak with Sautéed Greens (see page 227) served with broccoli mash and a green salad

- Lemon Herb Fish in a Bag (see page 227)

- San choy bau with filling of choice (see page 224)

- Sashimi salad with avocado, grated carrot, cucumber and a Miso Salad Dressing (see page 297)

- Tuna Pasta Bake (see page 205)

- Healthy Fish Tacos (see page 225)

- Harissa Chicken with Cauliflower Steaks (see page 211) served with a green salad

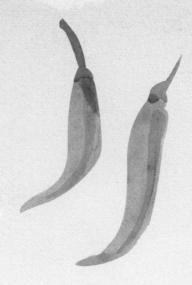

# DINNER PARTY IDEAS

*I love to entertain. Nothing beats cooking while chatting and sipping on a glass of vino. It brings me so much joy to invite my besties to my home to enjoy a wholesome meal (and gives me the added bonus of sharing the healthy life with people, and showing them how good it can taste!).*

*First create a healthy ambience – light some candles, dim the lights, get the cooking smell going, have some healthy snacks laid out and enjoy it rather than stress about it. Otherwise, what's the point?*

## HEALTHY SNACKS

* Fresh sashimi served with Rosemary Chilli Crackers (see page 251)
* Rosemary Chilli Cashews (see page 270)
* Lemon Tahini Kale Chips (see page 257)
* Carrot sticks dipped into Green Tahini Dressing (see page 296)
* Sesame-coated Carrot Chips (see page 237) dipped in healthy Chilli & Lime Guacamole (see page 290)

## HEALTHY STARTERS

* Tomato & Red Pepper Soup (see page 195) served with Rosemary Chilli Cashews (see page 270)
* Green Detox Soup (see page 196) served with Rosemary Chilli Cashews (see page 270)
* Burrata cheese, basil and tomato salad
* Healthy bruschetta – top flaxseed crackers with diced tomatoes and olive oil and some optional shaved parmesan
* Fresh ricotta served on Rosemary Chilli Crackers (see page 251)
* Quinoa sushi

## HEALTHY MAINS

* Broccoli Pizza night (see page 216) – everyone can add their choice of topping!
* Chilli & Rosemary Steak with Sautéed Greens (see page 227) served with Truffle Cauliflower Purée (see page 242) and a large rocket and parmesan salad
* Teriyaki Salmon Bowl (see page 206) served with roasted cauliflower and sautéed garlic greens
* Lemon Herb Fish in a Bag (see page 227)
* Barramundi with Baked Asparagus (see page 221) and Fried Kale with Almonds (see page 236)
* San choy bau night (see page 224) – this is so much fun!

## HEALTHY SIDES

* Healing Aubergine Bruschetta (see page 244)
* Miso Aubergine (see page 234)
* Roasted vegetables

## HEALTHY DESSERTS

* Salted Chocolate & Rosemary Tarts (see page 282)
* Fig & Pistachio Chocolate Bark (see page 276) or dark chocolate
* Berry Breakfast Crumble (see page 175) served as dessert with coconut milk yoghurt or coconut ice-cream
* Cacao Sea Salt Truffles (see page 268)
* Greek-style yoghurt served with raspberries or blueberries, topped with raw honey and homemade granola (see pages 140–1)

# CUMIN-SPICED LENTILS WITH SHAVED BRUSSELS SPROUTS

2–3 tablespoons virgin
  organic coconut oil or
  olive oil
½ leek, pale part only,
  trimmed and sliced
½ red onion, diced
Himalayan pink rock salt
  and ground pepper
300 g brussels sprouts,
  trimmed and thinly sliced
2–3 tablespoons filtered
  water
50 g tinned organic lentils,
  drained and rinsed
1 teaspoon ground cumin
1 teaspoon chilli powder,
  or to taste
hulled tahini, for drizzling
  (optional)
chilli flakes and flat-leaf
  parsley leaves, to serve
  (optional)

*This warming vegan main meal makes me feel so good, though it's delicious with chicken or fish too. It's also the perfect affordable meal for any students out there! I love to make extra so I can have it again for lunch the next day.*

Heat 1 tablespoon of the oil in a large frying pan over medium heat.

Add the leek and onion, season with salt and pepper and cook until softened and lightly coloured.

Increase the heat to medium–high, add the sprouts and a little more oil and sauté for a further 5–7 minutes or until golden. Add the water to help the ingredients cook nicely without sticking to the pan.

Stir in the lentils, cumin, chilli powder and remaining oil and sauté until the lentils are tender and warmed through.

Plate up and finish with a drizzle of tahini, if you wish. Scatter over chilli flakes and parsley, if using, and serve.

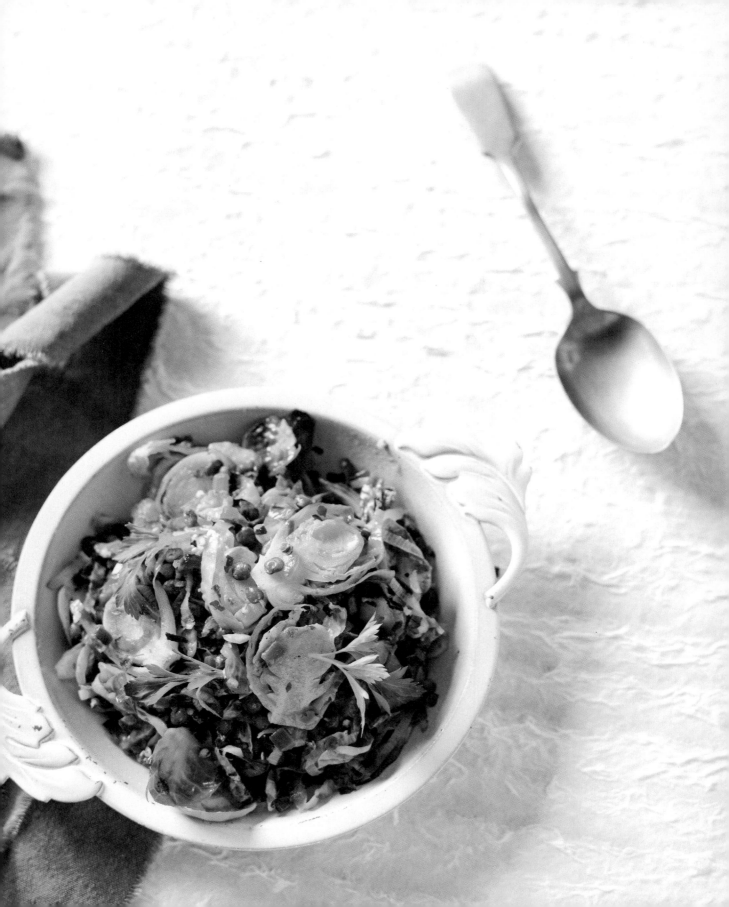

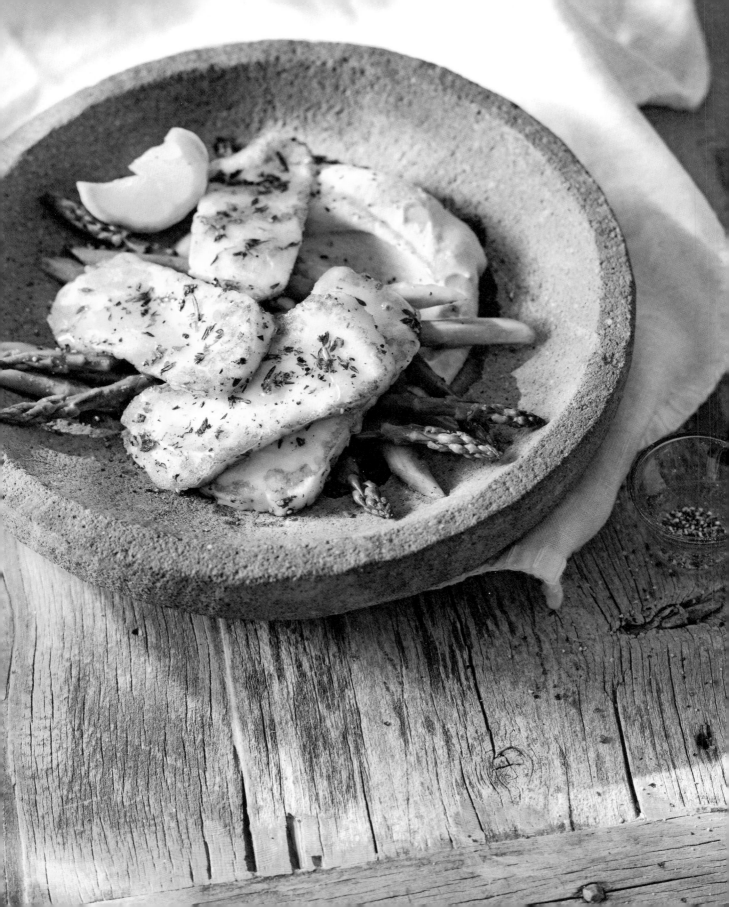

# CRISPY HALLOUMI WITH ASPARAGUS & HUMMUS

SERVES 4
PREP TIME: 25 minutes, including cooking

2–3 tablespoons good-quality hummus
juice of ½ lemon
Celtic sea salt (optional)

CRISPY HALLOUMI:
2 tablespoons finely chopped thyme or rosemary
250 g halloumi, cut lengthways into 1 cm thick
  slices
Celtic sea salt
1 tablespoon olive oil
1 garlic clove, crushed

GARLIC ASPARAGUS:
1 tablespoon olive oil or virgin organic coconut oil
1 garlic clove, crushed
2 bunches asparagus, trimmed and cut into short
  lengths
1 teaspoon ground cumin
1 teaspoon mixed spice
Celtic sea salt

To make the crispy halloumi, sprinkle the herbs
evenly over the halloumi and season with salt. Heat
the olive oil in a frying pan over medium heat, add
the garlic and cook until lightly golden. Take care
not to let it burn otherwise it will be bitter. Add the
halloumi and fry on both sides until golden and
warmed through.

Meanwhile, to make the garlic asparagus, heat the oil
in a frying pan over medium heat, add the garlic and
cook until lightly golden. Add the asparagus, cumin,
mixed spice and a pinch of salt and sauté until just
cooked.

To serve, spread the hummus over a platter. Top with
the asparagus and then the halloumi, then finish with
a squeeze of lemon juice and a final sprinkling of salt,
if you like. Serve immediately.

# TUNA PASTA BAKE

*This dish (the unhealthy version!) was a much-
loved part of my childhood in South Africa. Here's
my nutritious interpretation dedicated to my bestie,
Kira, who loves it.*

SERVES 4
PREP TIME: 40 minutes, including cooking

6–7 large courgettes
1–2 tablespoons olive oil
Celtic sea salt and ground pepper
375 ml good-quality tomato-based sauce (without
  additives or sugar)
1 x 425 g tin tuna in olive oil, drained (you can
  mix it with a little mayo if you wish)
½ red onion, diced
2 tablespoons pesto (see page 292)
20 g chopped basil, plus extra to garnish
chilli flakes, to taste (optional)
3 tablespoons grated parmesan or cashew cheese,
  plus extra to garnish (optional)

Preheat the oven to 180°C (160°C fan/gas 4) and
line a baking tray with baking paper.

Leave the skin on the courgettes and, using a
vegetable spiraliser or peeler, make noodle-like strips.
The vegetable peeler will give you fettuccine-like
pasta. Weigh as you go – you'll need about 500 g
in total.

Spread out the courgette noodles on the prepared
tray, then drizzle over the olive oil and season with
salt and pepper. Spoon the tomato sauce evenly over
the noodles, then top with the tuna, onion, pesto,
basil and chilli and parmesan or cashew cheese (if
using). (You can add any greens of your choice too –
spinach and broccoli are delicious here.)

Season to taste, then bake for 20 minutes or until
the topping is crisp and golden.

Garnish with extra basil and, if you like, a final
sprinkling of parmesan or cashew cheese.

# TERIYAKI SALMON BOWL

*I am a big fan of teriyaki, but many of the dishes found in restaurants and ready-made meals are high in sugar and preservatives. Obviously I felt I had to make a clean version. The salmon can be grilled, poached or steamed before you flake it into bite-sized pieces. A great way to use leftover salmon.*

SERVES 1
PREP TIME: 20 minutes, including cooking

70 g cooked brown rice
1 x 180 g salmon fillet, bones removed and skin on, cooked and flaked into bite-sized pieces
50 g mangetout, thinly sliced
½ red pepper, seeded and julienned
½ avocado, diced
½ Lebanese or ridge cucumber, diced
¼ red onion, thinly sliced
1 teaspoon black or white sesame seeds, roasted
½ spring onion, thinly sliced on the diagonal
thinly sliced nori seaweed, to serve
pickled ginger, to serve (optional)

TERIYAKI DRESSING:
4 tablespoons tamari
2 teaspoons sesame oil
2 teaspoons raw honey
½ garlic clove, crushed
1 teaspoon finely grated ginger
½ spring onion, finely chopped
Celtic sea salt and ground pepper

To make the teriyaki dressing, whisk together all the ingredients in a small bowl.

Place the rice, salmon, mangetout, red pepper, avocado, cucumber and red onion in a bowl. Add 1 tablespoon of the teriyaki dressing and gently toss together. Sprinkle the sesame seeds, spring onion and nori over the top and serve with pickled ginger, if desired. Store the remaining dressing in a jar in the fridge for up to 5 days.

# PONZU SESAME SALMON WITH ASIAN GREENS

SERVES 4
PREP TIME: 1 hour, including marinating and cooking

4 x 180 g salmon fillets, bones removed and skin on

MARINADE:
75 ml tamari
1 tablespoon ponzu sauce
1 tablespoon raw honey
1 tablespoon sesame oil
½ teaspoon chilli flakes

ASIAN GREENS:
1 tablespoon virgin organic coconut oil
2 bunches pak choi, sliced
½ white cabbage, shredded or grated
1 teaspoon grated ginger or ground ginger
Celtic sea salt
olive oil or sesame oil, for drizzling
1 tablespoon sesame seeds
2 tablespoons thinly sliced spring onion

To make the marinade, mix together all the ingredients in a shallow dish.

Add the salmon and turn to coat in the marinade, then leave to marinate for up to 30 minutes.

Preheat the oven to 200°C (180°C fan/gas 6) and line a baking tray with baking paper. Transfer the salmon to the prepared tray and bake for 12–15 minutes or until just cooked through.

Meanwhile, to make the Asian greens, melt the coconut oil in a wok or frying pan over high heat. Add the pak choi, cabbage, ginger, salt and a drizzle of oil and toss until cooked through. Sprinkle the sesame seeds and spring onion over the greens and serve with the salmon.

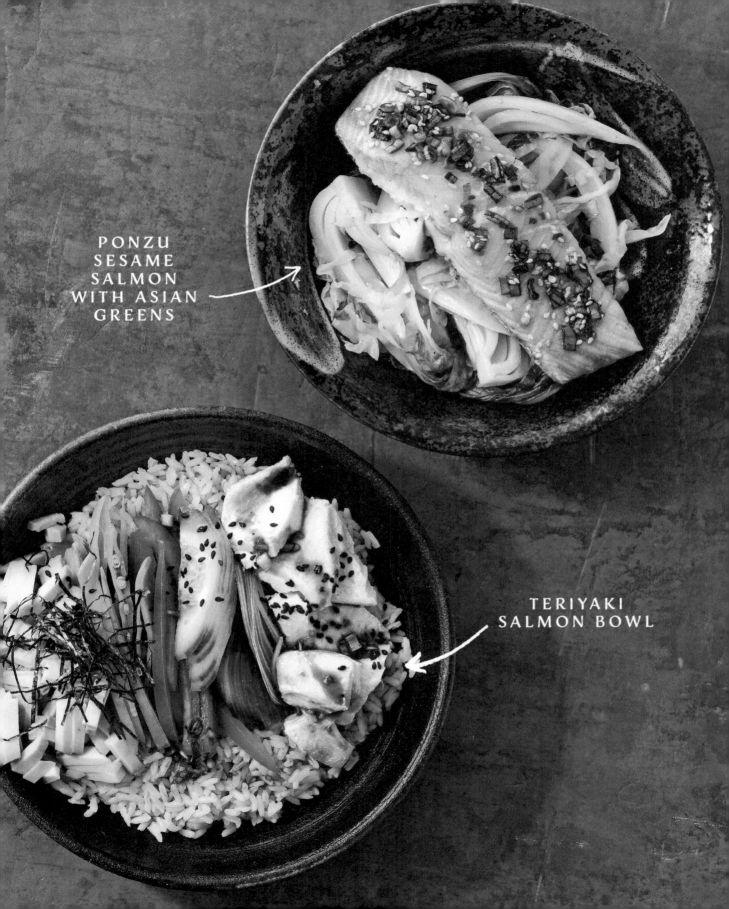

PONZU
SESAME
SALMON
WITH ASIAN
GREENS

TERIYAKI
SALMON BOWL

# WAYS WITH CHICKEN

**HEALTHY BBQ CHICKEN**

*Chicken is such a versatile protein! What's not to love? Barbecued, stir-fried, roasted or poached, pair a chicken breast with some sautéed veggies and you have a quick, easy and nourishing dinner or lunch in 15 minutes flat. Healthy eating doesn't have to be complicated! Recipes overleaf.*

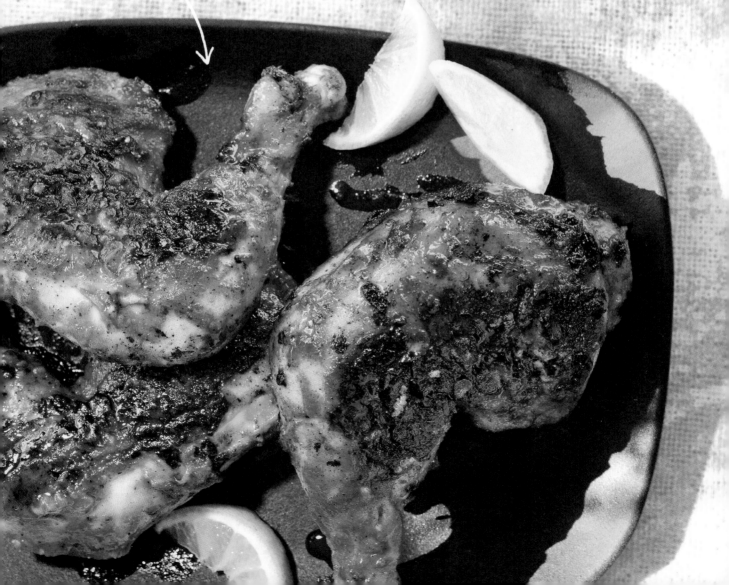

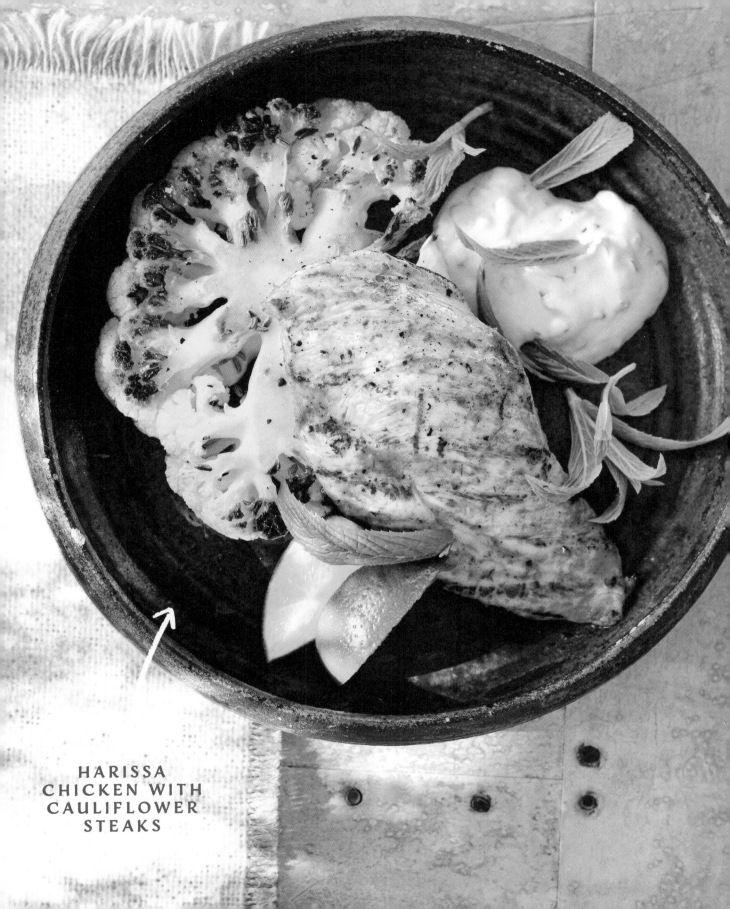

HARISSA
CHICKEN WITH
CAULIFLOWER
STEAKS

# HEALTHY BBQ CHICKEN

*A recipe by my lovely mum, Nicky Sepel. This household staple always made my sisters and me very excited for dinner! Always cook with organic free-range chicken – it makes such a difference.*

SERVES 6
PREP TIME: 50 minutes, including cooking + overnight marinating (optional)

6 chicken breasts
250 ml chicken stock
mixed salad and/or steamed asparagus and lemon wedges, to serve

MARINADE:
finely grated zest of 1 orange
½ teaspoon chilli flakes
2 teaspoons smoked paprika
2 tablespoons organic Dijon mustard
4 tablespoons raw honey or maple syrup
125 ml puréed tomatoes
2 teaspoons olive oil
Celtic sea salt and ground pepper
1 garlic clove, crushed
1 teaspoon grated ginger (optional)

Gently poach the chicken pieces in the stock for 15–20 minutes or until just cooked through.

To make the marinade, mix together all the ingredients in a non-metallic bowl or dish. Remove the chicken pieces from the poaching liquid while still warm and add to the marinade. Turn to coat well. The chicken may be cooked straight away or you can leave it in the fridge overnight to allow the flavours to intensify.

Barbecue the chicken on medium–high heat for 15–20 minutes or until golden and slightly charred, turning occasionally.

Serve with a mixed salad or steamed asparagus and lemon wedges, if desired.

# QUICK CHICKEN DINNERS

## MOROCCAN CHICKEN SKEWERS

Cut chicken thigh or breast fillets into 3 cm pieces. Coat in Moroccan spice mix, finely grated lemon zest and thyme leaves, thread onto skewers and chargrill until tender. Serve with lemon wedges on the side and a baby spinach, chickpea, cherry tomato and courgette ribbon salad.

## CHICKEN & GINGER STIR-FRY

Stir-fry chicken fillets or chicken breast strips in virgin organic coconut oil or olive oil, a good splash of tamari, crushed garlic, sliced leek, grated ginger and chilli flakes. Add some broccoli florets and pak choi and cook until just tender. Serve with brown rice.

# HARISSA CHICKEN WITH CAULIFLOWER STEAKS

SERVES 4
PREP TIME: 40 minutes,
including cooking

2 tablespoons olive oil
2 small cauliflowers, cut
  into 4 × 1.5 cm thick
  steaks (reserve the leftover
  florets for another recipe)
1 teaspoon fennel seeds,
  lightly crushed
Celtic sea salt and ground
  pepper
2 chicken breast fillets,
  fat trimmed, halved
  horizontally
2 tablespoons harissa paste
finely grated zest and juice
  of 1 lime
mint sprigs, to garnish
lime wedges, to serve
  (optional)

MINTED YOGHURT:
1 garlic clove, crushed
75 ml Greek-style yoghurt
2 tablespoons finely
  chopped mint
Celtic sea salt and ground
  pepper

*I adore the flavours and textures in this dish. I love cauliflower steak as an alternative to potato or rice – it's much more nutritious.*

Preheat the oven to 220°C (200°C fan/gas 7) and line a large baking tray with baking paper.

Heat half the olive oil in a large non-stick frying pan over medium–high heat. Sprinkle the cauliflower steaks with the fennel seeds, then add to the pan, in batches if necessary, and cook for 2–3 minutes on each side or until golden. Transfer the cauliflower to the prepared tray and season with salt and pepper.

Place the cauliflower in the oven and roast for 12–15 minutes or until tender.

Meanwhile, pour the remaining oil into a large ziplock bag, add the chicken, harissa paste and lime zest and juice. Season, then seal the bag and rub to coat the chicken.

Heat a griddle pan or barbecue to medium–high heat and cook the chicken for 3–4 minutes on each side or until lightly charred and cooked through.

To make the minted yoghurt, combine the garlic, yoghurt and mint in a small bowl. Season and mix well.

Serve the chicken with the cauliflower steaks and minted yoghurt. Garnish with mint sprigs and serve with lime wedges, if you like.

# BOLOGNESE WITH ZOODLES

SERVES 4
PREP TIME: 45 minutes,
including cooking

1 tablespoon olive oil
1 red onion, finely diced
1 garlic clove, crushed
1 stick celery, finely
 chopped
1 carrot, finely diced
400 g lean organic minced
 beef
150 g button mushrooms,
 sliced
3 vine tomatoes, finely
 diced or 1 x 400 g tin
 organic diced tomatoes
250 ml vegetable stock
75 ml organic tomato
 passata
1 teaspoon Worcestershire
 sauce
1 dried bay leaf
4 thyme sprigs
Celtic sea salt and ground
 pepper
4 large zucchini
 (courgettes)
shaved parmesan and small
 basil leaves, to serve

*Love your pasta? Me too! Here is the nutritious alternative that leaves you feeling satisfied – minus the bloat. Zoodles are simply zucchini (courgettes) spiralised into strips like spaghetti, and I am convinced they actually taste better than pasta! The kids won't even notice that you're sneaking in extra veggies.*

Heat the olive oil in a large non-stick frying pan over medium heat. Add the onion, garlic, celery and carrot and cook for 5 minutes or until softened. Add the mince and cook for a further 5 minutes or until browned, breaking up any lumps with the back of a wooden spoon.

Add the mushrooms and cook for 1 minute, then add the tomato, stock, tomato passata, Worcestershire sauce, bay leaf and thyme. Stir well and bring to the boil, then reduce the heat and simmer gently for 15–20 minutes or until the sauce has thickened. Season to taste.

Meanwhile, using a vegetable spiraliser or vegetable peeler and knife, cut the courgette (skin on) into thin, noodle-like strips (zoodles). Set aside in a sieve over a large bowl.

To serve, toss the zoodles through the bolognese sauce and top with parmesan and basil leaves.

## NEED SOME MORE HEALTHY SWAPS?

* *Refined white bread:* **wholegrain/rye/ gluten-free bread**

* *Refined cereal:* **homemade granola** (see pages 140–1)

* *Refined sugar:* **stevia, fruit, raw honey or raw maple syrup**

* *White pasta:* **brown rice pasta or courgette noodles**

* *Potato crisps:* **Sesame-coated Carrot Chips or Kale Chips** (see pages 237 and 256)

* *Vegetable oils:* **virgin organic coconut oil or olive oil**

* *Refined salt:* **Celtic sea salt or Himalayan pink rock salt**

* *Processed dairy:* **organic dairy/nut milks**

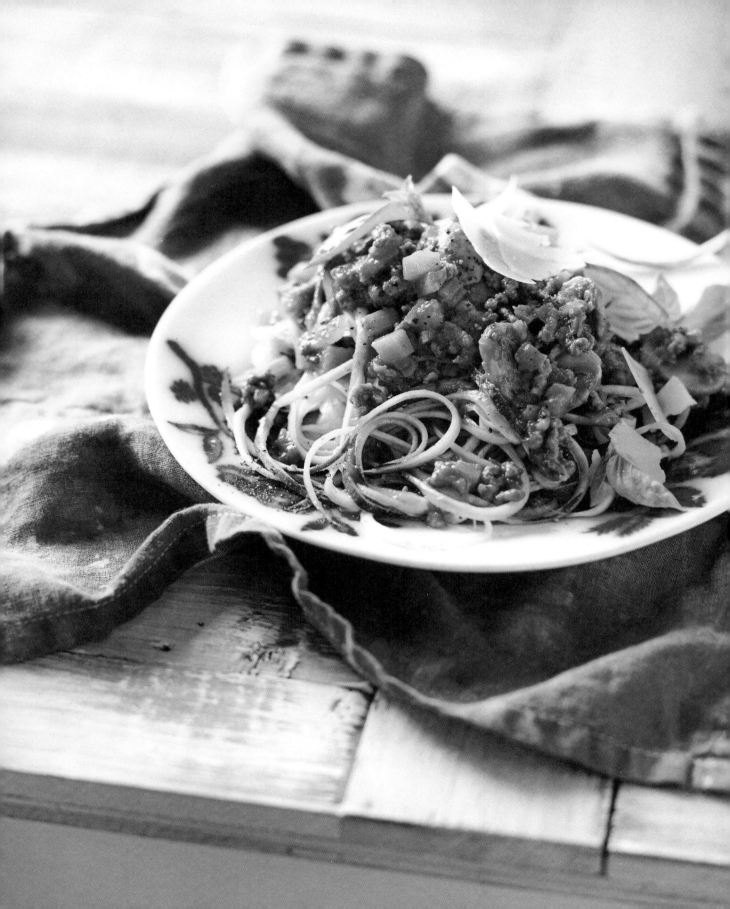

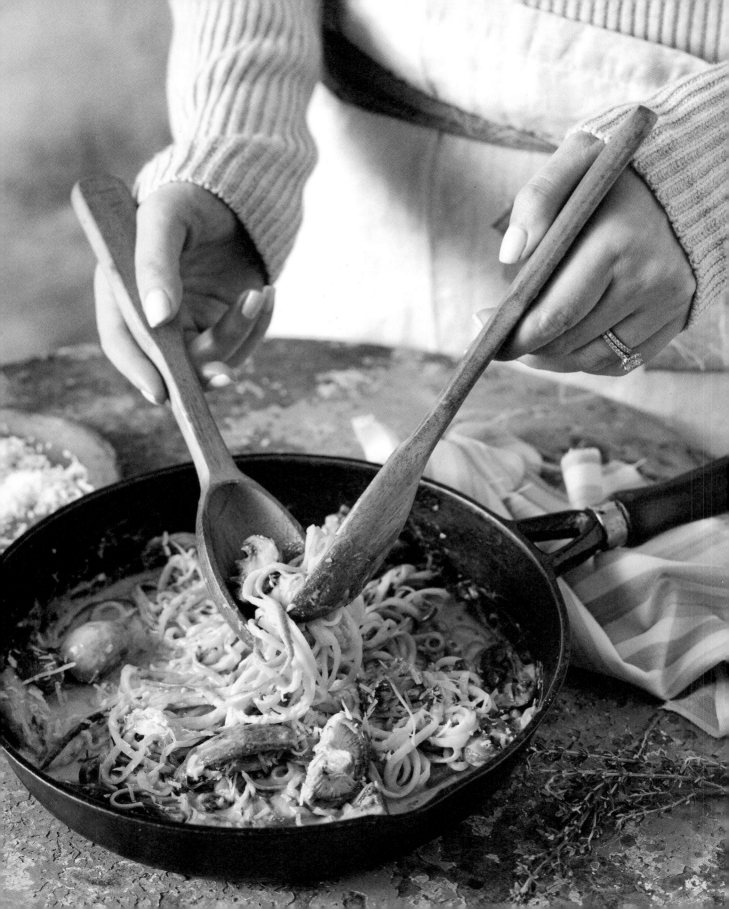

# COURGETTE MUSHROOM ALFREDO

SERVES 4
PREP TIME: 20 minutes,
including cooking

4 large courgettes
1 tablespoon virgin organic
  coconut oil
2 garlic cloves, crushed
400 g mixed mushrooms,
  sliced
125 ml coconut cream
a handful of thyme leaves
Celtic sea salt and ground
  pepper
grated parmesan, to serve
  (optional)

*The perfect vegetarian dish for those chilly evenings when you are dreaming of creamy pasta. Leave out the parmesan for a vegan dish, or go the other way and pair it with your protein of choice: chicken breast and poached or fried egg all go really well here.*

To make the 'pasta', leave the skin on the courgettes and, using a vegetable spiraliser or peeler, make noodle-like strips.

Melt the coconut oil in a frying pan over medium heat, add the garlic and cook gently until softened.

Add the mushrooms, coconut cream and thyme and sauté until the mushrooms are golden and cooked.

Add the courgette pasta and toss it through the mushroom sauce.

Season with salt and pepper and sprinkle with parmesan, if desired.

## OTHER VEGAN MEAL IDEAS

❋ *Mung bean/black bean pasta with pesto (see page 292), rocket and pumpkin seeds*

❋ *Brown rice bowl with steamed broccoli, avocado, sesame seeds and tempeh, finished with a drizzle of tamari/olive oil*

❋ *Tempeh veggie lentil burger*

❋ *Quinoa/brown rice sushi with avocado, cucumber, carrot and lettuce, served with tamari*

❋ *Thai-style Fried 'Rice' (see page 247)*

❋ *Healing Aubergine Bruschetta (see page 244)*

❋ *Lentil, avocado and roasted beetroot salad*

❋ *Mixed green salad with roasted cauliflower, pumpkin seeds, quinoa and a tahini dressing*

❋ *Roasted stuffed pepper, filled with herbs, tomato sauce, quinoa, seeds and veggies of choice, finished with a drizzle of olive oil*

❋ *Cauliflower & Brazil Nut Soup (see page 192)*

❋ *Gluten-free pizza topped with veggies of choice or Broccoli Pizza (see page 216)*

# BROCCOLI PIZZA

SERVES 2
PREP TIME: 45 minutes,
including cooking

olive oil spray
1 large or 2 small heads
  broccoli, cut into florets
½ red onion, diced
Celtic sea salt and ground
  pepper
1 egg
1 egg white
2 tablespoons olive oil
30 g ground flaxseed
2–3 tablespoons psyllium
  husk
1 garlic clove, crushed
½ teaspoon ground cumin
½ teaspoon mixed spice

## TOPPINGS

*Pesto (see page 292),
courgette slices and chopped
basil*

*Rosemary, Celtic sea salt and
olive oil – like a focaccia*

*Mozzarella and cherry tomato
halves*

*Parmesan, pesto (see page
292), flaked almonds and
rocket leaves (add the rocket
after the pizza is cooked)*

*This is just fabulous, and a great alternative to pizza. Packed with
fibre and nutrients, you can even use it as a breakfast toast! I think
this will become a book favourite!*

Preheat the oven to 180°C (160°C fan/gas 4). Line a large baking tray with
baking paper (or use two smaller trays) and spray with olive oil.

Pulse the broccoli, onion and a good pinch of salt in a food processor until it
reaches the texture of a fine crumb.

Whisk the egg and egg white in a mixing bowl. Add the broccoli crumb, olive oil,
flaxseed, psyllium husk, garlic and spices, season with salt and pepper and mix
well with a wooden spoon.

Add the broccoli mixture to the prepared tray, forming it into two mounds.
Spread them out into rounds and press down so they are as thin as possible.

Dab the rounds with paper towel to absorb any excess moisture.

Spray lightly with olive oil and season with salt.

Bake for 15–20 minutes or until firm and golden.

Remove from the oven and top with your choice of toppings (see left). Spray
the toppings with olive oil, then return to the oven for 5–10 minutes or until
warmed through and any cheese has melted.

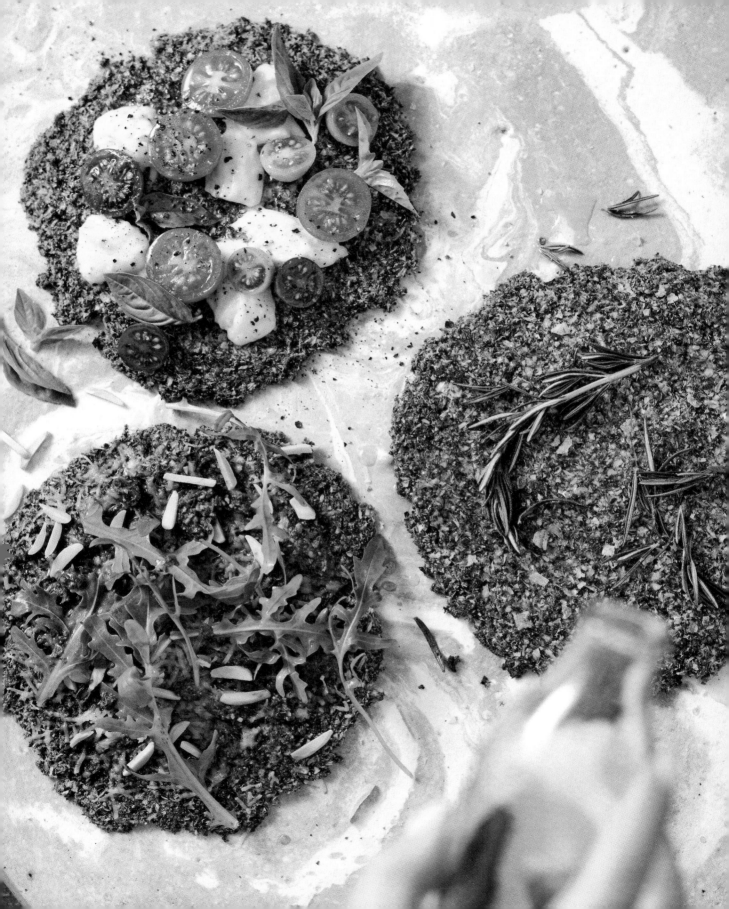

# COMFORTING VEGGIE CURRY

**SERVES 4-6**
**PREP TIME:** 1 hour
10 minutes, including
cooking

75 ml olive oil
1 onion, thinly sliced
1 garlic clove, crushed
1 leek, pale part only,
    trimmed and thinly sliced
2 carrots, sliced
4 sticks celery, sliced
1 head cauliflower, cut into
    florets
250 g green beans, topped
    and tailed, halved
2 heads broccoli, cut into
    florets
½ teaspoon chilli flakes, or
    to taste
3 tablespoons curry powder,
    plus extra if needed
Celtic sea salt and ground
    pepper
1 x 400 g tin organic diced
    tomatoes
400 ml organic tomato
    passata
500 ml vegetable stock or
    filtered water
30 g roughly chopped flat-
    leaf parsley or coriander
steamed brown rice, quinoa
    or lentils, to serve

*This delicious winter warmer is packed with nutritious herbs and
spices that act as anti-inflammatories in the body, making it great for
the immune system. It's so versatile too – enjoy it as a side dish or light
veggie main, or add your choice of protein to make it more substantial.
Beans and lentils make a welcome addition, but chicken is also a good
choice for the non-vegetarians out there.*

Heat the olive oil in a large non-stick frying pan over medium–high heat.
Add the onion, garlic, leek, carrot and celery and cook until softened and
lightly golden.

Add the cauliflower, beans, broccoli, chilli flakes, curry powder, salt and pepper,
diced tomatoes, tomato passata and stock or water.

Bring to the boil, then reduce the heat and simmer for 35–40 minutes or until
the vegetables are tender and the sauce has thickened.

Taste and add more curry powder if needed, then sprinkle with parsley
or coriander and serve with brown rice, quinoa or lentils.

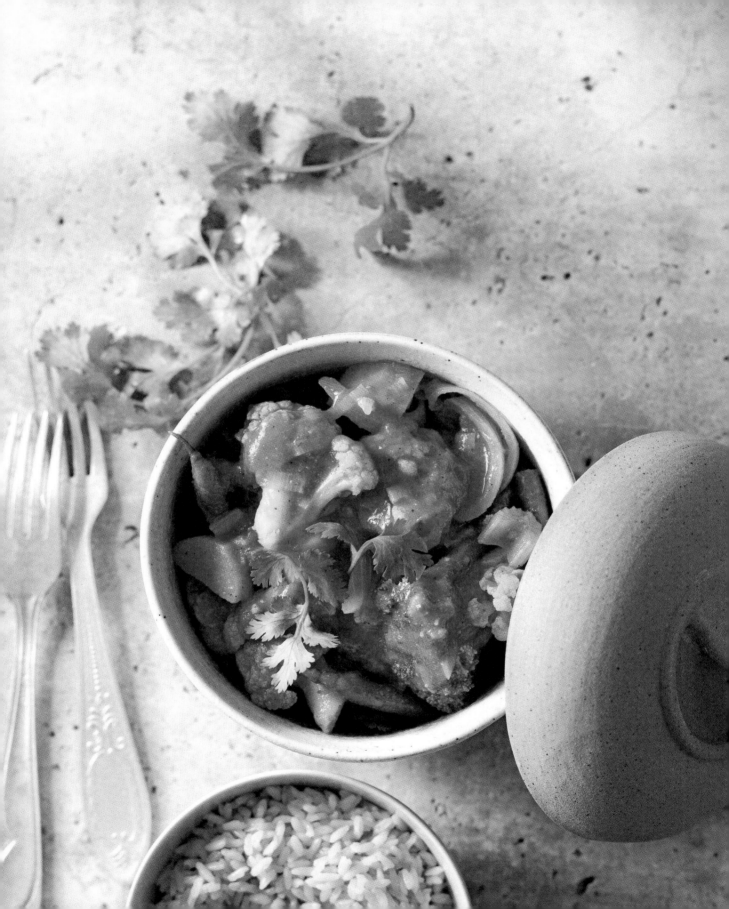

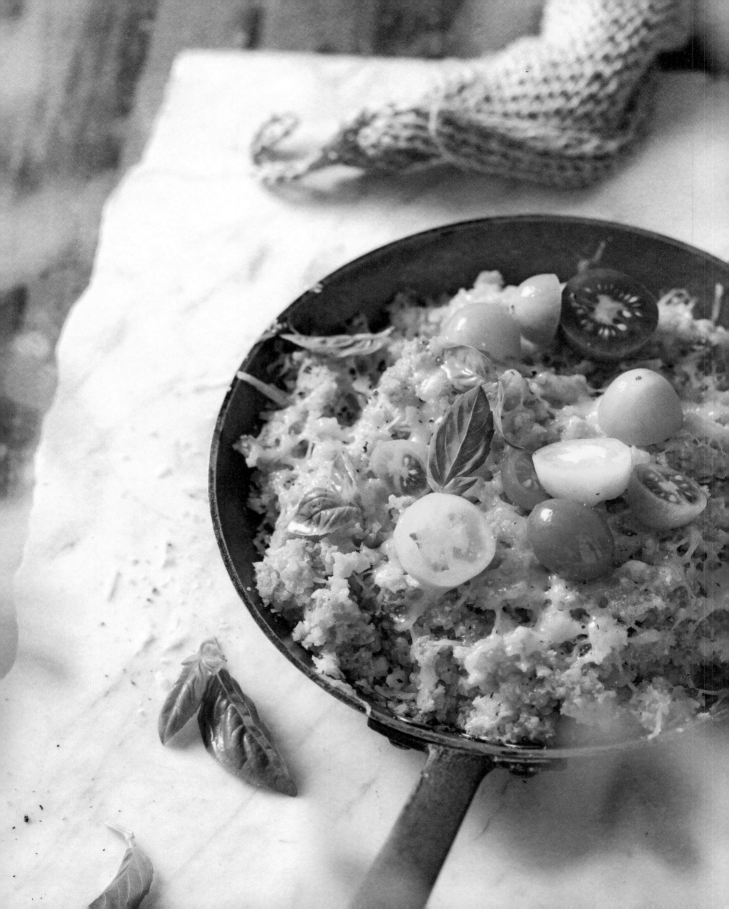

# CAULIFLOWER PARMIGIANA

*The result of a serious craving! I adore tomato sauce with my number one veggie: cauliflower. Full of goodness and easy to prepare, this dish is so warm and nourishing when you need a little coddling. Add some grilled chicken and avocado for your protein boost or vegans can swap cheese for crushed cashews or vegan cheese.*

SERVES 4
PREP TIME: 25 minutes, including cooking

1 head cauliflower, roughly cut into florets
1 tablespoon virgin organic coconut oil
1 small onion, chopped
2 tablespoons olive oil
Celtic sea salt
125 ml good-quality tomato-based sauce (without additives or sugar)
50 g grated parmesan
250 g baby heirloom tomatoes, halved
baby basil leaves, to serve

Pulse the cauliflower in a food processor until it reaches a rice-like consistency.

Melt the coconut oil in a large saucepan over medium–high heat. Add the onion and cook until softened and starting to colour. Gradually add the cauliflower rice.

Drizzle over the olive oil and sprinkle with salt, then cook, stirring, for 4–5 minutes.

Pour in the tomato sauce and stir gently to coat the cauliflower. Remove the pan from the heat and sprinkle over the parmesan, baby tomato halves and basil. Enjoy!

# FISH WITH BAKED ASPARAGUS

*As with most simple recipes, this is all about the quality of your ingredients. Make it when asparagus is at its seasonal best, and talk to your fishmonger about what is good on the day, or you can even replace the fish with chicken if you prefer.*

SERVES 2
PREP TIME: 35 minutes, including cooking

2 x 180 g white fish fillets, skin and bones removed
coconut oil or olive oil spray
2 heaped tablespoons pesto (see page 292)
1–2 bunches asparagus, trimmed
1–2 tablespoons olive oil
Celtic sea salt and ground pepper
chilli flakes, to taste (optional)

Preheat the oven to 200°C (180°C fan/gas 6) and line a baking tray with baking paper.

Place the fish fillets on the prepared tray and spray the fillets with oil. Spoon an even layer of pesto over each fish fillet.

Bake for 20–25 minutes or until cooked through.

Line another baking tray with baking paper. Spread the asparagus over the tray and drizzle with enough of the olive oil to coat well. Season to taste with salt and pepper, and add a sprinkling of chilli flakes, if you like.

Place in the oven and bake for 15–20 minutes or until just tender.

Remove the fish and asparagus from the oven and serve immediately.

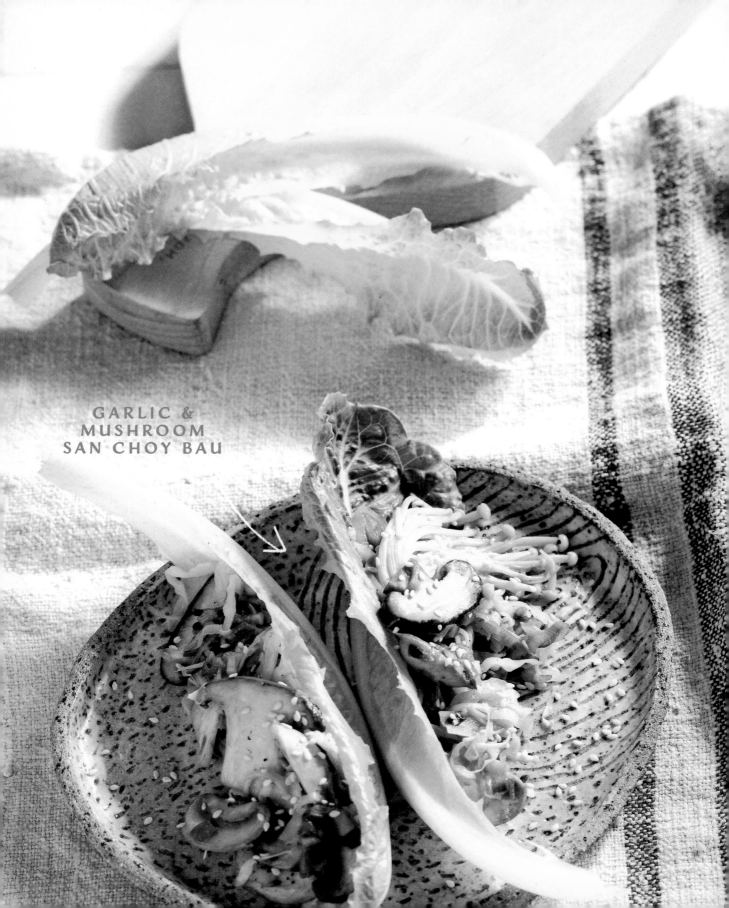

GARLIC &
MUSHROOM
SAN CHOY BAU

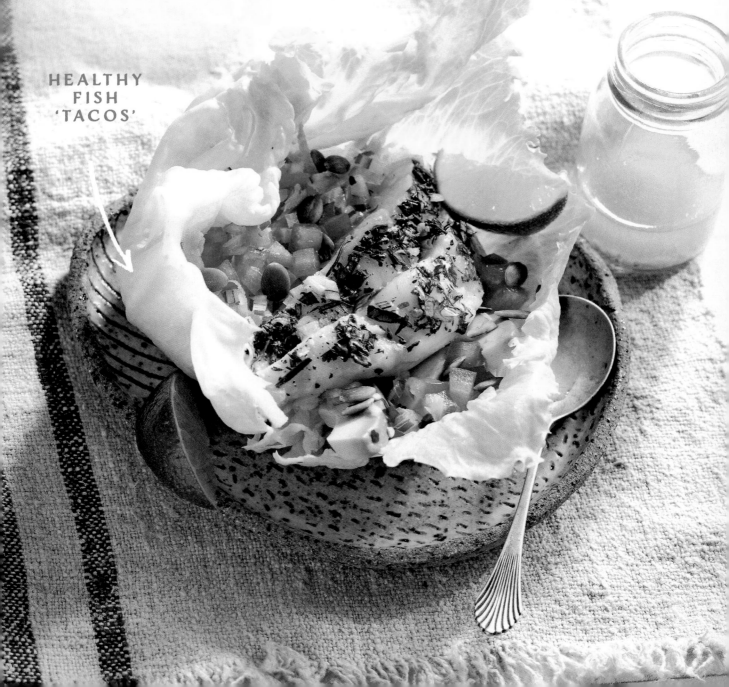

*San choy bau is a great option for lunch or dinner, and it's fun to make! Sometimes when I have friends over I set up a 'san choy bau station', offering lettuce leaves and all the filling ingredients in bowls so my guests can tailor their lettuce cups to their own taste. I also love this variation on the san choy bau: the healthy fish 'taco'. Recipes overleaf.*

# WAYS WITH SAN CHOY BAU

**HEALTHY FISH 'TACOS'**

## GARLIC & MUSHROOM SAN CHOY BAU

SERVES 4
PREP TIME: 15 minutes, including cooking

1 garlic clove, crushed
1 leek, thinly sliced
1 small red onion, diced
½ cabbage, shredded
400 g mixed mushrooms (chopped if large)
1½ tablespoons olive oil
Celtic sea salt and ground pepper
1 iceberg or cos lettuce, leaves removed intact
2 tablespoons tamari
2 teaspoons sesame oil
sesame seeds, to sprinkle

Sauté the garlic, leek, onion, cabbage and mushrooms in the olive oil in a large non-stick frying pan over medium–high heat for 5 minutes or until tender.

Season, then spoon the filling into the lettuce cups.

Drizzle with the tamari and sesame oil, toss over the seeds and serve.

## TEMPEH SAN CHOY BAU

Sauté crushed garlic, sliced tempeh, thinly sliced leek and mixed mushrooms in olive oil over medium–high heat. Season with Celtic sea salt and ground pepper. Spoon into lettuce cups and serve.

## SHREDDED CHICKEN SAN CHOY BAU

Fill the lettuce cups with shredded leftover cooked chicken and top with diced avocado, grated carrot and chopped fresh tomato. Drizzle with Lemony Tahini Dressing (see page 297) and season to taste with Celtic sea salt, ground pepper and chilli flakes.

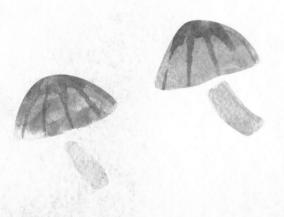

## TIP

*The basic steps for san choy bau are always the same: get yourself a nice, big round iceberg or long cos lettuce, choose a protein (tuna, marinated shredded chicken, sliced steak, sliced tempeh, lentils or sliced boiled egg), chop up your veggies of choice, pile it all into the lettuce leaves and top with your favourite dressing. Then roll it up and chomp away – yum!*

# HEALTHY FISH 'TACOS'

SERVES 2
PREP TIME: 30 minutes,
including cooking

2 x 180 g firm white fish
fillets, skin and bones
removed

20 g chopped mixed herbs
(such as flat-leaf parsley,
dill, coriander and
rosemary)

Himalayan pink rock salt
and ground pepper

1 teaspoon chilli flakes, or
to taste (optional)

1 tablespoon olive oil (or
use olive oil spray)

1 iceberg or cos lettuce,
leaves removed intact

½ red onion, diced

1 tomato, chopped

½ avocado, cut into chunks

1 carrot, grated

1–2 tablespoons sunflower
seeds or pumpkin seeds

1 tablespoon organic Dijon
mustard

juice of 1 lemon or lime,
plus extra to serve
(optional)

*When I visited Mexico, fish tacos were by far my favourite dish – lying on the beach with a delicious taco and a lime mojito was heaven. This healthy version is a great one for dinner parties. You should allow three or four lettuce cups per person.*

Preheat the oven to 200°C (180°C fan/gas 6) and line a baking tray with baking paper.

Place the fish fillets on the prepared tray and top with the chopped herbs, salt, pepper, chilli flakes (if using) and olive oil. Bake the fish for 12–15 minutes or until cooked through.

Meanwhile, fill each lettuce cup with the onion, tomato, avocado, carrot and seeds.

Once the fish is cooked, take it out of the oven and allow it to cool. Flake the fish into strips and add to the lettuce cups.

Mix together the mustard and lemon juice and drizzle over the lettuce tacos. (Alternatively, serve with the Green Tahini Dressing on page 296.) Finish with an extra squeeze of lemon or lime juice, if liked, and serve.

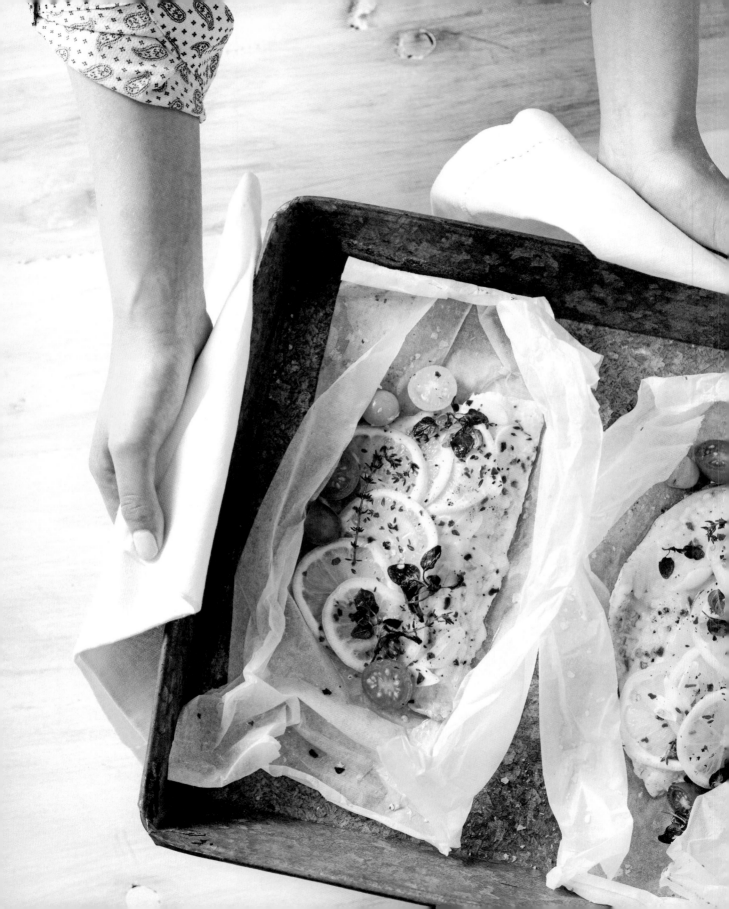

# LEMON HERB FISH IN A BAG

SERVES 2
PREP TIME: 35 minutes, including cooking

2 x 180 g white fish fillets, skin and bones
  removed
1 lemon, thinly sliced
a handful of mixed rosemary, oregano and thyme
  leaves or 1–2 tablespoons mixed dried rosemary,
  oregano, thyme and parsley
2 tablespoons olive oil
Celtic sea salt and ground pepper
chilli flakes, to taste (optional)
8 baby tomatoes, halved
1 garlic clove, sliced

Preheat the oven to 180°C (160°C fan/gas 4)
and line a baking tray with baking paper.

Tear off a 30 cm piece of baking paper and lay it
flat on the prepared tray. Place the fish fillets in the
middle of the paper.

Top the fish with the lemon slices, fresh herbs, olive
oil, salt, pepper and chilli flakes (if using). Scatter
over the tomatoes and garlic.

Take each corner of the paper and fold into the
centre to form a bag, then seal it.

Bake for 15–20 minutes or until the fish is cooked
through. Break open the bag just before serving so
you and your dinner date can enjoy the fragrances it
releases. Spoon all the wonderful juices over the
fish – you don't want to miss a drop.

# CHILLI & ROSEMARY STEAK WITH SAUTÉED GREENS

*If I had to choose my last meal on earth this would
be it!*

SERVES 4
PREP TIME: 25 minutes, including cooking

olive oil spray
4 x 200 g beef fillet steaks, fat trimmed
1 tablespoon finely chopped rosemary
½ teaspoon chilli flakes, or to taste
Celtic sea salt and ground pepper
1 tablespoon olive oil
1 garlic clove, crushed
1 leek, pale part only, trimmed and thinly sliced
1 bunch tenderstem broccoli, blanched, cut into
  thirds
finely grated zest and juice of 1 lemon
3 tablespoons finely chopped flat-leaf parsley
2 tablespoons roughly chopped hazelnuts, roasted
Truffle Cauliflower Purée (see page 242), to serve

Lightly spray a griddle pan or barbecue with olive
oil and heat to medium–high. Sprinkle the steaks
with rosemary and chilli flakes and season. Cook for
4–5 minutes on each side for medium-rare or until
cooked to your liking. Set aside, covered with foil
for 10 minutes.

Meanwhile, heat the olive oil in a large non-stick
frying pan over medium heat, add the garlic and
cook for 1 minute. Add the leek and cook for
2–3 minutes, then add the broccoli and cook for a
further 1–2 minutes.

Add the lemon zest and juice and toss to coat.
Remove from the heat and stir through the parsley
and hazelnuts.

Serve the steaks with the sautéed greens and truffle
cauliflower purée.

# SALMON & QUINOA CAKES WITH LEMON & TAHINI YOGHURT

SERVES 4
PREP TIME: 50 minutes,
including cooking

55 g quinoa, rinsed
2 x 180 g salmon fillets,
 skin and bones removed,
 roughly chopped
35 g almond meal
2 spring onions, thinly
 sliced
1 egg, lightly beaten
1 teaspoon fennel seeds,
 lightly crushed
1 garlic clove, crushed
1½ tablespoons finely
 chopped dill
½ teaspoon chilli flakes
 (optional)
Celtic sea salt and ground
 pepper
1 tablespoon virgin organic
 coconut oil
lemon wedges, to serve
sliced baby fennel, sliced
 radish or rocket leaves, to
 serve

LEMON & TAHINI
YOGHURT:
finely grated zest and juice
 of ½ lemon
75 ml Greek-style yoghurt
1 tablespoon hulled tahini
1 garlic clove, crushed
1½ tablespoons finely
 chopped dill
Celtic sea salt and ground
 pepper

*When I was growing up in South Africa I became a little obsessed with a gorgeous little patisserie that served the best salmon fish cakes. I've never forgotten them so of course I had to make a healthy version to satisfy the craving! These are so delicious for lunch or dinner and, as a bonus, they're gluten-free too.*

Cook the quinoa according to the packet instructions or until just tender. Drain well and set aside to cool.

Place the salmon, almond meal, spring onion, egg, fennel seeds, garlic, dill and chilli flakes (if using) in a food processor and process until just combined. Transfer to a large bowl and stir in the quinoa. Season well with salt and pepper.

Melt the coconut oil in a large non-stick frying pan over medium heat. Using damp hands, shape the mixture into 12 patties. Add to the pan (in batches if necessary) and cook for 3–4 minutes on each side or until golden and cooked through. Transfer to a tray lined with paper towel.

Meanwhile, to make the lemon and tahini yoghurt, combine all the ingredients in a small bowl.

Serve three fish cakes per person with the lemon and tahini yoghurt, lemon wedges and your choice of fennel, radish or rocket (or all three!).

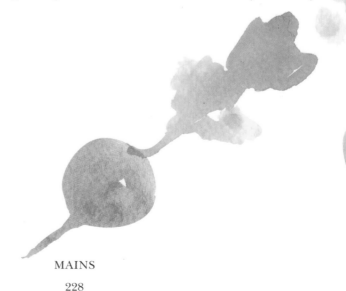

MAINS

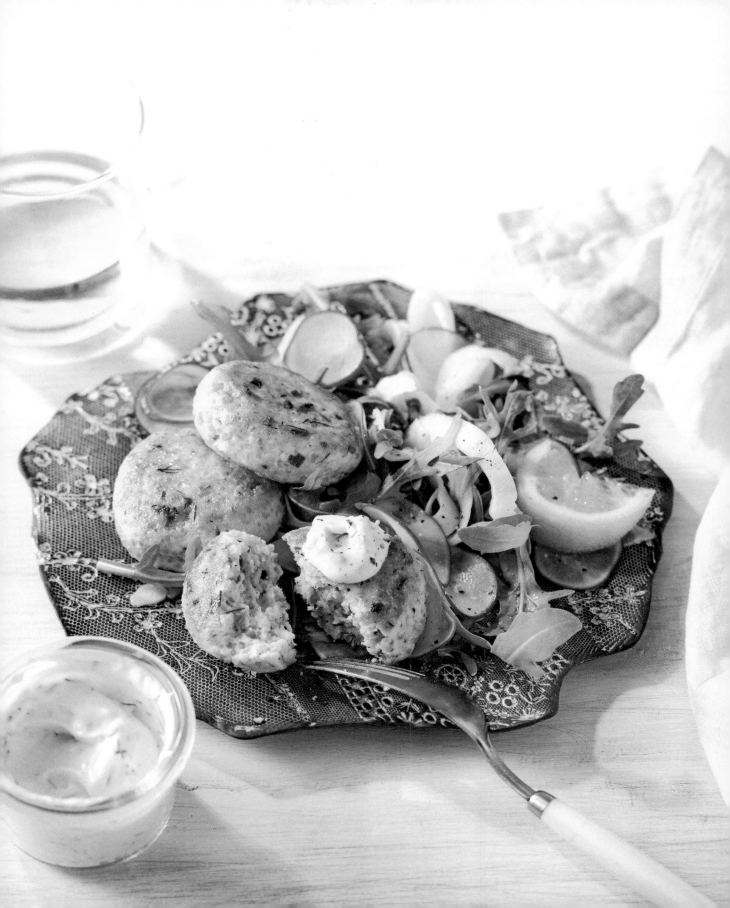

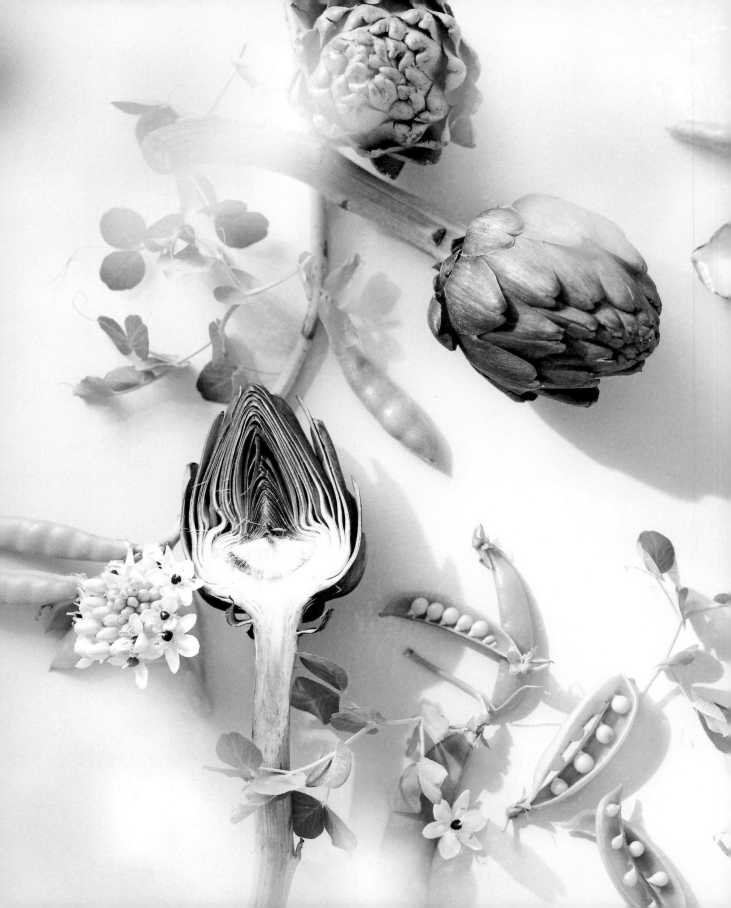

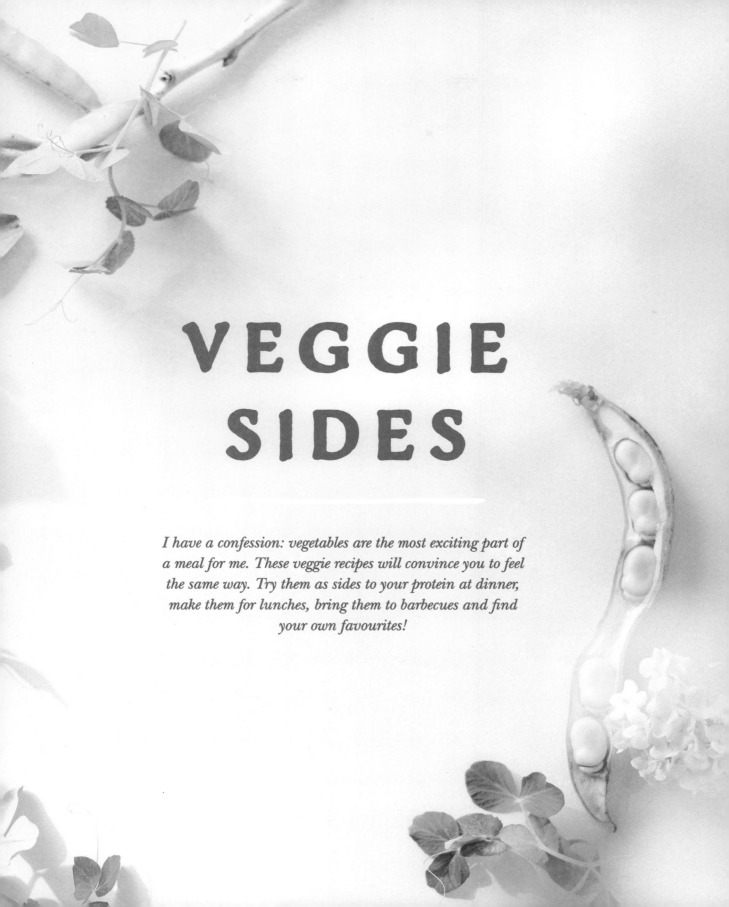

# VEGGIE SIDES

*I have a confession: vegetables are the most exciting part of a meal for me. These veggie recipes will convince you to feel the same way. Try them as sides to your protein at dinner, make them for lunches, bring them to barbecues and find your own favourites!*

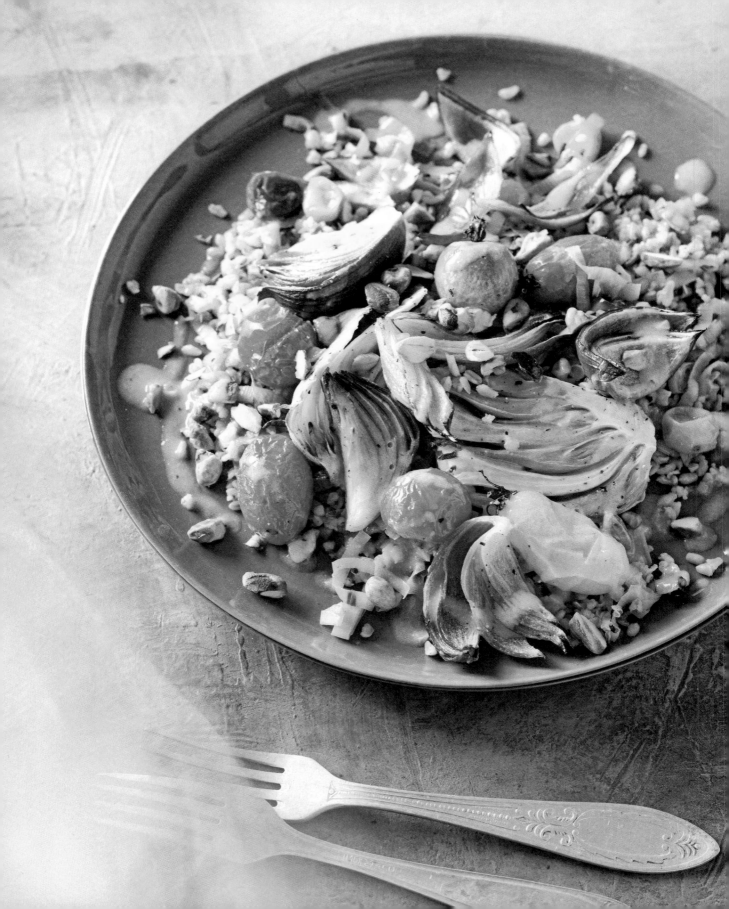

# ROASTED VEGETABLE & FREEKEH SALAD

SERVES 4
PREP TIME: 50 minutes,
including cooking

250 g cherry tomatoes
3 bulbs baby fennel, cut
 into wedges
2 red onions, cut into
 wedges
75 ml olive oil
Celtic sea salt and ground
 pepper
170 g freekeh
1 teaspoon curry powder
1 leek, pale part only,
 trimmed and thinly sliced
40 g pistachio kernels,
 roughly chopped
shaved parmesan, to serve
 (optional)

CUMIN TAHINI DRESSING:
2 tablespoons hulled tahini
125 ml olive oil
125 ml white balsamic
 vinegar
1 teaspoon ground cumin

*I first made this on a sunny Sunday for our weekly family lunch. Big hit! This salad is full of rich flavours and aromas, is incredibly satisfying and goes well with any protein dish. And it looks really beautiful plated up too. If you decide not to use all the dressing, keep the leftovers in a mason jar in your fridge and use it in other meals over the next few days.*

Preheat the oven to 200°C (180°C fan/gas 6) and line a baking tray with baking paper.

Spread out the tomatoes, fennel and onion on the prepared tray, drizzle with 2 tablespoons of the olive oil and season well with salt. Roast for 25–30 minutes or until tender. Remove from the oven and set aside to cool for 10 minutes.

Meanwhile, bring a saucepan of water to the boil, add the freekeh and cook for about 20 minutes or until tender. Drain and set aside to cool slightly.

Tip the cooled freekeh into a bowl and drizzle with 1 tablespoon of the oil. Toss through the curry powder.

Heat the remaining oil in a large non-stick frying pan over medium–high heat, add the leek and cook until softened and slightly golden.

Add the leek to the freekeh, then toss through the pistachios and shaved parmesan (if using).

Top the freekeh with the roasted vegetables.

To make the dressing, whisk together the tahini, olive oil, vinegar and cumin.

Drizzle the dressing over the salad, season to taste and serve.

# MISO AUBERGINE

*I am a true lover of Japanese cuisine. However sometimes this dish can be quite high in sugar, so I created a healthy version with my JSHealth team. These aubergines are delicious as a side to any Japanese-inspired dish or on their own with some sautéed greens and brown rice. It's my go-to recipe for last-minute dinner guests – guaranteed to impress!*

SERVES 6
PREP TIME: 30 minutes, including cooking

3 aubergines, halved lengthways
3 tablespoons sesame oil
4 tablespoons white miso paste
2 tablespoons raw honey or maple syrup
1 tablespoon soy sauce or tamari
1 teaspoon white wine vinegar
2 tablespoons sesame seeds, roasted
2 tablespoons chopped spring onions

Preheat the oven to 200°C (180°C fan/gas 6) and line a baking tray with baking paper.

Lightly score the cut surface of the aubergine halves in a criss-cross pattern and place on the prepared tray. Brush with 2 tablespoon of the sesame oil and roast for 15 minutes or until browned and softened.

Meanwhile, combine the miso, honey or maple syrup, soy sauce or tamari, vinegar and remaining sesame oil to make a smooth paste.

Remove the aubergine from the oven and brush with a thick layer of the miso glaze. Return to the oven for 6–8 minutes or until the glaze is toasted and fragrant.

Scatter sesame seeds and spring onion over the top and serve.

# ALMOND & HERB-STUFFED MUSHROOMS

*This is another dinner side I make often. It's all about the texture with this one, and it goes so well with salmon or steak. Even if you don't particularly love mushrooms I'd encourage you to give these a go!*

SERVES 4
PREP TIME: 35 minutes, including cooking

4 large portobello mushrooms, wiped clean, stems removed
4 tablespoons olive oil
Himalayan pink rock salt and ground pepper
100 g flaked almonds
2 large handfuls of basil leaves
2 large handfuls of flat-leaf parsley leaves
chilli flakes (optional)
basil leaves, to garnish

Preheat the oven to 180°C (160°C fan/gas 4) and line a baking tray with baking paper.

Place the mushrooms on the prepared tray and drizzle with half the olive oil. Season with salt.

Pulse the almonds, basil, parsley, remaining oil and a good pinch of salt in a food processor until it forms a rough crumb.

Fill the mushrooms with the stuffing and sprinkle with chilli flakes, if desired.

Bake for 20–25 minutes or until the mushrooms are cooked and the stuffing is golden. Garnish with basil leaves. Serve and enjoy.

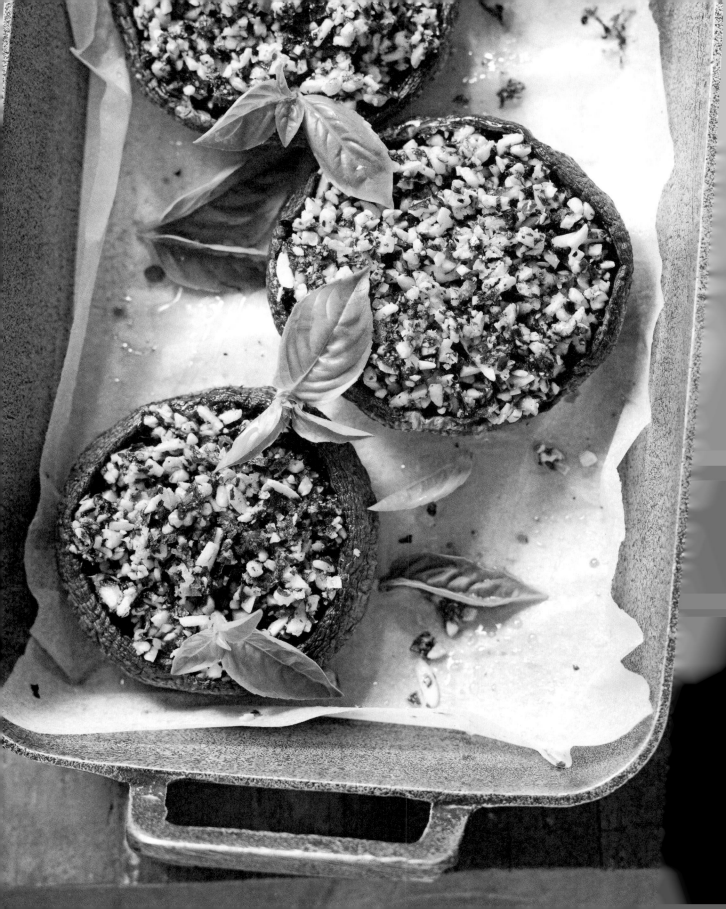

# FRIED KALE WITH ALMONDS

*This delicious side is very quick to make and pairs beautifully with any protein at your table. Mix it up to suit your own taste; for instance, you can swap the kale for Swiss chard, and the almonds with a sprinkling of sesame seeds.*

SERVES 4
PREP TIME: 15 minutes, including cooking

3–4 tablespoons olive oil or virgin organic
  coconut oil
1 garlic clove, crushed
½ leek, pale part only, trimmed and sliced
1 large bunch kale, stalks removed and leaves torn
1–2 teaspoons chilli flakes
Celtic sea salt and ground pepper
50 g flaked almonds

Heat 2 tablespoons of the oil in a large frying pan over medium heat, add the garlic and leek and cook until just softened.

Add the kale and sauté for 1–2 minutes.

Add the chilli and remaining oil, and season to taste with salt and pepper.

Top with the almonds and serve.

# FRIED GARLIC & CHILLI BROCCOLI

*I really love this paired with grilled salmon or chicken. I make this at least twice a week.*

SERVES 2
PREP TIME: 15 minutes, including cooking

2–3 tablespoons olive oil
1 garlic clove, crushed or thinly sliced
1 head broccoli, cut into florets
1–2 teaspoons chilli flakes, to taste
Himalayan pink rock salt and ground pepper

Heat 1 tablespoon of the olive oil in a large frying pan over medium heat, add the garlic and cook until just softened. Add the broccoli florets and sauté briefly. Add the chilli and remaining oil and season to taste with salt and pepper. Pour in a splash of boiling water if needed to stop the broccoli sticking to the pan.

Cook until the broccoli is just tender, then serve immediately.

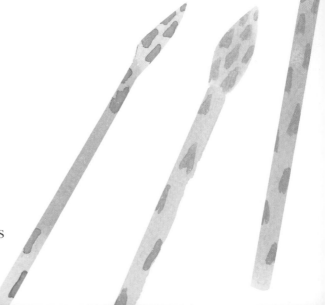

# SESAME-COATED ASPARAGUS

*This brilliant recipe comes from my aunty Renee, who showed me how to make it on a recent trip to London. It was so easy and good that I had to include it in the book. Thanks Ren!*

SERVES 2
PREP TIME: 15 minutes, including cooking

8–10 asparagus spears, trimmed
75 ml olive oil
Celtic sea salt and ground pepper
4 tablespoons sesame seeds, plus extra to serve
  (optional)
finely grated lemon zest, to garnish (optional)

Wash the asparagus spears and pat dry with paper towel.

On a plate or board, coat the spears in 2 tablespoons of the olive oil and season well with salt and pepper.

Sprinkle the sesame seeds over the spears, then roll them on the plate to coat all over in the seeds.

Heat a griddle or frying pan and pour in the remaining olive oil.

Add the asparagus and cook for about 5 minutes or until tender and slightly charred.

Plate up and enjoy. If you like, sprinkle over some lemon zest and extra sesame seeds.

# SESAME-COATED CARROT CHIPS

*I love serving these as a snack when guests come over for dinner – they're amazing with guacamole or you can make a quick dipping sauce by mixing 2 heaped tablespoons of hulled tahini and a good squeeze of lemon juice.*

SERVES 4
PREP TIME: 50 minutes, including cooking

5 large carrots, cut lengthways into 1 cm thick
  'chips'
3–4 tablespoons olive oil (or use olive or coconut
  oil spray)
40 g mixed black and white sesame seeds
Himalayan pink rock salt and ground pepper
Chilli & Lime Guacamole (see page 290)
  or tahini dip, to serve

Preheat the oven to 200°C (180°C fan/gas 6) and line a baking tray with baking paper.

Spread the carrot chips over the prepared tray and drizzle with enough oil to coat well – toss with your hands to make sure they are well coated.

Sprinkle over the sesame seeds and season with salt and pepper.

Bake for 30–40 minutes or until golden and cooked through.

Remove from the oven and leave them to cool slightly, then serve with guacamole or tahini dip.

# CRISPY BRUSSELS BY CAYLEY

*My bestie, Cayley Meyer, makes the best crispy brussels sprouts ever and I'm thrilled that she's allowed me to share her recipe with my lovely readers. You won't be sorry!*

SERVES 4
PREP TIME: 40 minutes, including cooking

20 brussels sprouts, trimmed and cut into quarters
olive oil, for drizzling
Celtic sea salt and ground pepper
3–4 pickled chillies, diced, to taste
½ red onion, diced
1 teaspoon raw honey
2 splashes of red wine vinegar
1 tablespoon sesame seeds

Preheat the oven to 200°C (180°C fan/gas 6) and line a large baking tray with baking paper.

Spread the brussels sprouts over the prepared tray and drizzle with olive oil. Season to taste with salt and pepper.

Bake for 25 minutes or until crispy.

Remove from the oven and toss through the pickled chilli and onion.

Drizzle the honey over the sprouts, followed by a splash or two of the vinegar.

Sprinkle with the sesame seeds and serve.

# SWEET POTATO SALAD WITH GREEN TAHINI DRESSING

*Vegans can enjoy this salad by simply swapping the goat's cheese for cashew cheese.*

SERVES 4
PREP TIME: 1 hour 15 minutes, including cooking and cooling

800 g sweet potatoes, scrubbed and cut into 4 cm pieces
3 red onions, cut into wedges
2 tablespoons olive oil
½ teaspoon chilli flakes, or to taste, plus extra for serving (optional)
3 rosemary sprigs, leaves stripped
Celtic sea salt and ground pepper
200 g green beans, topped and tailed, cut into thirds
150 g baby rocket leaves
1 x 400 g tin organic lentils, drained and rinsed
Green Tahini Dressing (see page 296)
80 g goat's cheese, crumbled (optional)

Preheat the oven to 200°C (180°C fan/gas 6) and line a large baking tray with baking paper. Spread out the sweet potato and onion on the prepared tray. Drizzle the olive oil over the top, and sprinkle with the chilli flakes and rosemary. Season with salt and pepper and toss to coat. Roast for 35–40 minutes or until golden and tender. Remove from the oven and allow to cool for 20 minutes.

Blanch the beans in a saucepan of boiling water for 1–2 minutes. Remove and refresh in cold water, then drain well.

Toss the rocket and beans in a large bowl. Top with the roasted sweet potato and onion and the lentils. Drizzle with the green tahini dressing and finish with goat's cheese and extra chilli, if desired.

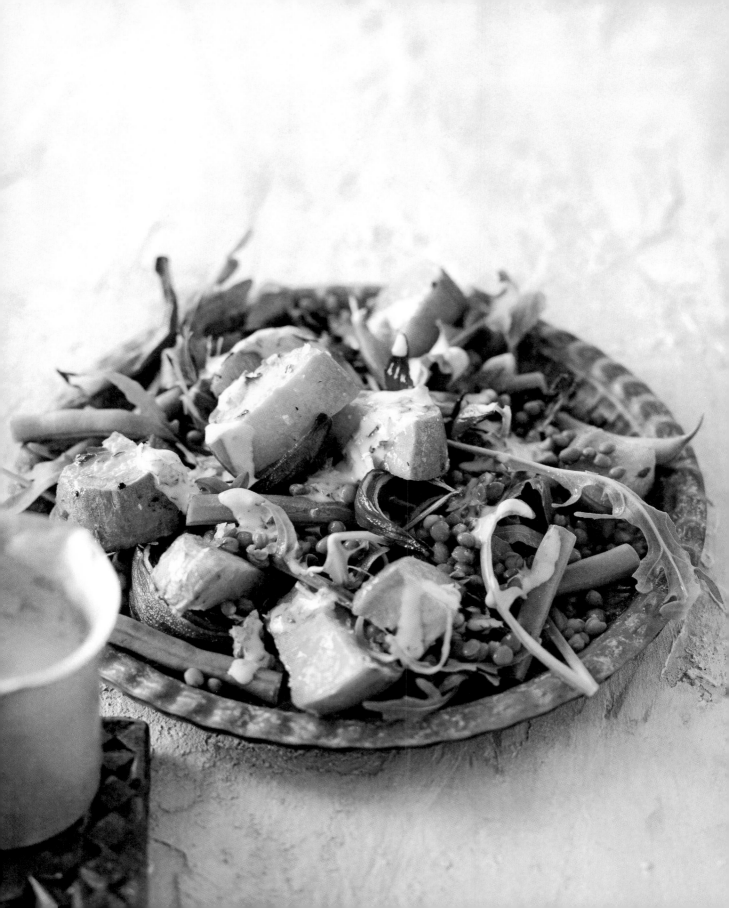

# COCONUT & ROSEMARY WEDGES

*You won't miss unhealthy fried potato wedges after trying these. The almond meal adds a lovely flavour but if you don't have any just use coconut flour.*

SERVES 4
PREP TIME: 50 minutes, including cooking

750 g sweet potatoes, scrubbed and cut into wedges
coconut oil spray
50 g mixed coconut flour and/or almond meal
5 rosemary sprigs, leaves stripped
Celtic sea salt and ground pepper
1 teaspoon chilli flakes, or to taste
hulled tahini, to serve

Preheat the oven to 200°C (180°C fan/gas 6) and line a large baking tray with baking paper.

Spread out the sweet potato on the prepared tray and spray generously with coconut oil.

Sprinkle the coconut flour and/or almond meal evenly over the sweet potato and scatter with the rosemary leaves. Season to taste with salt, pepper and chilli flakes.

Bake for about 35 minutes or until golden.

Remove from the oven and allow to cool slightly.

Serve with tahini as a dipping sauce.

# ZA'ATAR COURGETTE CHIPS

*Swap your potato fries for courgette chips. Great as a side, but they are also delicious to enjoy as a starter snack at dinner parties, dunked into some hummus or tahini.*

SERVES 6
PREP TIME: 15 minutes, including cooking

1 tablespoon virgin organic coconut oil
1 garlic clove, crushed
4 courgettes, thinly sliced on the diagonal
1 tablespoon za'atar
1 teaspoon Celtic sea salt, or to taste

Melt the coconut oil in a large non-stick frying pan over medium heat. Add the garlic and cook until just softened.

Sprinkle the courgette slices with the za'atar and salt.

Add the courgette slices to the pan (you may need to do this in batches) and fry on each side for 1 minute or until golden. Serve hot!

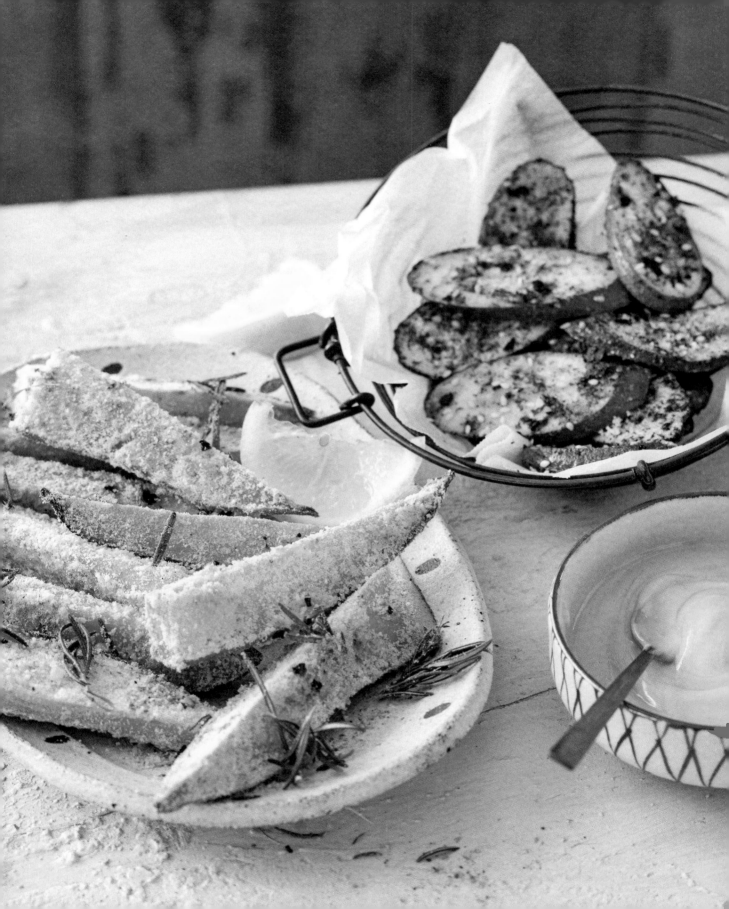

# TRUFFLE CAULIFLOWER PURÉE

*This is the most nourishing and wholesome side dish, yet it tastes rich and decadent. It goes so well with a grass-fed steak and a glass of organic vino. In fact, I have to admit that it is my ultimate comfort meal. Just typing it is making me drool!*

SERVES 4
PREP TIME: 30 minutes, including cooking

1 head cauliflower, trimmed and cut into florets
1 red onion, roughly chopped
500 ml chicken or vegetable stock
125 ml almond milk or milk of your choice
3 tablespoons walnuts, crushed.
2 tablespoons truffle oil, plus extra for drizzling
  (optional)
filtered water, if needed
Himalayan pink rock salt and ground pepper
1 tablespoon chopped flat-leaf parsley

Place the cauliflower, onion and stock in a large saucepan over high heat.

Bring to the boil, then reduce the heat and simmer, covered, for about 15 minutes or until the vegetables are tender.

Stir in the milk and walnuts.

Purée the cauliflower mixture with a stick blender or in a food processor until smooth and creamy. With the motor running, gradually add the truffle oil. The mixture should be runnier than mash – add a little water if it is too thick for your liking.

Season well with salt and pepper.

Finish with a sprinkling of parsley and an extra drizzle of truffle oil, if desired.

# SPICED CAULIFLOWER ON CARROT HUMMUS

*This dish came about by accident when I was trying to work out what to do with all the carrots in my fridge. It works so well at dinner parties, and the carrot dip has become a household staple. I often have a batch in the fridge to eat with my veggie sticks.*

SERVES 4
PREP TIME: 1 hour, including cooking

1 head cauliflower, trimmed and quartered
2 tablespoons olive oil (or use olive oil spray)
Celtic sea salt and ground pepper
2 teaspoons chermoula spice mix
1 teaspoon chilli flakes, or to taste
chopped flat-leaf parsley, to garnish

CARROT HUMMUS:
4 carrots, roughly chopped and steamed
2 tablespoons olive oil
1 teaspoon Himalayan pink rock salt
1 garlic clove
75 g hulled tahini
1 teaspoon raw honey
¼ teaspoon chilli flakes, or to taste
2–3 tablespoons filtered water

Preheat the oven to 200°C (180°C fan/gas 6) and line a baking tray with baking paper.

Place the cauliflower on the prepared tray. Drizzle with the olive oil and season with salt and pepper, then sprinkle over the chermoula and chilli flakes.

Roast for 45 minutes or until tender and a little crispy. Remove from the oven and set aside to cool slightly.

To make the carrot hummus, place all the ingredients in a food processor and pulse until well combined but still a little chunky. Spread out the hummus on a serving platter and arrange the cauliflower on top. Garnish with chopped parsley and serve.

# CURRIED ALMOND CAULIFLOWER

*Hands down, this is my favourite side in the entire book. It tastes like unhealthy deep-fried cauliflower but of course is so much better for you.*

SERVES 6
PREP TIME: 35 minutes, including cooking

4 tablespoons olive oil or virgin organic coconut
  oil
1 garlic clove, crushed
1 red or brown onion, diced
2 heads cauliflower, cut into florets and chopped
  into smaller pieces
2 teaspoons ground cumin
1–2 teaspoons fennel seeds, to taste
2 teaspoons mild curry powder, or to taste
½ teaspoon ground turmeric
1 teaspoon chilli flakes, or to taste
Himalayan pink rock salt and ground pepper
a few splashes of filtered water
2 spring onions, chopped
40 g raw almonds, crushed

Heat 1 tablespoon of the oil in a large frying pan or wok over medium–high heat, add the garlic and onion and cook until softened.

Add the cauliflower and sprinkle with the cumin, fennel seeds, curry powder, turmeric, chilli flakes and 1 teaspoon salt.

Pour in the remaining oil and a few splashes of water to help the cauliflower steam. Cover the pan to encourage steaming, if you like.

Add most of the spring onion (save a little for garnish) and continue to cook until the cauliflower becomes soft and golden – this will take about 20–25 minutes all up.

Taste and adjust the seasoning to suit you. Plate up and top with the crushed almonds and remaining spring onion. Yum!

# SESAME CAULIFLOWER WITH CRISPY LEEKS

*As you can probably tell by now, I really love my cauliflower! This is another irresistible way to enjoy it.*

SERVES 4
PREP TIME: 1 hour, including cooking

1 head cauliflower, cut into 4 × 1.5 cm thick steaks
  (reserve the leftover florets to stir-fry with your
  eggs in the morning!)
½ leek, pale part only, trimmed and thickly sliced
4 tablespoons sesame seeds
1–2 tablespoons olive oil (or use olive oil spray)
2 tablespoons white wine vinegar
Himalayan pink rock salt
1 teaspoon chilli flakes, or to taste
a handful of flat-leaf parsley, chopped

Preheat the oven to 180°C (160°C fan/gas 4) and line a baking tray with baking paper.

Place the cauliflower steaks on the prepared tray and top evenly with the leek and sesame seeds.

Drizzle the olive oil and vinegar over the steaks and season to taste with salt and chilli flakes.

Roast for 45 minutes or until cooked through and golden.

Sprinkle with fresh parsley and serve.

# SESAME & LEEK ROASTED FENNEL

*I love fennel, to the point of chomping on it raw as I chop it up, but it seems to be a most underrated vegetable. Apart from its unique flavour, it acts as a digestive calmer, which is a decided bonus. This side is fresh and tasty and very quick and easy to make – delicious with fish or lentils.*

SERVES 4
PREP TIME: 50 minutes, including cooking

4 bulbs fennel, trimmed and quartered
½ leek, pale part only, trimmed and thinly sliced
2 tablespoons olive oil (or use olive oil spray)
1 tablespoon fennel seeds
2 teaspoons ground cumin
2 tablespoons sesame seeds
Celtic sea salt and ground pepper
shaved parmesan, to serve (optional)

Preheat the oven to 180°C (160°C fan/gas 4) and line a large baking tray with baking paper.

Spread the fennel and leek over the prepared tray and add the olive oil, fennel seeds, cumin, sesame seeds and plenty of salt and pepper.

Mix well with your hands or a spoon so the fennel is well coated in the oil and flavourings.

Roast for 30 minutes or until golden and tender.

Finish with shaved parmesan (if using) and serve.

# HEALING AUBERGINE BRUSCHETTA

*A great alternative to bread-based bruschetta and much more nutritious. Win win!*

SERVES 4
PREP TIME: 1 hour 15 minutes, including standing and cooking

2 large aubergines, cut lengthways into 2 cm thick slices
Himalayan pink rock salt
olive oil or olive oil spray, to coat
thinly sliced mozzarella, parmesan or cashew cheese, to cover (optional)
a handful of small basil leaves, to garnish

BRUSCHETTA MIX:
250 g cherry tomatoes, quartered
1 red onion, diced
1 garlic clove, crushed
1 tablespoon olive oil
1 tablespoon balsamic vinegar

Arrange the aubergine slices on a plate or tray and sprinkle generously with salt. Set aside for 30 minutes or so until the aubergine has softened. Pat dry with paper towel.

Preheat the oven to 200°C (180°C fan/gas 6) and line a large baking tray with baking paper.

Drizzle or spray the aubergine with olive oil so that each slice is lightly oiled on both sides. Arrange on the prepared tray and top with cheese slices, if desired.

To make the bruschetta mix, combine all the ingredients in a bowl. Spoon the bruschetta mix evenly over the aubergine slices.

Bake for 25–30 minutes or until cooked through and crispy. Garnish with basil leaves. Serve warm or at room temperature.

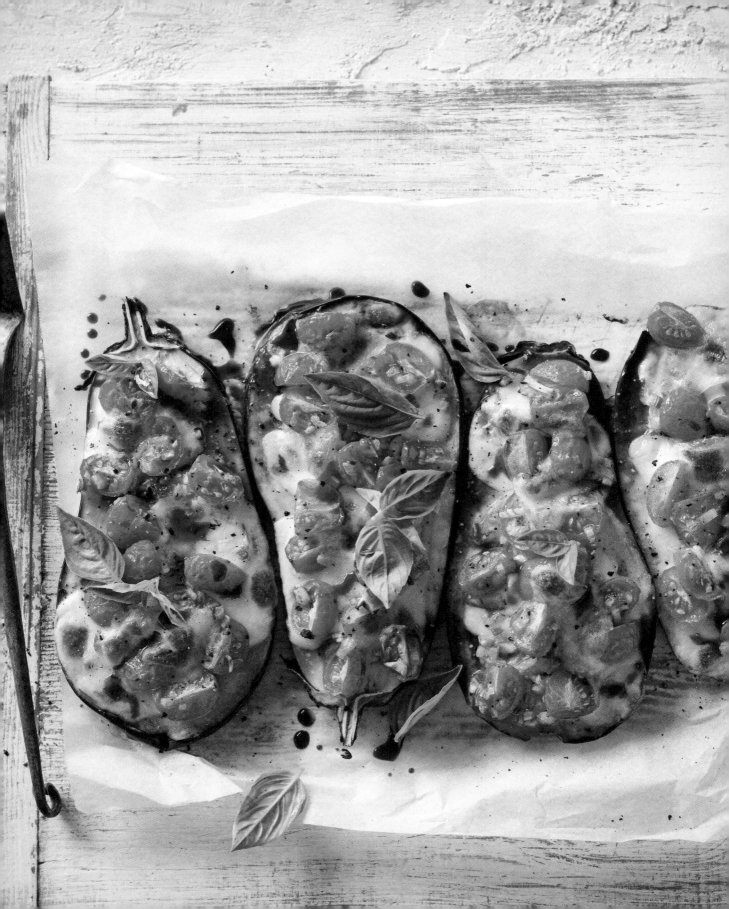

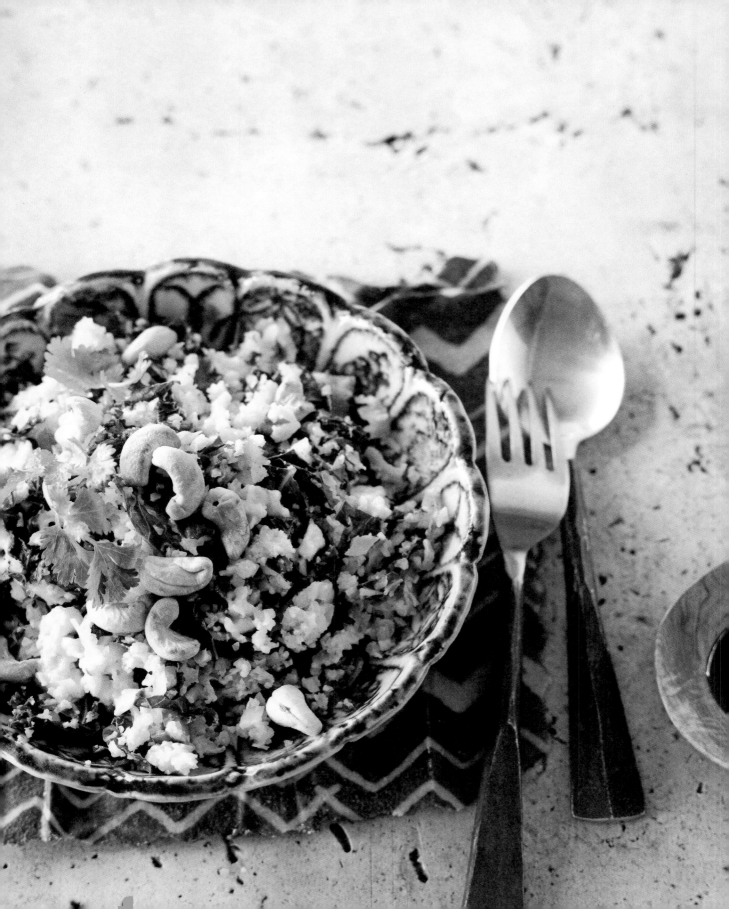

# THAI-STYLE CAULIFLOWER FRIED 'RICE'

*When I go to Thailand, fried rice is my favourite dish, so I created this healthier version. Top each serve with an extra poached or boiled egg.*

SERVES 2
PREP TIME: 30 minutes, including cooking

2 tablespoons virgin organic coconut oil
1 leek, pale part only, trimmed and sliced
1 garlic clove, finely chopped
1 head cauliflower, cut into florets
½ teaspoon chilli powder, or to taste
1 teaspoon curry powder or ground cumin (optional)
2 spring onions, thinly sliced, plus extra to garnish
2 handfuls of kale, stalks removed and leaves shredded (or any other green veggies of your choice)
2 eggs, lightly beaten
1 tablespoon tamari
Celtic sea salt and ground pepper
4 tablespoons cashews, chopped
coriander sprigs, to garnish

Heat 1 tablespoon of the coconut oil in a large frying pan over medium heat. Add the leek and garlic and cook until softened.

Pulse the cauliflower in a food processor until it reaches a rice-like consistency. Add to the leek mixture. Stir in the chilli powder and curry powder or ground cumin (if using) and the remaining coconut oil. Add the spring onion and kale.

Create two indents in the middle of the mixture. Crack the eggs into the indents, add the tamari and stir-fry until the egg is cooked and the cauliflower is golden. Season with salt and pepper.

Serve the 'rice' garnished with the cashews and coriander sprigs.

# BAKED ONION & TOMATO BRUSSELS SPROUTS

*Two words for this dish: warming and nourishing. That's all you need to know!*

SERVES 4
PREP TIME: 1 hour, including cooking

20 brussels sprouts, trimmed and halved or quartered
6 small vine tomatoes or about 12 cherry tomatoes
3 red onions, sliced
3–4 tablespoons olive oil (or use olive oil spray)
1 tablespoon mixed spice
Himalayan pink rock salt and ground pepper
Green Tahini Dressing (see page 296), for drizzling (optional)

Preheat the oven to 200°C (180°C fan/gas 6) and line a baking tray with baking paper.

Combine the sprouts, tomatoes and onion in the baking tray.

Add enough of the olive oil to coat well and the mixed spice and season with salt and pepper, then toss everything together.

Bake for 45 minutes or until cooked through and crisp. Drizzle with green tahini dressing, if desired, and serve.

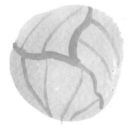

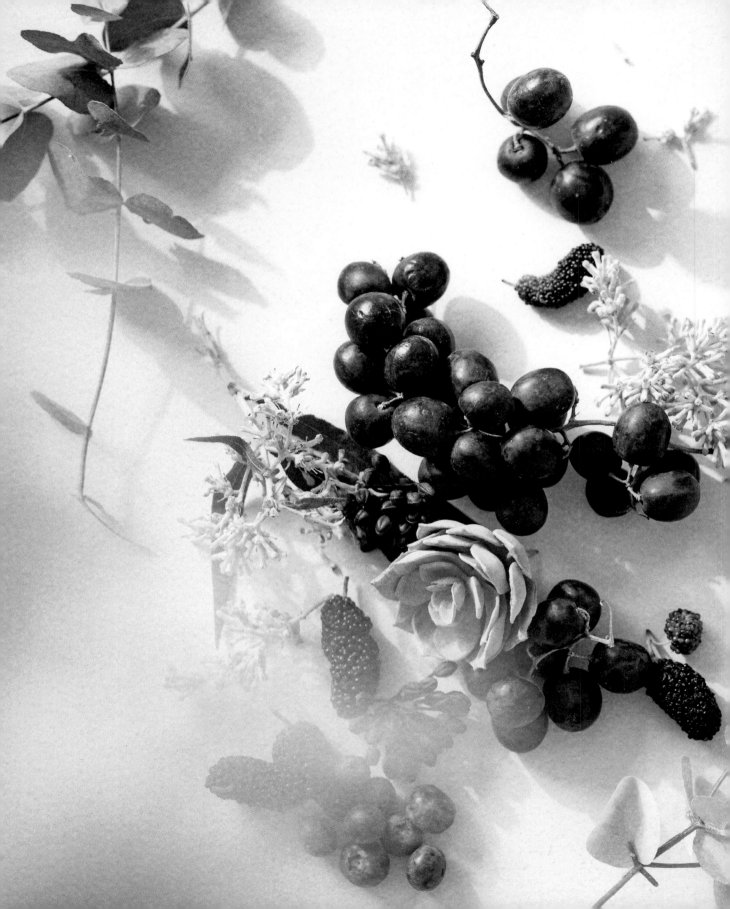

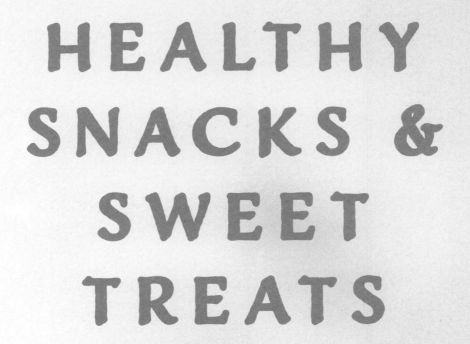

# HEALTHY SNACKS & SWEET TREATS

*It's 4 pm and your cravings have kicked in. Why pick up a processed snack at the supermarket when you can create so many delicious treats and portable snacks at home? It may seem daunting, but the results are cheaper, often just as quick and much better for you — your body will thank you.*

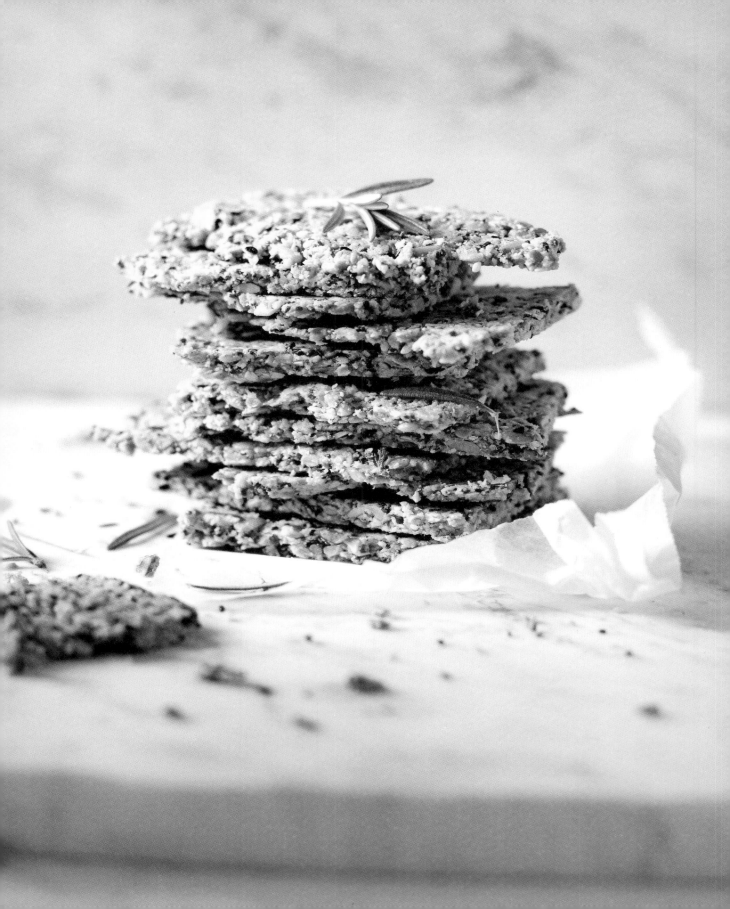

# ROSEMARY CHILLI CRACKERS

*These are gluten-free and packed with flavour. They're nice as a side, and they go well with dips and Sweet Baked Rosemary Ricotta (see page 259).*

MAKES about 20
PREP TIME: 50 minutes, including cooking

100 g almond meal
70 g sunflower seeds, ground
70 g pumpkin seeds, ground
2 tablespoons chia seeds
2 tablespoons black or white sesame seeds
   (or a combination of both)
3 tablespoons finely chopped rosemary
2 tablespoons finely grated parmesan
1 teaspoon chilli flakes
1 garlic clove, crushed
Himalayan pink rock salt and ground pepper
finely grated zest and juice of ½ lemon
3 tablespoons olive oil
3 tablespoons filtered water

Preheat the oven to 170°C (150°C fan/gas 3) and line a large baking tray with baking paper.

Combine the almond meal, seeds, rosemary, parmesan, chilli flakes and garlic in a medium bowl. Season to taste with salt and pepper.

In a jug combine the lemon zest and juice, olive oil and water. Gradually pour the wet ingredients into the bowl and whisk to combine. The mixture should be sticky but not too wet, making it easy to spread. Spread the mixture evenly and thinly on the prepared tray.

Bake for 15–20 minutes. Remove from the oven and cut into rectangular crackers while the mixture is warm and pliable. Turn the crackers over and cook for another 10–15 minutes or until crisp. Remove and cool on the tray. The crackers can be stored in an airtight container for up to 5 days.

# MAPLE & CARDAMOM ALMONDS

*Flavour bomb! These are absolutely incredible served with some coconut milk yoghurt or creamy Greek-style yoghurt. Serve as a snack when friends come over.*

MAKES about 135 g
PREP TIME: 20 minutes, including cooking

135 g raw almonds
coconut oil or olive oil spray
1 tablespoon maple syrup
1 teaspoon ground cinnamon
¼ teaspoon ground cardamom
¼ teaspoon grated nutmeg

Preheat the oven to 200°C (180°C fan/gas 6) and line a large baking tray with baking paper.

Spread out the almonds on the prepared tray and spray with oil.

Combine the maple syrup, cinnamon, cardamom and nutmeg in a bowl, then drizzle evenly over the nuts.

Bake for 10–15 minutes or until dry and lightly golden. Remove from the oven and set aside to cool before serving.

# HIGH-PROTEIN CARROT CAKE SNACK

*I often turn to this snack in the afternoon when I'm craving something sweet but satisfying. It keeps me full until dinner.*

SERVES 1
PREP TIME: 10 minutes

1 carrot, roughly chopped
2–3 tablespoons almond milk
2 tablespoons walnuts
1 teaspoon ground cinnamon, plus extra to serve (optional)
3–4 drops stevia or 1 teaspoon stevia granules
a pinch of grated nutmeg (optional)
1 serve vanilla pea protein powder
1 tablespoon Greek-style yoghurt or hulled tahini (optional)

Blend the carrot, almond milk, walnuts, cinnamon, stevia and nutmeg (if using) in a food processor or blender. Don't make it too smooth – it's good to have some chunks in there!

Spoon into a bowl and mix through the protein powder.

Top with a dollop of yoghurt or tahini and a sprinkling of extra cinnamon if you wish.

Enjoy!

# MANGO CHIA ICE-CREAM

*One weekend my mum came up with this amazing concoction. We couldn't get over how delicious it tasted – like summer in a bowl! Enjoy it as a healthy dessert on a hot day or try it for breakfast.*

SERVES 4
PREP TIME: 1 hour 10 minutes, including soaking

75 g chia seeds
coconut milk, almond milk or filtered water, for soaking, plus extra if needed
350 g frozen mango cubes
2 tablespoons Greek-style yoghurt or coconut milk yoghurt
1 teaspoon ground cinnamon, plus extra to serve
1 tablespoon maple syrup or raw honey, plus extra to serve
mint sprigs, mango cubes and chopped raw almonds, to garnish (optional)

Soak the chia seeds in enough milk or water to just cover for 30–60 minutes or even overnight.

Place the soaked chia seeds, mango, yoghurt, cinnamon and maple syrup or honey in a food processor and blend until smooth, with the consistency of a soft ice-cream. You may need to add more milk or water to make it really smooth.

Drizzle with a little extra maple syrup or honey and add a sprinkle of cinnamon. Garnish with mint sprigs and chopped almonds, if desired.

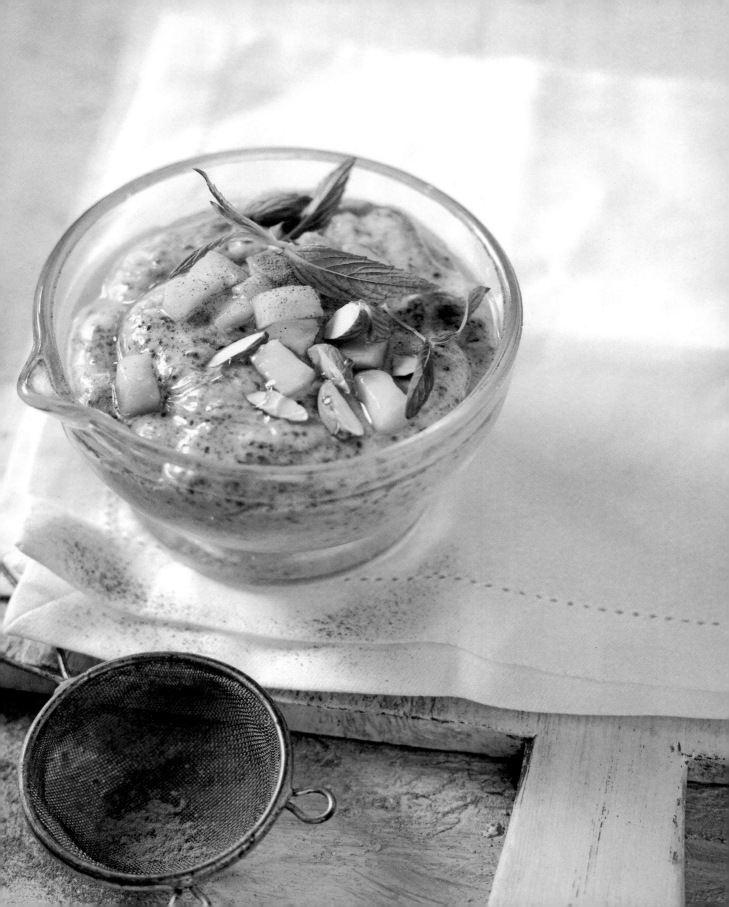

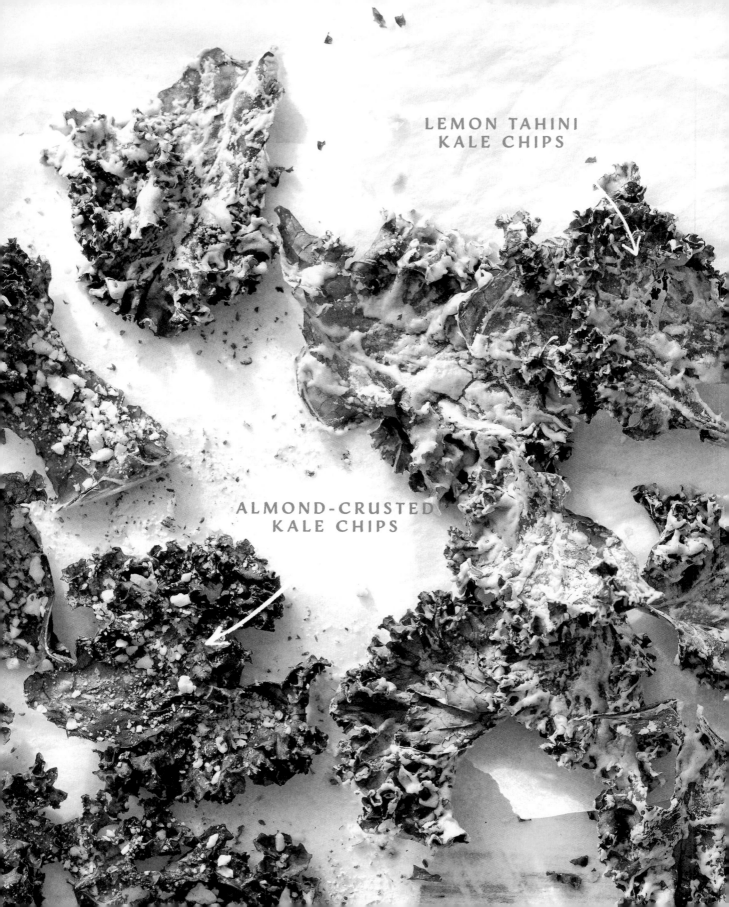

LEMON TAHINI
KALE CHIPS

ALMOND-CRUSTED
KALE CHIPS

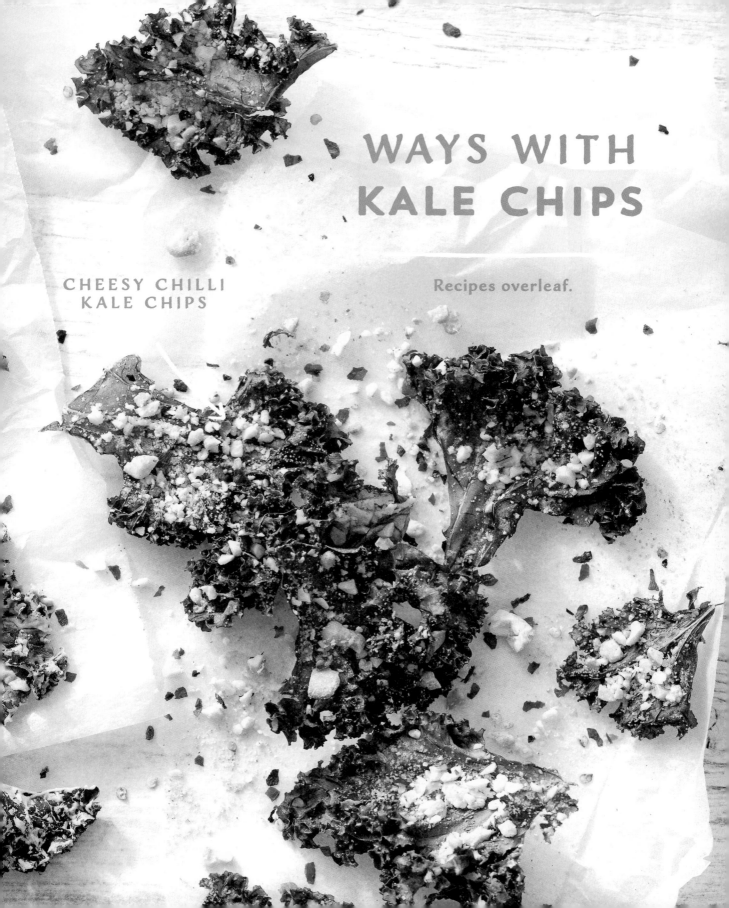

# WAYS WITH
# KALE CHIPS

CHEESY CHILLI
KALE CHIPS

Recipes overleaf.

# KALE CHIPS

SERVES 4
PREP TIME: 25 minutes,
including cooking

1 bunch kale, stalks
  removed and leaves torn
1 tablespoon virgin organic
  coconut oil, melted (or
  use olive oil or coconut
  oil spray)
Himalayan pink rock salt
  and ground pepper
your choice of ground
  spices (I like cumin,
  paprika, turmeric and
  sumac)

*Whenever I have guests over for dinner, I love to serve chips and dip!
By this I mean kale chips with a tahini or hummus dip – so yummy
and perfect with a glass of vino.*

Preheat the oven to 150°C (130°C fan/gas 2) and line a large baking tray
with baking paper.

Place the kale leaves in a large bowl and drizzle or spray with oil. Season well
with salt and pepper and sprinkle over your choice of spices.

Mix with your hands to make sure all the leaves are coated in the oil and
seasonings.

Spread the kale evenly over the prepared tray and bake for about
10–12 minutes or until crisp. Keep a close eye on them as they can burn
easily, even with the oven at such a low temperature.

Remove from the oven and leave to cool completely on the tray. They will
crisp up on cooling.

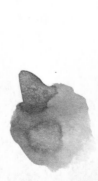
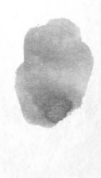

# 5 WAYS WITH KALE CHIPS

- **SESAME KALE CHIPS:** Sprinkle white sesame seeds, Himalayan pink rock salt and virgin organic coconut oil over your kale leaves before baking.

- **CHILLI KALE CHIPS:** Sprinkle chilli flakes, virgin organic coconut oil and a dash of cayenne pepper over your kale leaves before baking.

- **ALMOND-CRUSTED KALE CHIPS:** Sprinkle crushed almonds, olive oil and Himalayan pink rock salt over your kale leaves before baking.

- **CHEESY CHILLI KALE CHIPS:** Sprinkle nutritional yeast flakes, chilli flakes, garlic powder and chopped cashews over your kale leaves before baking.

- **LEMON TAHINI KALE CHIPS:** In a mixing bowl, mix together 3 tablespoons hulled tahini, juice of ½ lemon, 3 tablespoons warm water and a pinch or two of ground cumin. Massage into the kale leaves before baking. They taste cheesy!

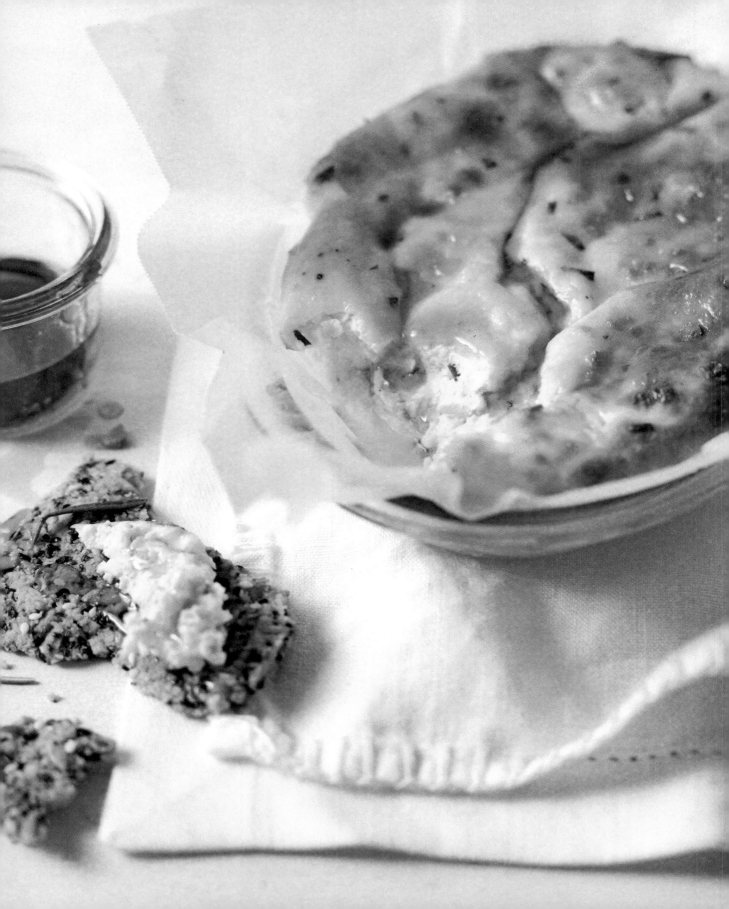

# SWEET BAKED ROSEMARY RICOTTA

*This is divine spread over Rosemary Chilli Crackers (see page 251) or over my Gluten-free Green Bread (see page 156).*

SERVES 4-6
PREP TIME: 1 hour, including cooking

coconut or olive oil spray
500 g fresh full-fat ricotta
3 rosemary sprigs, leaves stripped and finely chopped, plus extra sprigs to serve
1 tablespoon raw honey or maple syrup, plus extra to serve
2 eggs, lightly beaten
2 tablespoons milk of choice (I use almond milk)
Celtic sea salt and ground pepper
Rosemary Chilli Crackers (see page 251), to serve

Preheat the oven to 180°C (160°C fan/gas 4). Spray a small baking dish or ramekin with oil and line with baking paper.

Mix together the ricotta, chopped rosemary, honey or maple syrup, eggs, milk, salt and pepper in a bowl.

Transfer the mixture to the prepared dish or ramekin and smooth the surface. Bake for 45–50 minutes or until set and golden brown.

Drizzle with extra honey or maple syrup and garnish with extra rosemary sprigs. Serve warm or at room temperature with Rosemary Chilli Crackers.

# CARROT & ROSEMARY LOAF

MAKES 1 loaf
PREP TIME: 1 hour, including cooking

olive or coconut oil spray
200 g almond meal
50 g LSA or ground flaxseed
75 g chia seeds
4 tablespoons pumpkin seeds
4 tablespoons psyllium husk
1½ teaspoons baking powder
½ teaspoon ground cumin
1 teaspoon Himalayan pink rock salt
a handful of rosemary sprigs, leaves stripped
2–3 carrots, grated
1 garlic clove, crushed
3 eggs, lightly beaten
2 tablespoons olive oil or virgin organic coconut oil
4 tablespoons almond milk
olive oil, for drizzling

Preheat the oven to 180°C (160°C fan/gas 4) and spray a standard loaf tin with oil.

Place the almond meal, LSA or flaxseed, seeds, psyllium husk, baking powder, cumin, salt and rosemary in a bowl and mix to combine.

Make a well in the centre, add the carrot, garlic, egg, oil and milk and mix together well.

Pour into the prepared tin and bake for 35–45 minutes or until a skewer inserted in the centre of the loaf comes out clean. If it's not quite ready and the top is starting to brown, cover with foil and continue baking until the loaf feels more solid than normal bread.

Remove the loaf from the oven and leave to cool in the tin. Cut into slices and serve with a drizzle of olive oil and a sprinkle of salt, if desired.

This loaf will keep covered in the fridge for up to 1 week. It also freezes well.

## BERRY ICE-BLOCKS

*Healthy living doesn't mean deprivation, especially for the kiddies. These are the perfect treat on a hot summer's day!*

MAKES 6–8
PREP TIME: about 4 hours, including freezing

150 ml freshly squeezed orange juice
1 small ripe pear, peeled, cored and roughly chopped
50 g frozen blueberries
60 g frozen raspberries
8 strawberries, hulled and halved

Blend all the ingredients in a high-powered blender or food processor until smooth and well combined. Pour into six to eight ice-block moulds (about 100 ml capacity).

Place the lids on the moulds or carefully insert lolly sticks into the ice-blocks. Freeze for 4 hours or until solid.

Take the ice-blocks out of the freezer 1–2 minutes before removing from the moulds.

## CHOCOLATE ALMOND COCONUT NICE-CREAM

*I am an ice-cream lover – I crave it – so I am grateful to have found a very healthy and clean alternative to appease my cravings! This is my personal vegan favourite and out of this world. Keep peeled bananas in the freezer so you always have some on hand to whip this up.*

SERVES 2

1½ frozen bananas
2 tablespoons almond butter or 100% peanut butter
1 heaped tablespoon raw cacao powder
a pinch of Celtic sea salt
3 tablespoons desiccated coconut
ground cinnamon, to taste
3–4 tablespoons filtered water
a handful of chopped or flaked almonds

Put the bananas, nut butter, cacao powder, salt, coconut, cinnamon and water in a food processor and pulse to the consistency of a soft ice-cream (you may not need all the water – just enough to make it creamy without being runny). Scrape into a bowl or container and freeze for 20–30 minutes. Top with almonds, then enjoy the most indulgent healthy dessert ever.

## TIRAMISU NICE-CREAM

SERVES 2

2 frozen bananas
1 tablespoon hulled tahini
1 teaspoon ground cinnamon
1 teaspoon organic instant coffee or ½ shot espresso
1 tablespoon raw cacao powder
a pinch of Celtic sea salt
250 ml coconut milk
a small handful of ice (optional)
crushed peanuts and dark choc bits, to garnish

Put the bananas, tahini, cinnamon, coffee, cacao powder, salt, coconut milk and ice (if using) in a food processor and pulse to the consistency of a soft ice-cream. Scrape into a bowl or container and freeze for 20–30 minutes. Top with crushed peanuts and dark choc bits and serve.

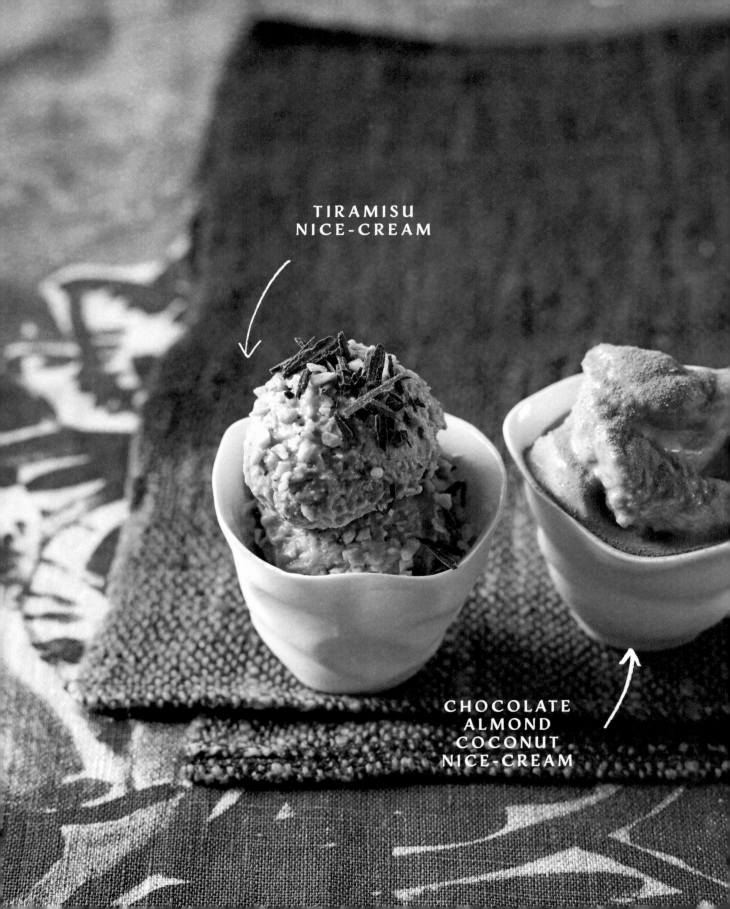

TIRAMISU
NICE-CREAM

CHOCOLATE
ALMOND
COCONUT
NICE-CREAM

## CHOC CINNAMON YOGHURT

*This blissful combination knocks any complaints from my sweet tooth away – it's so good. The kids will love it too.*

SERVES 1
PREP TIME: 5 minutes, plus freezing (optional)

200 g Greek-style yoghurt or
  100 g coconut milk yoghurt
1 tablespoon raw cacao powder
ground cinnamon, to taste
1 tablespoon raw honey, stevia
  granules or rice malt syrup
1 tablespoon almond butter
raw cacao nibs, to garnish
  (optional)

Place the yoghurt in a cup and mix through the cacao powder, cinnamon and sweetener.

Enjoy as is or put it in the freezer for 30 minutes for froyo!

## ALMOND DREAM YOGHURT

*If you love creamy kinda things and go nuts for those sugar-laden yoghurts – try this instead! Just as delicious and so much better for you.*

SERVES 1
PREP TIME: 5 minutes, plus freezing (optional)

200 g Greek-style yoghurt
  or 100 g coconut milk
  yoghurt
4 drops vanilla stevia
  (or 1 tablespoon sweetener
  of choice)
ground cinnamon, to taste
1 tablespoon almond butter

Place the yoghurt in a cup and mix through the stevia and cinnamon.

Drizzle the almond butter through and on top of the yoghurt.

Enjoy as is or put it in the freezer for 30 minutes for froyo!

## HEALTHY BERRY COCOWHIP

SERVES 1–2
PREP TIME: 5 minutes, plus freezing

200 g coconut milk yoghurt
115 g frozen berries
½–1 frozen banana, cut into
  chunks
½ teaspoon vanilla powder
1 tablespoon maple syrup
  or stevia granules
filtered water, if needed
berries, pumpkin or sunflower
  seeds and desiccated coconut,
  to garnish

Put the yoghurt, frozen berries, banana, vanilla and sweetener in a food processor and pulse to the consistency of a soft ice-cream. (Add a little water if needed – just enough to make it creamy without being runny.) Scrape into a bowl or container and freeze for 10 minutes

Garnish with berries, seeds and coconut and serve. Drizzle the almond butter through and on top of the yoghurt and garnish with cacao nibs (if using).

## ALMOND BUTTER CINNAMON BANANA HALVES

*Cut a banana in half lengthways and spread the cut sides generously with almond butter. Sprinkle with shredded or desiccated coconut, ground cinnamon and raw cacao nibs and finish with a drizzle of raw honey. A heavenly snack for kids of all ages!*

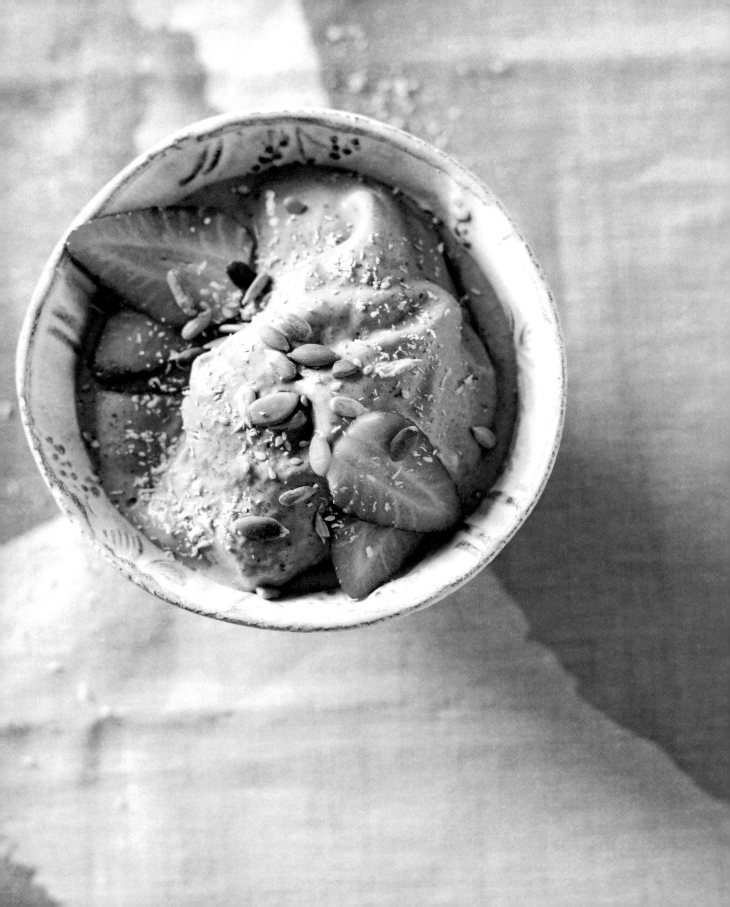

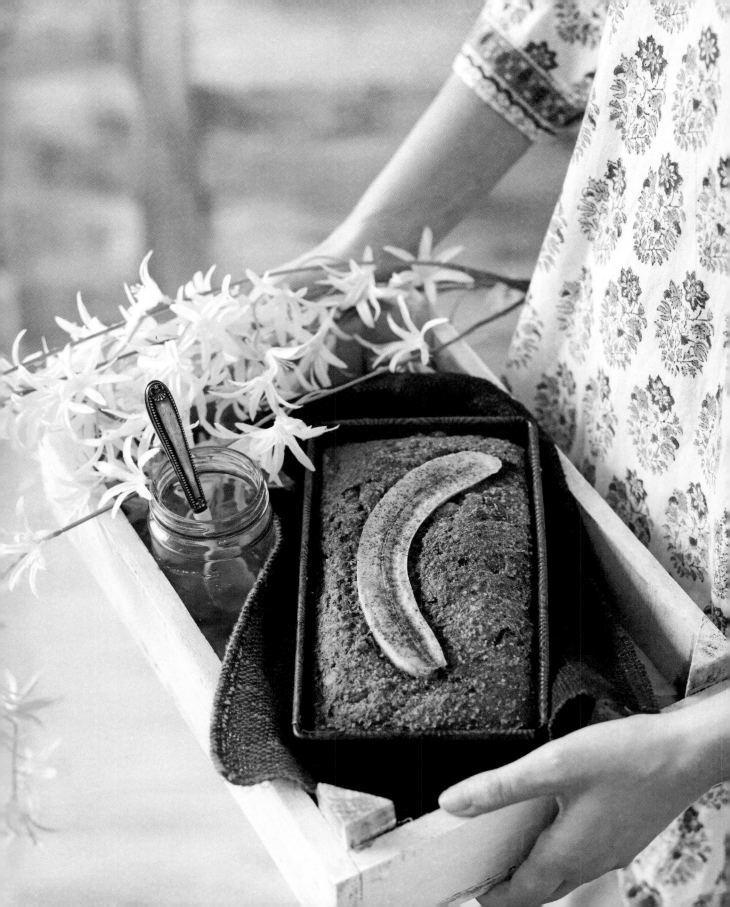

# BANANA HAZELNUT CHOCOLATE BREAD

MAKES 1 loaf
PREP TIME: 1 hour
15 minutes, including
cooking

coconut oil spray
almond meal, for coating
200 g hazelnut meal, plus
    extra if needed
50 g LSA or ground
    flaxseed
3 tablespoons psyllium
    husk (for a fibre hit, but
    optional)
2 heaped tablespoons raw
    cacao powder
40 g hazelnuts, skins
    removed, crushed or
    chopped
2 teaspoons ground
    cinnamon
1½ teaspoons baking
    powder
75 g roughly chopped dark
    chocolate or raw vegan
    chocolate chunks
3 ripe bananas, mashed
3 eggs
90 g medjool dates, pitted
    and roughly chopped
3 tablespoons almond milk
    (or milk of your choice),
    plus extra if needed
2 tablespoons virgin organic
    coconut oil, melted
2 tablespoons stevia
    granules, raw honey or
    maple syrup
½ banana, extra, sliced
almond butter, raw honey
    and raw cacao powder,
    extra, to serve

*The JSHealth community so adored the banana bread in my first book that I felt I really should include a variation of it in this book. And I have to tell you, it could be my favourite sweet treat in this chapter. A slice of this with a smear of almond butter and a cup of chai and I'm in heaven.*

Preheat the oven to 180°C (160°C fan/gas 4). Lightly spray a standard loaf tin with coconut oil and coat generously with almond meal, tipping out the excess.

Combine the hazelnut meal, LSA or flaxseed, psyllium husk (if using), cacao powder, hazelnuts, cinnamon, baking powder and chocolate in a large mixing bowl.

In a jug, whisk together the mashed banana, eggs, dates, milk, coconut oil and sweetener.

Pour the banana mixture into the dry ingredients and mix until well combined. If the batter is too wet, add extra hazelnut meal; if it is too dry, add more milk.

Spoon the batter into the prepared tin and decorate the top with the sliced banana.

Bake for 45–60 minutes or until a skewer inserted in the centre comes out clean.

Remove and allow to cool in the tin.

Gently tip the cooled loaf out of the tin and cut into slices. This is delicious served with almond butter, honey and a sprinkle of cacao powder.

Store in an airtight container in the fridge for up to a week, or wrap individual slices and store in the freezer for a month.

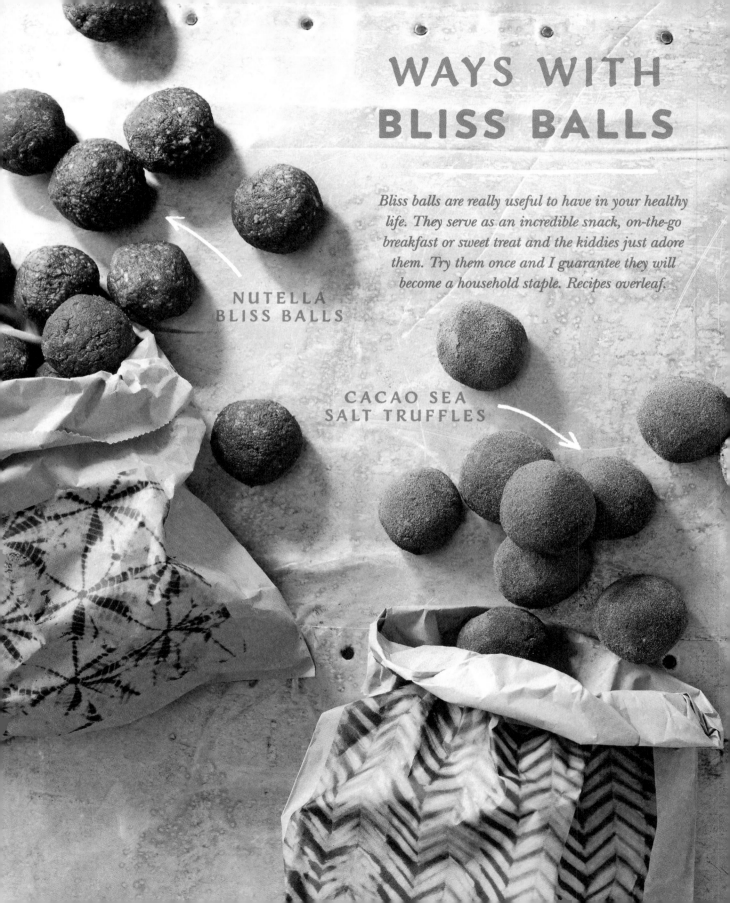

# WAYS WITH BLISS BALLS

*Bliss balls are really useful to have in your healthy life. They serve as an incredible snack, on-the-go breakfast or sweet treat and the kiddies just adore them. Try them once and I guarantee they will become a household staple. Recipes overleaf.*

NUTELLA
BLISS BALLS

CACAO SEA
SALT TRUFFLES

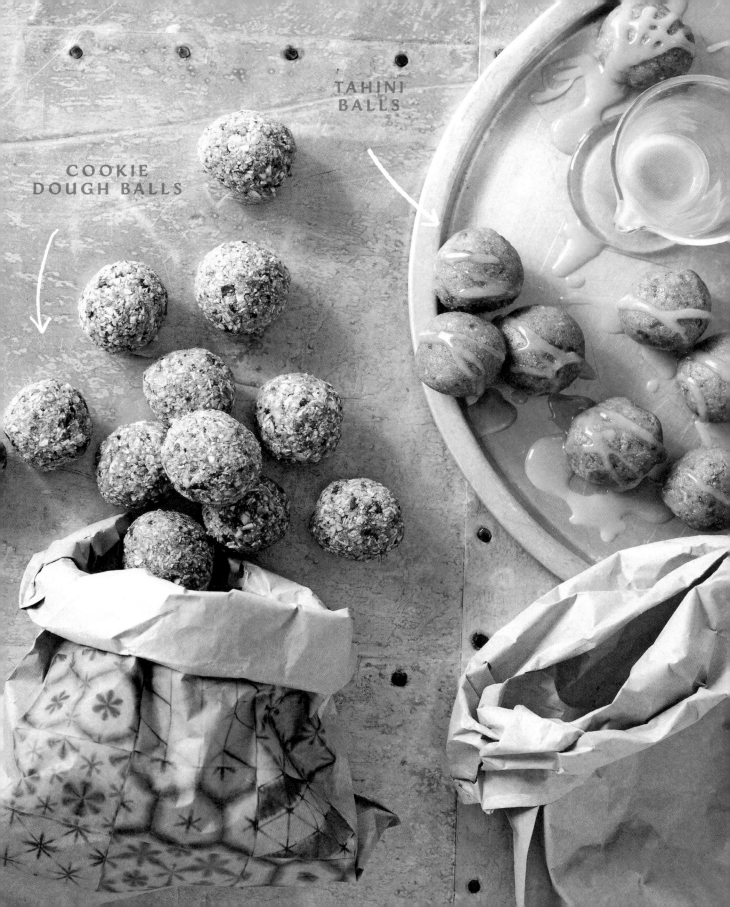

COOKIE
DOUGH BALLS

TAHINI
BALLS

# NUTELLA BLISS BALLS

MAKES about 10
PREP TIME: 40 minutes,
including refrigeration

175 g medjool dates, pitted
2 heaped tablespoons hazelnut
    or almond butter
70 g hazelnuts, skins removed
1 tablespoon raw cacao powder
a pinch of Celtic sea salt
½ teaspoon ground cinnamon,
    plus extra to coat
2–3 tablespoons filtered water

Line a small tray or plate with
baking paper.

Blend the dates, nut butter,
hazelnuts, cacao powder,
salt and cinnamon in a food
processor until well combined.

Gradually add enough water to
make the mixture chunky and
sticky but not wet.

Roll tablespoons of the mixture
into balls – you should have
enough to make 10 all up. Put
them on the prepared tray
or plate.

Coat the balls in a little extra
cinnamon and place in the
fridge for 30 minutes to set.
Refrigerate for up to 7 days
in an airtight container.

# CACAO SEA SALT TRUFFLES

MAKES about 12
PREP TIME: 50 minutes,
including refrigeration

135 g raw cashews
175 g medjool dates, pitted
¼ teaspoon Himalayan pink
    rock salt
2 heaped tablespoons raw
    cacao powder, plus extra to
    coat (optional)
2 tablespoons nut butter (I use
    almond butter)
3–4 tablespoons filtered water

Line a small tray or plate with
baking paper.

Blend the cashews, dates, salt,
cacao powder and nut butter
in a food processor until well
combined. Gradually add
enough water to make the
mixture well combined but
still a little chunky. The texture
needs to be a little softer than
normal bliss balls. You want
'chocolate chunks' as opposed
to smooth chocolate balls.

Roll teaspoons of the mixture
into chunky balls. Put them on
the prepared tray or plate and
sprinkle a little extra cacao over
each ball if you like.

Place in the fridge for
30–40 minutes to set.
Refrigerate for up to 7 days
in an airtight container.

# COOKIE DOUGH BALLS

MAKES about 12
PREP TIME: 40 minutes,
including refrigeration

100 g organic or gluten-free oats
70 g raw almonds
40 g desiccated coconut
3 tablespoons raw cacao chocolate
    or roughly chopped dark
    chocolate
2 tablespoons hulled tahini
2 tablespoons rice malt syrup or
    maple syrup
1–2 pinches of Celtic sea salt
1 teaspoon ground cinnamon
1 teaspoon vanilla powder
2–3 tablespoons filtered water

Line a small tray or plate with
baking paper.

Blend the oats, almonds, coconut,
chocolate, tahini, syrup, salt,
cinnamon and vanilla in a food
processor until well combined.
Gradually add enough water to
make the mixture chunky and sticky
but not wet.

Roll heaped tablespoons of the
mixture into balls. Put them on the
prepared tray or plate.

Place in the freezer for 10 minutes
or in the fridge for 30 minutes to
set. Refrigerate for up to 7 days
in an airtight container.

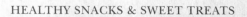

# TAHINI BALLS

MAKES about 8
PREP TIME: 45 minutes,
including refrigeration

50 g almond meal
2 heaped tablespoons hulled
  tahini
2 tablespoons desiccated
  coconut
5 medjool dates, pitted and
  roughly chopped
1 teaspoon ground cinnamon
2 tablespoons maple syrup or
  raw honey
a pinch of Celtic sea salt
2–3 tablespoons filtered water

SWEET TAHINI DRIZZLE:
1 tablespoon hulled tahini
3–4 drops stevia
1 teaspoon raw honey
1–2 tablespoons filtered water

Line a small tray or plate with
baking paper.

Blend the almond meal, tahini,
coconut, dates, cinnamon,
maple syrup or honey and salt
in a food processor until well
combined. Gradually add the
water to make the mixture sticky
but not wet.

Roll heaped tablespoons of the
mixture into balls. Put them on
the prepared tray or plate.

To make the sweet tahini drizzle,
combine all the ingredients in
a bowl and stir until smooth.
Drizzle evenly over the balls.
Place in the freezer for 10 minutes
or in the fridge for 30 minutes to
set. Refrigerate for up to 7 days
in an airtight container.

# JSHEALTH SUGAR-FREE PROTEIN BALLS

MAKES 10
PREP TIME: 5 minutes

4 heaped tablespoons LSA or
  chocolate protein powder
2 tablespoons mixed seeds (I
  like pumpkin and sunflower
  seeds)
1 heaped tablespoon raw cacao
  powder
2 heaped tablespoons almond
  butter or 100% peanut butter
1 teaspoon ground cinnamon
1 tablespoon chia seeds or
  psyllium husk
2 tablespoons stevia granules or
  3–4 drops stevia liquid
4 tablespoons warm filtered
  water

Combine all the ingredients
in a high-powered blender or
food processor and blend until
smooth.

If the mixture is too wet, add
more LSA; if the mixture is
too dry, add a splash of warm
filtered water.

Roll into balls – you should have
enough mixture to make 10 all
up – and refrigerate for up to
7 days in an airtight container.

# NUT-FREE BLISS BALLS

MAKES about 12
PREP TIME: 45 minutes,
including refrigeration

100 g organic or gluten-free
  oats
3 tablespoons pitted and
  chopped medjool dates
3 tablespoons desiccated
  coconut
3 tablespoons white chia seeds
2 tablespoons pumpkin seeds
2 tablespoons sunflower seeds
2 tablespoons goji berries
2 tablespoons dried cranberries
1 tablespoon ground cinnamon
1–2 tablespoons hulled tahini
1 tablespoon raw honey
2 tablespoons virgin organic
  coconut oil, melted
2–3 tablespoons filtered water

Line a small tray or plate with
baking paper.

Blend the oats, dates, coconut,
seeds, berries, cinnamon, tahini,
honey and coconut oil in a food
processor until well combined.
Gradually add enough water to
make the mixture sticky but
not wet.

Roll heaped tablespoons of the
mixture into balls. Put them on
the prepared tray or plate.

Place in the freezer for
10 minutes or in the fridge for
30 minutes to set. Refrigerate
for up to 7 days in an airtight
container.

# ROSEMARY CHILLI CASHEWS

*Cashews and rosemary are made for each other. These are great to nibble on as they are or sprinkle them over soups or salads for extra crunch and flavour.*

MAKES about 140 g
PREP TIME: 20 minutes, including cooking

135 g raw cashews
coconut or olive oil spray
a handful of rosemary sprigs, leaves stripped
1 teaspoon chilli flakes, or to taste
½–1 teaspoon Himalayan pink rock salt

Preheat the oven to 200°C (180°C fan/gas 6) and line a large baking tray with baking paper.

Spread out the cashews on the prepared tray and spray with oil.

Combine the rosemary leaves, chilli flakes and salt and scatter evenly over the nuts.

Bake for 10–15 minutes or until dry and lightly golden.

Remove from the oven and set aside to cool.

# CHOCOLATE SKIN-GLOW MOUSSE

*This vegan mousse filled with nutrients will feed your skin for the glow factor! The key ingredients are the good fats found in the cashews and coconut, which are so important for glowing skin and hormonal balance. Don't be afraid of good fats! In addition, goji berries are high in antioxidants which will help fight wrinkles by protecting skin cells. Indulge with confidence and moderation – it's all good!*

SERVES 4
PREP TIME: 10 minutes

140 g cashews
2 tablespoons chia seeds
250 ml coconut milk
2 tablespoons raw cacao powder
1 teaspoon virgin organic coconut oil, melted and cooled
2 tablespoons coconut sugar or maple syrup
¼ teaspoon Himalayan pink rock salt
¼ teaspoon vanilla powder

TOPPING:
115 g roughly chopped dark or raw cacao chocolate
a handful of desiccated coconut
a handful of goji berries or fresh berries

Combine the cashews, chia seeds, milk, cacao powder, coconut oil, sugar or maple syrup, salt and vanilla powder in a blender or food processor. Blend or pulse until nice and smooth.

Spoon the mousse into four bowls or one large serving bowl.

Sprinkle the topping ingredients over the mousse and serve. This mousse keeps well in the fridge for up to 2 days so can be made in advance if you like.

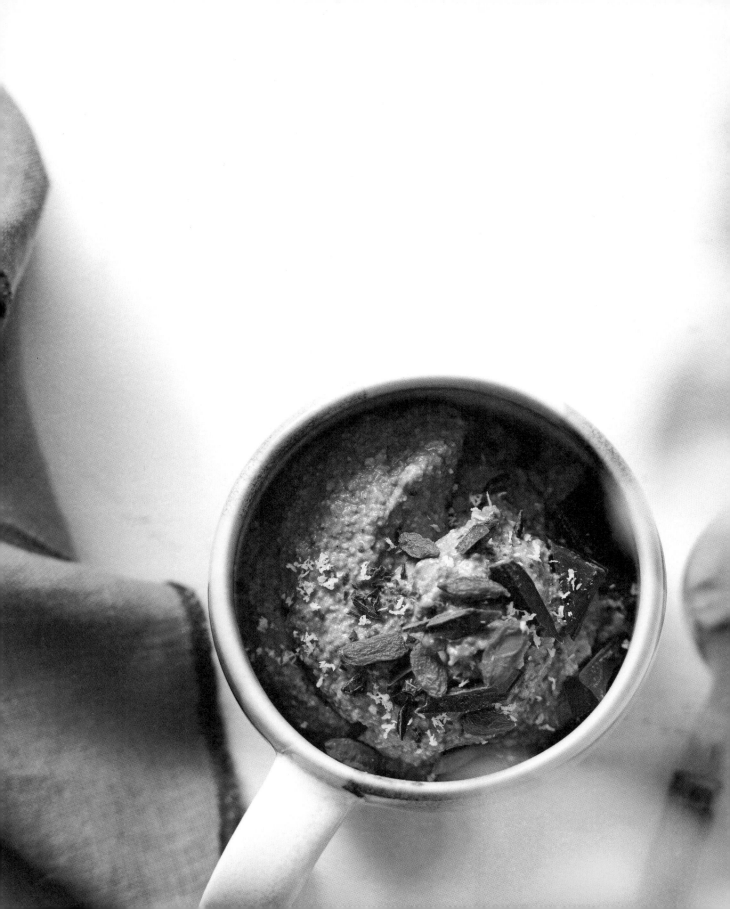

# CHOC DATE ALMOND COOKIES

*I love making these on a Sunday afternoon to dunk into warm cinnamon almond milk. And they happen to be vegan! They disappear quickly so double the quantities if you have a crowd to feed.*

MAKES about 6 medium cookies
PREP TIME: 30 minutes, including cooking

8 medjool dates, pitted and chopped
50 g raw cacao powder, plus extra for sprinkling
100 g almond meal
2 tablespoons almond butter or cashew butter
a pinch of Celtic sea salt
½ teaspoon vanilla powder
½ teaspoon ground cinnamon
3 tablespoons filtered water, plus extra if needed
3 tablespoons raw cacao nibs or dark choc bits

Preheat the oven to 180°C (160°C fan/gas 4) and line a baking tray with baking paper.

Place the dates, cacao powder, almond meal, nut butter, salt, vanilla powder and cinnamon in a food processor. Pulse the ingredients while gradually adding the water – you want the mixture to be gooey, but solid.

Roll the mixture into six balls and place on the prepared tray, then flatten gently with a fork.

Top the cookies with the cacao nibs or choc bits and finish with an extra sprinkling of cacao powder.

Keep them raw and eat straight away or bake them for 10–15 minutes. Cool on the tray before serving.

# COCONUT ROUGH SNACK SLICE

*I absolutely love a slice of this with a cup of chai in the late afternoon, but it goes just as well with a big glass of milk for the kiddies.*

MAKES 6–8 pieces
PREP TIME: 1 hour 15 minutes, including refrigeration

coconut oil spray
70 g raw cashews
40 g shredded coconut
3 tablespoons sunflower seeds
90 g medjool dates, pitted and torn
2 tablespoons chia seeds
¼ teaspoon Celtic sea salt
2 tablespoons maple syrup
3 tablespoons filtered water

Spray a 20 cm square cake tin or baking dish with coconut oil and line with baking paper.

Place all the remaining ingredients in a food processor and blend until well combined.

Spoon the mixture into the prepared tin or dish and smooth the surface.

Place in the fridge for 45–60 minutes or in the freezer for 20 minutes until set. Cut into pieces and serve.

## TIP

*I often add a pinch of salt to my sweet recipes because it makes food taste sweeter and more decadent. Himalayan pink rock salt and Celtic sea salt contain minerals that are essential for good health and adrenal function – but of course, in moderation.*

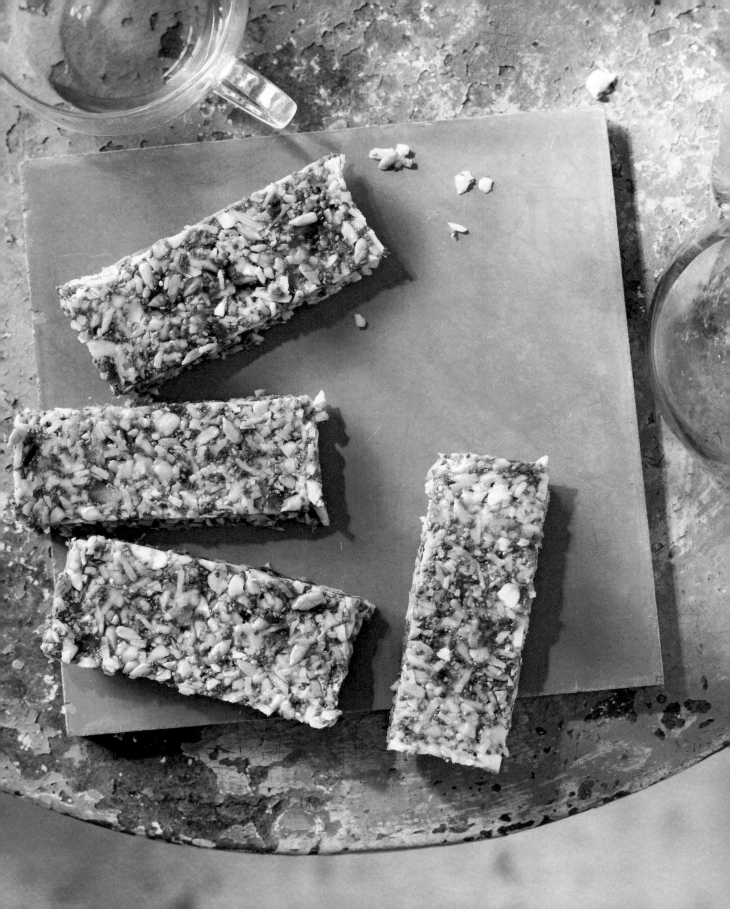

## FOODS TO TAKE TO THE MOVIES

- An organic raw bar from your local health-food shop or a homemade breakfast bar (see pages 166–7)
- Natural popcorn – most health-food shops stock them
- Homemade bliss balls (see pages 266–9)
- A raw cacao chocolate bar, a few pieces of dark chocolate or carob chocolate
- Chia, Blueberry & Banana Breakfast Muffins (see page 143)
- Healthy Chai Latte with cinnamon definitely hits the spot for me (see page 308)!

## HEALTHY KIDDIE TREATS

- Baked Banana with Tahini Caramel Sauce (see page 148)
- Choc Cinnamon Yoghurt (see page 262)
- Healthy flavoured milk (see page 298)
- Chia, Blueberry & Banana Breakfast Muffins (see page 143)
- Kale Chips (see pages 256)
- Almond butter-filled dates – taste like caramel!
- Berry Ice-blocks (see page 260)
- Carob chocolate

## MUM-ON-THE-GO SNACK IDEAS

- Raw nuts
- Kale Chips (see page 256)
- Greek-style yoghurt and ground cinnamon
- Green apples sprinkled with ground cinnamon
- Almond butter-filled dates
- Nutella Bliss Balls (see page 268)
- Raw cacao chocolate
- Natural popcorn
- Flaxseed crackers and carrot sticks with hummus

## TRAVEL SNACK IDEAS

My favourite healthy travel snacks include: raw almonds, dates stuffed with nut butter, sliced veggies with hummus, a green apple, rice cakes with almond butter, Greek-style yoghurt, a raw protein bar, bliss balls (see pages 266–69), Kale Chips (see pages 256–57) and a breakfast bar (see pages 166–69) (or some health-food shops make sugar-free ones now too).

NOTE: *If I am going to be at the airport or on a flight for a meal, I plan ahead as it can be very hard to find healthy food in the airport or on the plane itself. I stop at my local health-food shop or deli on the way and grab something to take with me – usually a hearty salad, brown rice sushi or a brown rice and veggie dish.*

# MY FAVOURITE SNACKS

*I am one of those people that just HAS to have that late-afternoon snack to avoid being HANGRY! But also it saves me from overeating at dinnertime. Here are some nutritionally balanced protein-rich snacks to curb your hunger and cravings.*

- Protein yoghurt, made with Greek-style yoghurt, vanilla pea protein powder, ground cinnamon and vanilla powder
- Boiled egg with veggie sticks or hummus
- JSHealth Protein Smoothie (see page 147) without the fruit

- JSHealth Sugar-free Protein Balls or homemade bliss balls (see pages 268–9)
- Cottage cheese mixed with ground cinnamon, walnuts and a little stevia granules or maple syrup
- Two brown rice cakes topped with almond butter, banana slices and ground cinnamon or smashed avocado with Celtic sea salt and ground pepper
- Sesame Kale Chips (see page 257) dipped in Lemony Tahini Dressing (see page 297)
- My High-protein Carrot Cake Snack (see page 252)

# VEGAN SNACK IDEAS

- Carrot and cucumber sticks with hummus/tahini
- Flaxseed crackers with hummus
- Brown rice cakes/corn thins with almond butter spread, banana slices and a sprinkling of ground cinnamon
- Coconut milk yoghurt with ground cinnamon and berries

- Raw nuts/seeds
- Fresh dates filled with nut butter
- Tahini and ground cinnamon spread onto brown rice cakes
- Handful of shredded coconut and raw almonds
- Chocolate Almond Coconut Nice-cream (see page 260)

# VEGAN PEANUT BUTTER BARS

*This recipe almost wrote itself, thanks to a jar of peanut butter sitting in my pantry. I've been snacking on these bars all week and wish I could hand them out virtually, but sharing the recipe is the next best thing! This treat is vegan, gluten-free, sugar-free and dairy-free, and it's high in fibre, too. What's not to love?*

MAKES 8–10
PREP TIME: 1 hour 10 minutes, including chilling

90 g medjool dates, pitted
50 g almond meal
2 tablespoons chia seeds
2 tablespoons 100% peanut butter
a pinch of Celtic sea salt
1–2 tablespoons filtered water, plus extra
  if needed

Line a small baking dish with baking paper.

Place all the ingredients in a food processor and pulse until the mixture forms a sticky, dough-like texture, adding a little more water if necessary.

Transfer the mixture to the prepared dish and gently press down to cover the base evenly.

Place in the fridge to set for 45–60 minutes, or in the freezer for 20 minutes. Cut into bars and serve chilled.

# FIG & PISTACHIO CHOCOLATE BARK

*This decadent bark is my favourite chocolatey thing to enjoy as a treat after dinner. And of course the great thing about bark is that you can break off a piece as little or as large as you like!*

SERVES 6
PREP TIME: 50 minutes, including freezing

100 g virgin organic coconut oil
50 g raw cacao powder
1 tablespoon hulled tahini
3–4 tablespoons maple syrup, rice malt syrup,
  raw honey or coconut sugar
1 teaspoon ground cinnamon, plus extra
  for sprinkling (optional)
a pinch of Celtic sea salt
50 g pistachio kernels, roughly chopped
70 g dried figs, cut into small chunks

Line a baking tray with baking paper.

Melt the coconut oil in a medium saucepan over medium heat. Reduce the heat to low and whisk in the cacao powder, tahini and sweetener of choice, whisking constantly to stop any lumps forming. Stir in the cinnamon and salt, then remove from the heat.

Set the pan aside for about 5 minutes so the mixture cools slightly and begins to set.

Pour the mixture evenly onto the baking paper – you want the bark to be about 5–8 mm thick.

Scatter the pistachios and figs over the chocolate mixture and finish with a sprinkle of extra cinnamon if you wish.

Cover with cling film and put it in the freezer for 30–40 minutes or until set firm. You can then break it into irregular shards. For the best texture, enjoy it straight from the freezer.

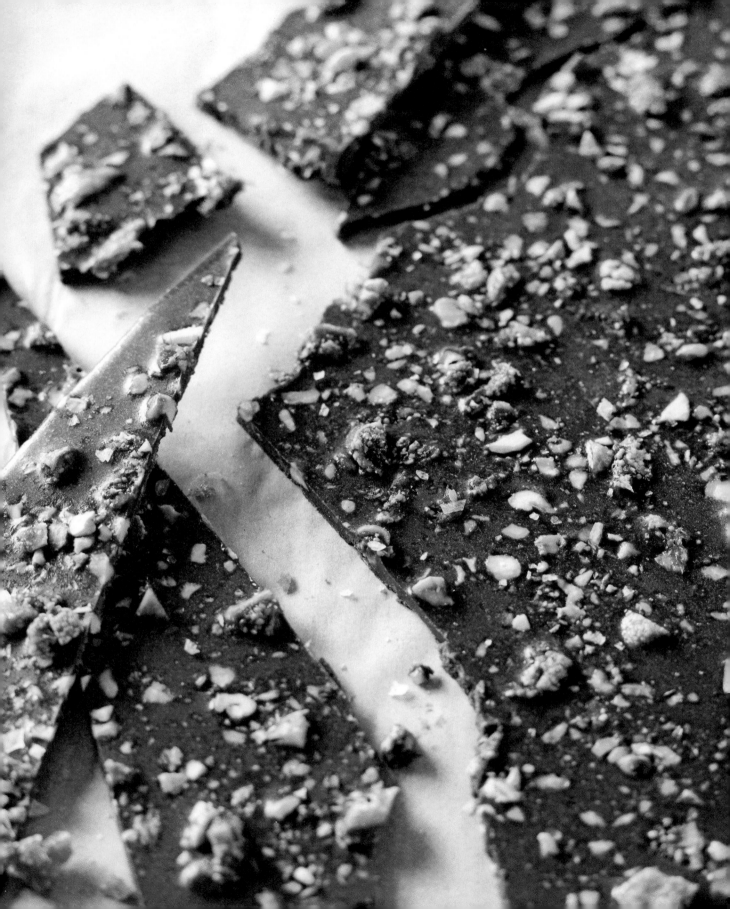

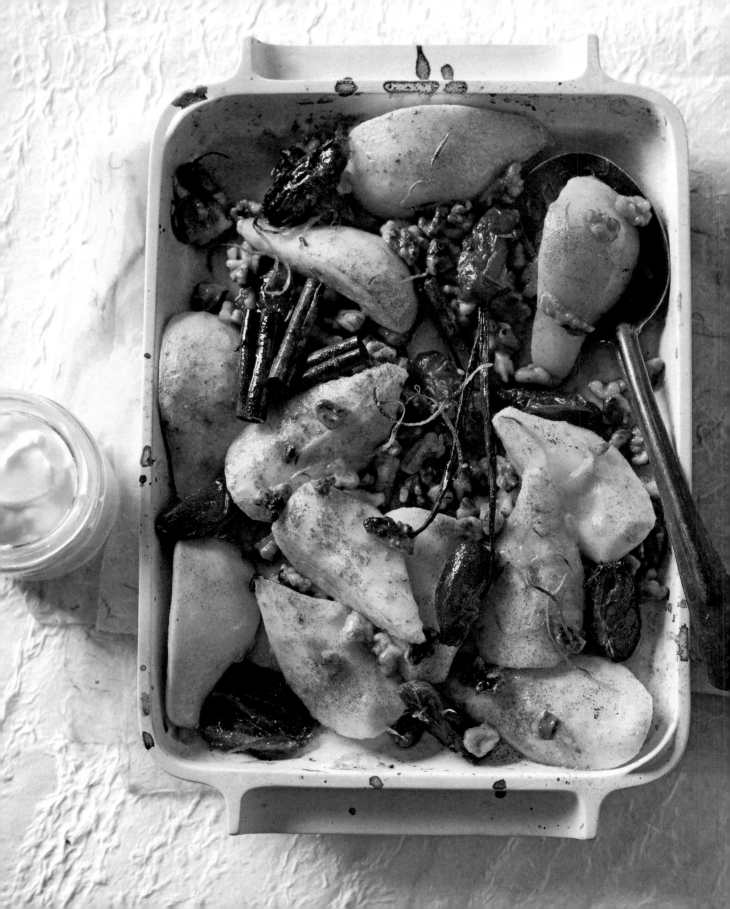

## HEALING WARM CINNAMON PEARS

*This is a stunning dessert but why stop there? I love it for breakfast and brunch too.*

SERVES 6
PREP TIME: 1 hour 15 minutes, including cooking

6 just-ripe pears
finely grated zest and juice of 2 oranges
1 teaspoon ground cinnamon
2 cinnamon sticks
2 vanilla pods, split and seeds scraped, or
   1 teaspoon vanilla powder
5 medjool dates, pitted and roughly chopped
115 g raw walnuts, chopped
Greek-style yoghurt or coconut milk yoghurt,
   to serve

Preheat the oven to 180°C (160°C fan/gas 4).

Cut the pears into wedges and remove the cores.

Place the pear wedges in a baking dish large enough to fit them in a single layer and toss with the orange zest and juice, ground cinnamon, cinnamon sticks and vanilla.

Add the dates and walnuts and toss again.

Cover the dish with foil and bake for 40–50 minutes or until fragrant and the pears are tender.

Remove the foil and place under the grill on medium–high heat for 10 minutes or until the top layer is golden and chewy.

Serve the pears and cooking juices with yoghurt.

## CARAMELISED FIGS WITH HAZELNUT CRUNCH

*This is the perfect dessert for a dinner party – people just love it. The coconut ice-cream is a delightful foil but if you prefer a little more contrast, try it with Greek-style yoghurt. Absolute heaven!*

SERVES 6
PREP TIME: 15 minutes, including cooking

6 fresh figs
1 tablespoon maple syrup
1½ teaspoons ground cinnamon
coconut oil spray
4 tablespoons hazelnuts, skins removed
1 tablespoon desiccated coconut
good-quality coconut ice-cream, to serve

Cut the figs in half, then drizzle evenly with the maple syrup and 1 teaspoon of the cinnamon.

Spray a small frying pan with coconut oil and place over medium heat. Add the figs, cut side down, and cook until lightly caramelised.

While the figs are cooking, pulse the hazelnuts and remaining cinnamon in a food processor until roughly chopped.

Remove the figs from the pan and arrange on a serving plate. Sprinkle over the hazelnut topping then the desiccated coconut.

Serve with coconut ice-cream.

# LEMON CURD TART

coconut oil spray
desiccated coconut, for
   sprinkling
60 g raw macadamias
50 g organic or gluten-free
   oats
4 tablespoons raw almonds
175 g medjool dates, pitted
   and torn
1 tablespoon rice malt
   syrup
a pinch of Celtic sea salt
finely grated lemon zest,
   to serve

LEMON CURD:
3 large eggs
1 tablespoon finely grated
   lemon zest
4 tablespoons raw honey
125 ml freshly squeezed
   lemon juice, strained
70 g virgin organic coconut
   oil
1 vanilla pod, split and
   seeds scraped, or
   1 teaspoon vanilla pod
   paste
1 tablespoon cacao butter
   (optional)

*You're going to love this gluten-free, dairy-free, refined sugar-free tart from model and lifestyle blogger Brooke Meredith. It's smooth, creamy and lemony, making it a wonderful dessert for a warm summer night, or enjoy it simply with a morning cup of tea when you feel like treating yourself.*

Spray the base and side of a tart tin with a removable base with coconut oil, then sprinkle a little desiccated coconut over the base to prevent the tart from sticking.

Place the macadamias, oats, almonds, dates, rice malt syrup and salt in a food processor and blend until well combined.

Spread the mixture over the base and up the side of the prepared tin and press firmly.

Place the tart base in the freezer to set.

Meanwhile, to make the lemon curd, place the eggs, lemon zest and honey in a small saucepan and whisk over low heat for about 1 minute.

Add the lemon juice, coconut oil, vanilla and cacao butter (if using) and whisk over medium heat for 5–10 minutes or until the mixture is smooth and starting to thicken. If it is taking a while to thicken, whisk off the heat briefly, then return to the heat and whisk until bubbles start to appear and the curd is creamy.

Pour the curd into the tart tin, covering the base mixture as evenly as possible. Any leftover curd may be stored in a jar in the fridge for up to 5 days.

Place in the fridge to set. This should take about 3 hours, but if you can, make the tart a day ahead so it can set in the fridge overnight.

Serve scattered with extra lemon zest.

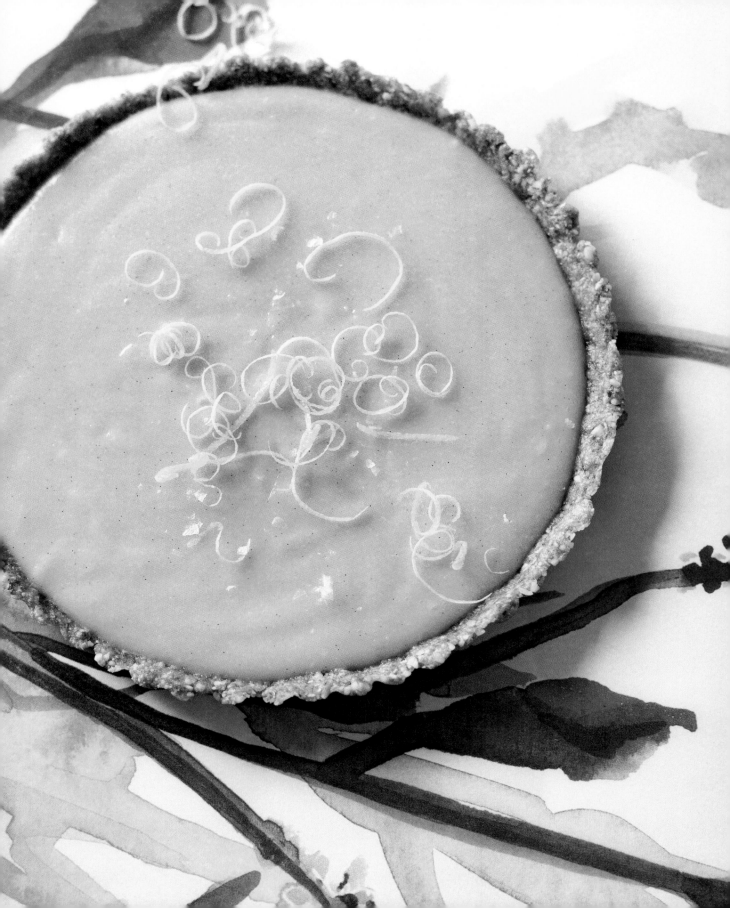

# SALTED CHOCOLATE & ROSEMARY TARTS

SERVES 4
PREP TIME: 1 hour
30 minutes, including
chilling and cooking

100 g hazelnuts, skins
   removed
2 tablespoons raw cacao
   powder
40 g shredded coconut
¼ teaspoon Celtic sea salt,
   plus extra for sprinkling
   (optional)
10 medjool dates, pitted
   and torn
2 tablespoons virgin organic
   coconut oil, melted
finely chopped hazelnuts,
   extra, and rosemary
   sprigs, to garnish
fresh strawberries or
   raspberries, to serve
   (optional)

FILLING:
4 tablespoons virgin organic
   coconut oil
50 g raw cacao powder
75 ml rice malt syrup
1 tablespoon hulled tahini
1 tablespoon finely
   chopped rosemary
¾ teaspoon Celtic sea salt

*Seriously, who would have thought chocolate and rosemary would make such a fantastic food combo? This recipe proves it. I absolutely go nuts for these. Speaking of nuts, you can replace the hazelnuts in the base with the same quantity of hazelnut meal, if preferred.*

Place the hazelnuts in a food processor and blitz until finely chopped. Add the cacao powder, coconut and salt and process again to combine. Add the dates one at a time and process until the mixture comes together.

Tip the mixture into a bowl and add the coconut oil, mixing well with a wooden spoon to combine.

Transfer the dough to a board lined with baking paper and roll it into a log shape. Cut the log into four even pieces and flatten each piece to form a round.

Press the rounds into four 8 cm tart tins using the back of a spoon – if the mixture is too sticky place it in the freezer for 5 minutes. Freeze the tart shells while you prepare the filling.

To make the chocolate filling, melt the coconut oil in a medium saucepan over low heat. Remove from the heat, add the remaining ingredients and whisk until smooth.

Remove the tart shells from the freezer. Carefully take the shells out of the tins and spoon in the filling. Place in the fridge for at least 1 hour to set.

To serve, decorate the tarts with extra hazelnuts, rosemary sprigs and a pinch of salt, if desired. Serve with berries, if you like.

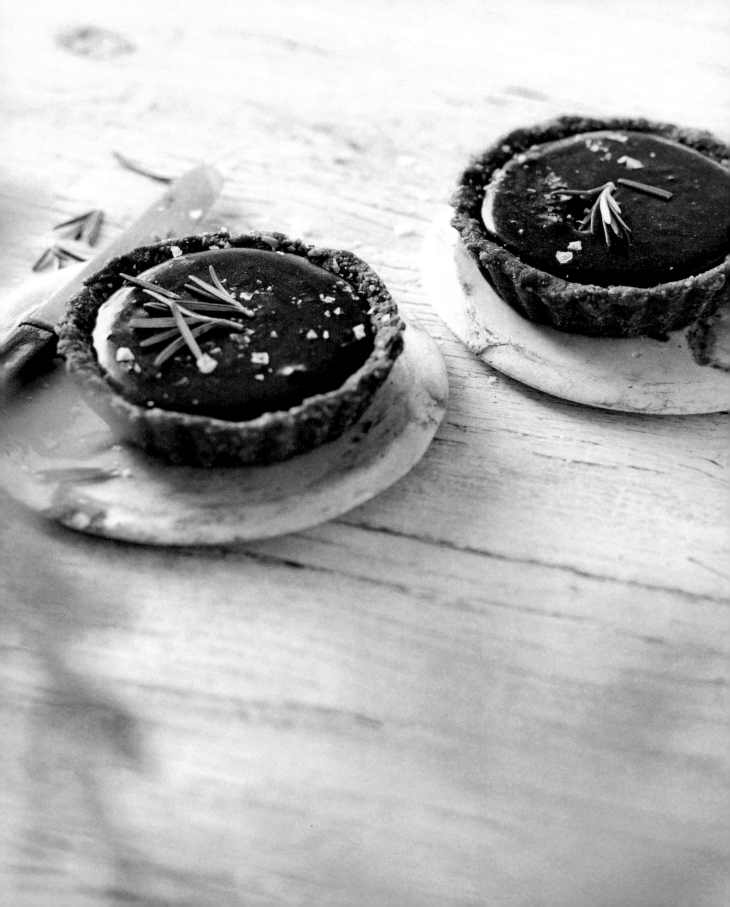

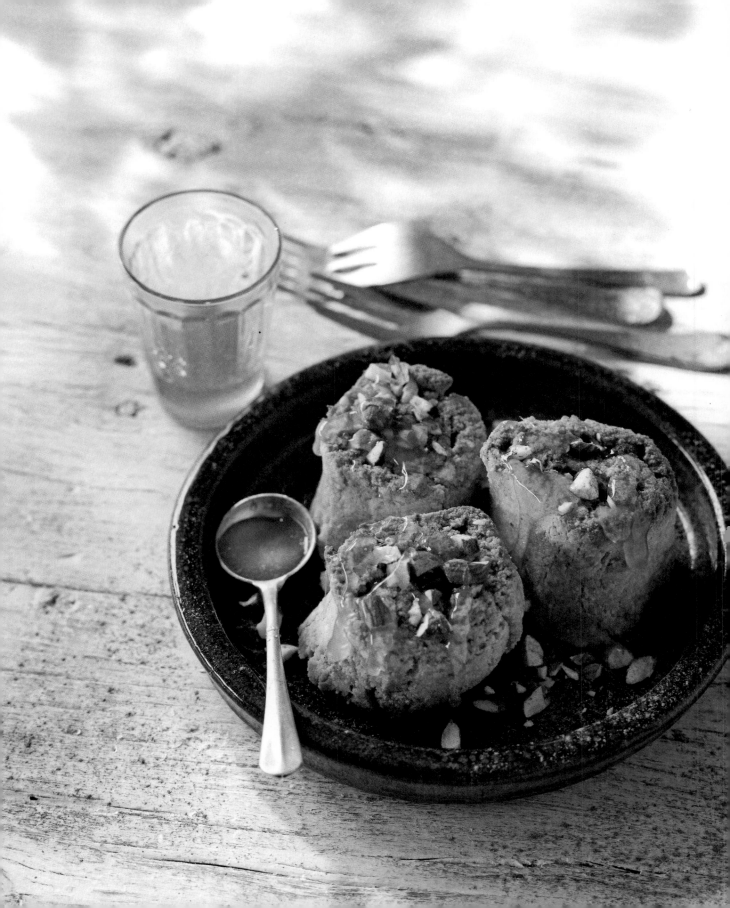

# HEALTHY CINNAMON SCROLLS

MAKES 8
PREP TIME: 1 hour,
including chilling and
cooking

250 g almond meal
4 tablespoons coconut flour
½ teaspoon baking powder
½ teaspoon Celtic sea salt
4 tablespoons coconut
 sugar
4 tablespoons virgin organic
 coconut oil, melted
2 tablespoons raw honey
2 eggs, lightly beaten
1 tablespoon vanilla extract
coconut oil spray
chopped raw almonds, to
 garnish
ground cinnamon, for
 sprinkling

FILLING:
3 tablespoons ground
 cinnamon
4 tablespoons virgin organic
 coconut oil
40 g raw almonds, chopped

GLAZE:
4 tablespoons raw honey,
 maple syrup or rice malt
 syrup (I use rice malt
 syrup)
1 teaspoon vanilla extract

*I grew up in a household that constantly smelt of cinnamon buns. My great grandmother made them, my grandmother made them … so I just had to create a healthy, non-bloating version so I could continue the family tradition. These are gluten-free too – yay!*

Combine the almond meal, coconut flour, baking powder, salt and coconut sugar in a medium bowl, stirring well to remove any lumps.

Whisk together the coconut oil, honey, egg and vanilla in a jug.

Pour the wet ingredients into the bowl with the dry ingredients and mix well. Place the dough in the fridge to chill for 15 minutes.

Preheat the oven to 180°C (160°C fan/gas 4). Lightly spray a baking tray with coconut oil.

Using a rolling pin, roll out the dough between two large sheets of baking paper to a rectangle with a thickness of about 1–1.5 cm. Remove the top sheet of baking paper. The dough is extremely delicate so handle it gently.

To make the filling, mix together all the ingredients in a small bowl.

Sprinkle the filling evenly over the flattened dough, then carefully roll up the dough using the baking paper to help you.

Cut the roll into eight even-sized rounds using a serrated knife. Place the rounds side by side on the prepared tray.

Bake for 20–25 minutes or until lightly golden and cooked through.

Meanwhile, to make the glaze, combine all the ingredients in a small bowl.

Drizzle the glaze over the cinnamon scrolls while they are still warm. Sprinkle with chopped almonds and a light dusting of cinnamon. These are best eaten on the day of baking – I'm sure you won't have any trouble with that. Invite friends over for tea!

# GLUTEN-FREE ROSEMARY & SESAME FOCACCIA

MAKES 1
PREP TIME: 50 minutes,
including cooking

2 tablespoons chia seeds
125 ml filtered water
310 g gluten-free flour
240 g oat flour
5 rosemary sprigs, leaves
  stripped and finely
  chopped
1 teaspoon finely chopped
  thyme
2 teaspoons Celtic sea salt
1 tablespoon baking
  powder
3 tablespoons psyllium husk
3 tablespoons raw honey
175 ml olive oil, plus extra
  if needed
2 eggs
1 egg white

TOPPING:
1 egg, lightly beaten
1 tablespoon sesame seeds
1 teaspoon chilli flakes
2 rosemary sprigs, leaves
  stripped
Celtic sea salt

*I can't believe I managed to create a healthy, nutritious, high-fibre focaccia bread. What a delicious bread to make for your Sunday family lunch!*

Preheat the oven to 180°C (160°C fan/gas 4) and line a baking tray with baking paper.

Soak the chia seeds in the filtered water for 10 minutes or until gel-like.

Sift the flours into a large bowl, then stir in the rosemary, thyme, salt, baking powder and psyllium husk.

Make a well in the middle and add the honey, olive oil, eggs, egg white and soaked chia seeds. Mix to combine with your hands. If it feels dry, add a little more oil.

Turn out the dough onto a lightly floured surface and knead for a few minutes until it comes together in a smooth ball. Form the dough into a large rectangle 2–3 cm thick and place on the prepared tray.

Brush the focaccia with the beaten egg, then sprinkle with the sesame seeds, chilli flakes, rosemary leaves and a little salt.

Bake for 30 minutes or until golden and cooked through.

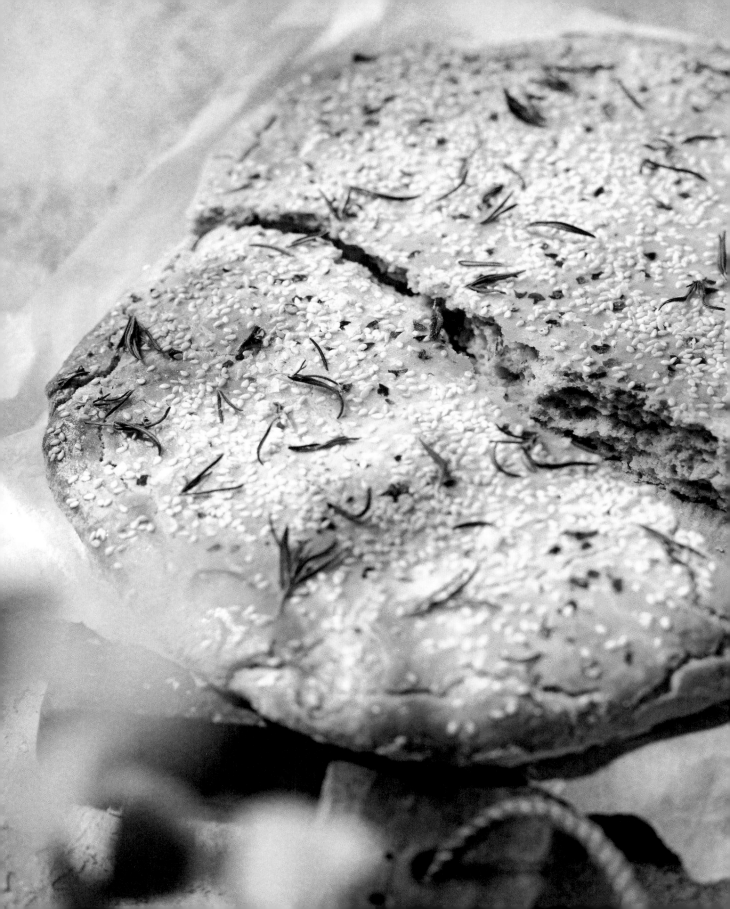

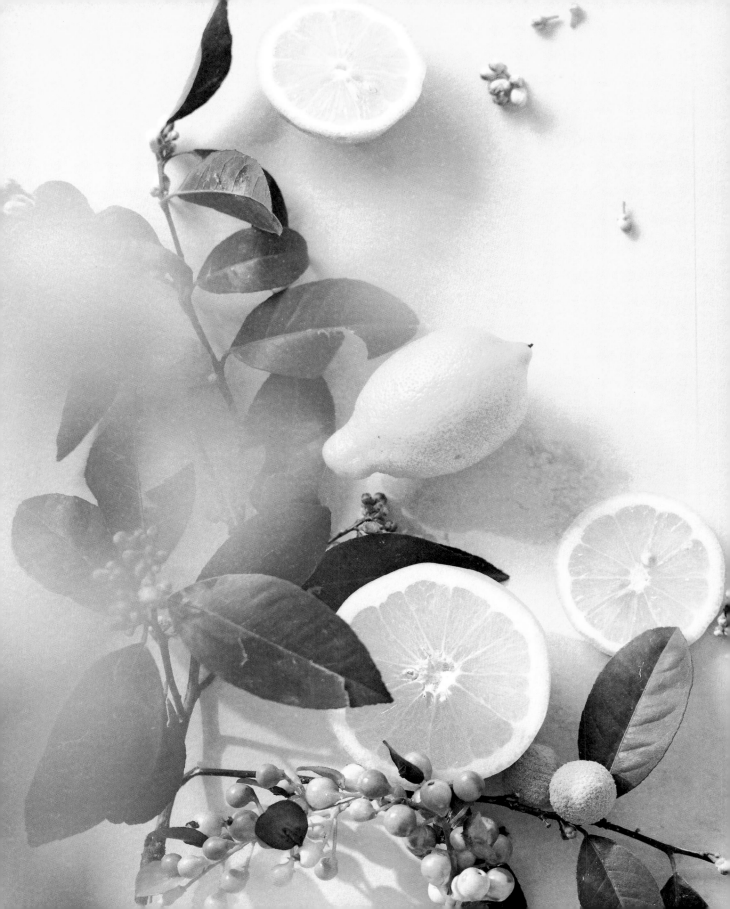

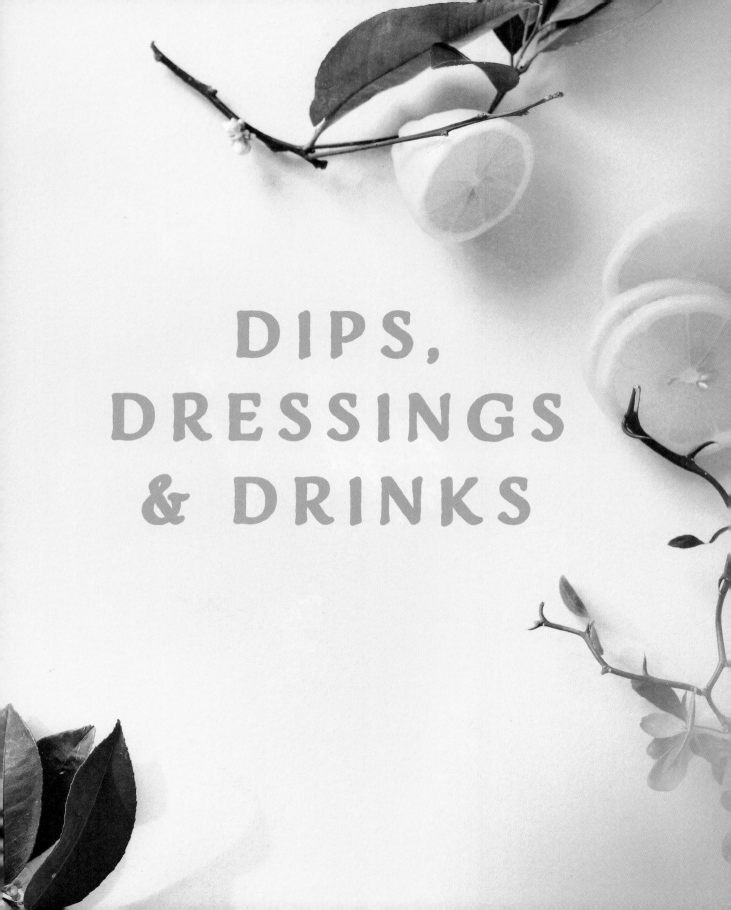

# DIPS,
# DRESSINGS
# & DRINKS

# SPINACH & ALMOND DIP

MAKES about 300 ml
PREP TIME: 10 minutes

100 g baby spinach leaves
135 g raw almonds
2 tablespoons olive oil
1 garlic clove
juice of ½ lemon
1–2 tablespoons filtered water
Celtic sea salt and ground pepper

Put the spinach, almonds, olive oil, garlic and lemon juice in a food processor and blend to combine. Add enough water to reach a smooth consistency, then season to taste with salt and pepper.

# ZA'ATAR CARROT DIP

MAKES about 750 ml
PREP TIME: 20 minutes, including cooking

6 carrots, peeled and roughly chopped
1 teaspoon Himalayan pink rock salt
2–3 tablespoons olive oil
1 teaspoon za'atar, plus extra to garnish
½ garlic clove (optional)
60–120 ml filtered water
2 heaped tablespoons coconut milk yoghurt or
    Greek-style yoghurt

Steam the carrots for 10 minutes or until soft. Place the steamed carrots in a food processor, add the salt, olive oil, za'atar, garlic (if using) and some of the water. Pulse to a smooth consistency, adding more water if needed. Spoon into a bowl, then top with the yoghurt and an extra sprinkle of za'atar.

# ROASTED BEETROOT HUMMUS

MAKES about 250 ml
PREP TIME: 1 hour 30 minutes, including cooking and cooling

1 beetroot, quartered
4 tablespoons olive oil
Celtic sea salt and ground pepper
1 rosemary sprig, leaves stripped and chopped
75 g hulled tahini
½–1 teaspoon dried chilli, to taste
½ teaspoon ground cumin

Preheat the oven to 200°C (180°C fan/gas 6) and line a small baking tray with baking paper. Place the beetroot on the prepared tray and drizzle with 1 tablespoon of the olive oil. Sprinkle with salt and rosemary and roast for 45–60 minutes or until tender. Set aside to cool, then transfer to a food processor, add the tahini, chilli, cumin and remaining olive oil and season well. Pulse until smooth and well combined.

# CHILLI & LIME GUACAMOLE

MAKES about 175 ml
PREP TIME: 10 minutes

1 avocado, flesh removed
2 spring onions, finely chopped
juice of 1 lime
1 tablespoon olive oil
1 teaspoon dried chilli
Himalayan pink rock salt and ground pepper

Mash all the ingredients together in a mixing bowl. Done!

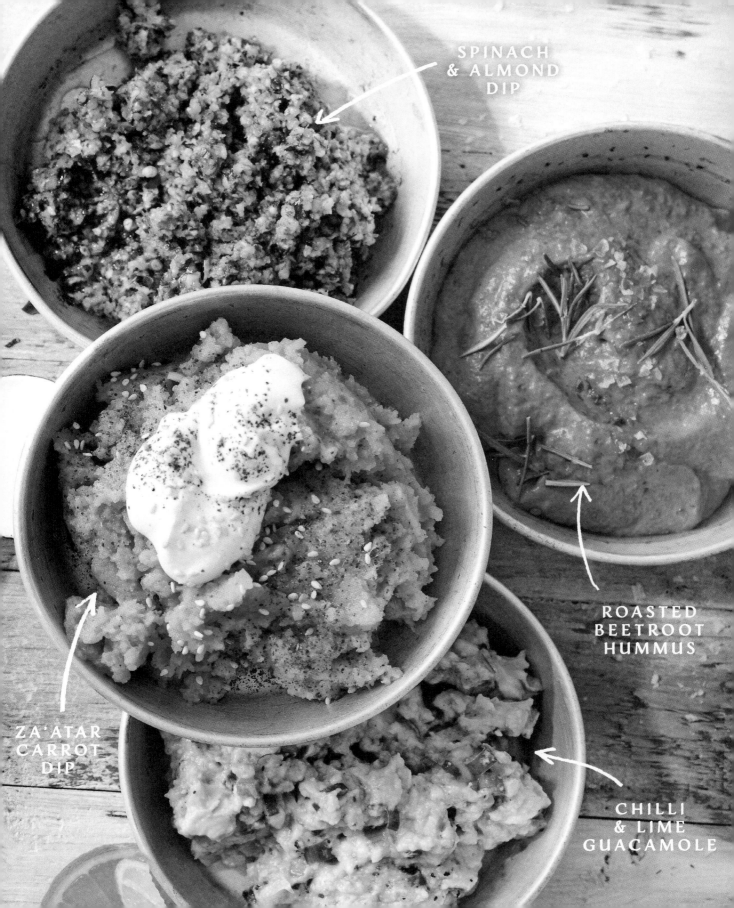

SPINACH
& ALMOND
DIP

ROASTED
BEETROOT
HUMMUS

ZA'ATAR
CARROT
DIP

CHILLI
& LIME
GUACAMOLE

# ROCKET & ALMOND PESTO

*I never get tired of pesto as it is so easy to vary the flavours. All you need to do is combine your choice of nuts and greens with olive oil, salt and garlic – too easy! This is my favourite combo. It's a dairy-free version but if you like your pesto with cheese you are welcome to add a few tablespoons of grated pecorino or parmesan at the end.*

MAKES about 375 ml
PREP TIME: 15 minutes

135 g raw almonds
60 g basil leaves, chopped
50 g rocket leaves
1 garlic clove, chopped
3 tablespoons olive oil, plus extra to serve
1 teaspoon chilli flakes, plus extra to serve
  (optional)
a squeeze of lemon juice (optional)
Himalayan pink rock salt and ground pepper
2–3 tablespoons filtered water

Combine the almonds, basil and rocket in a food processor and pulse until roughly chopped.

Add the garlic, olive oil and chilli, and lemon juice (if using). Season to taste with salt and pepper and pulse again.

With the motor running, gradually add the water until the pesto is well combined and reaches your desired consistency.

Spoon into a bowl and serve with an extra drizzle of olive oil and a sprinkling of chilli flakes, if you like.

# NUT-FREE SUNFLOWER SEED PESTO

*If you are trying to avoid nuts, here is the perfect alternative. You can't miss out on pesto, no matter what!*

MAKES about 375 ml
PREP TIME: 15 minutes

40 g coriander leaves
130 g sunflower seeds
2 garlic cloves, chopped
juice of 1 lemon
2 tablespoons filtered water
a pinch of chilli flakes (optional)
Himalayan pink rock salt and ground pepper
3 tablespoons olive oil, plus extra to serve
  (optional)
3 tablespoons grated parmesan or pecorino
  (optional)

Combine the coriander and sunflower seeds in a food processor and blend until the seeds are well ground and the coriander is finely chopped.

Add the garlic, lemon juice, water and chilli flakes (if using) and season to taste with salt and pepper.

With the motor running, gradually pour in the olive oil until the pesto is smooth and creamy.

Stir through the cheese, if desired.

Serve straight away, drizzled with a little extra olive oil, if desired. Otherwise, store in an airtight container in the fridge for up to 6 days.

# TOMATO SAUCE

*My husband loves tomato sauce so I just had to create a healthy version for him. This sauce is very versatile and is delicious with chicken, fish, mince, courgette 'noodles' and stir-fried veggies.*

MAKES about 1 litre
PREP TIME: 1 hour 50 minutes, including cooking and cooling

1 tablespoon olive oil
1 red onion, finely chopped
2 shallots, finely chopped
1 small carrot, finely diced
1 stick celery, finely diced
150 g button mushrooms, finely chopped
3 tomatoes, finely chopped
2 tablespoons organic tomato paste
700 ml organic tomato passata
1 tablespoon red wine vinegar
3 garlic cloves, crushed
1 tablespoon thyme leaves
3 tablespoons finely chopped flat-leaf parsley
1 teaspoon ground coriander
1 teaspoon ground cumin
1 teaspoon smoked paprika
a pinch of chilli powder
Himalayan pink rock salt and ground pepper

Heat the olive oil in a large non-stick frying pan over medium–high heat, add the onion and shallot and cook for 5 minutes or until softened. Add the carrot, celery and mushrooms and cook for 5 minutes.

Stir in the tomato, tomato paste, passata, vinegar, garlic, herbs and spices and season. Bring to the boil, then reduce the heat and simmer for 20 minutes or until slightly thickened.

Remove from the heat and let the sauce sit for 1 hour to allow the flavours to develop before using.

To store, pour into an airtight container and keep it in the fridge for up to 2 weeks, or several months in the freezer.

# SATAY SAUCE

*Similar in flavour to Healing Peanut Sesame Dressing (see page 297), this is more of a sauce or marinade. It's beautiful with stir-fries, chicken kebabs, grilled tempeh or sautéed greens.*

MAKES about 125 ml
PREP TIME: 10 minutes

1 tablespoon tamari
2 tablespoons crunchy 100% peanut butter
1 heaped tablespoon raw honey
1 tablespoon sesame oil
1 teaspoon grated ginger (optional, but amazing!)
a handful of sliced spring onion (optional)
chilli flakes, to taste (optional)
1 tablespoon warm filtered water

Place all the ingredients in a bowl and whisk until well combined.

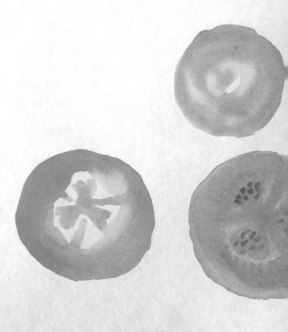

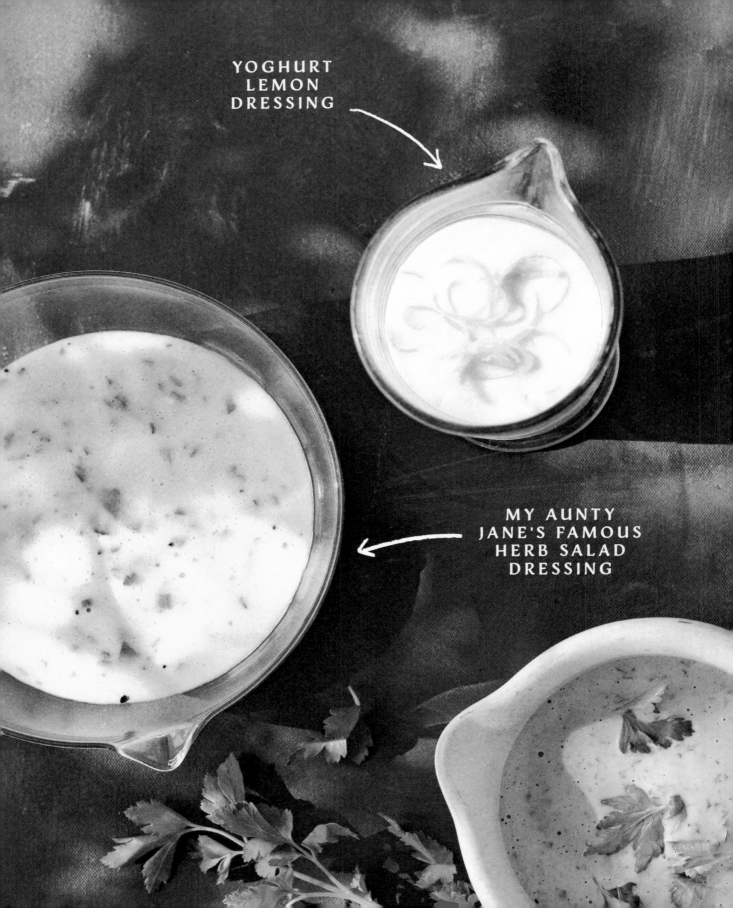

YOGHURT
LEMON
DRESSING

MY AUNTY
JANE'S FAMOUS
HERB SALAD
DRESSING

HEALING
PEANUT
SESAME
DRESSING

# WAYS WITH DRESSINGS

*Dressings are such a simple way to customise your salads without putting in much effort — or time. Play with dressing and salad combinations and your taste buds will sing! Recipes overleaf.*

GREEN TAHINI
DRESSING

### MY AUNTY JANE'S FAMOUS HERB SALAD DRESSING

*My aunty Jane just makes the best salad dressing ever so I simply had to share it with you. It makes quite a lot but you can halve the quantities if you like or, better still, make the full amount and store it in the fridge for the week. You'll find yourself reaching for it again and again.*

MAKES about 500 ml
PREP TIME: 10 minutes

1 garlic clove
juice of 2 lemons
2 heaped tablespoons organic
  Dijon mustard
2 tablespoons chopped mixed
  herbs (I love basil and flat-leaf
  parsley, with a touch of thyme)
Celtic sea salt and ground pepper
4 tablespoons apple cider vinegar
4 tablespoons white wine vinegar
2 teaspoons tamari
250 ml olive oil

Place all the ingredients in a blender and blend to combine.

Serve straight away or pour into a mason jar and store in the fridge for up to 5 days.

### YOGHURT LEMON DRESSING

*So simple, but absolutely delicious over sweet potato or a fresh salad.*

MAKES about 175 ml
PREP TIME: 10 minutes

2 tablespoons Greek-style yoghurt
juice of 1 lemon
1 tablespoon olive oil
1 tablespoon raw honey or maple
  syrup
3 tablespoons filtered water

Place all the ingredients in a mixing bowl and whisk to combine.

Serve straight away or pour into a mason jar and store in the fridge for up to 5 days.

### GREEN TAHINI DRESSING

*This is a dressing I come back to time and time again.*

MAKES about 250 ml
PREP TIME: 10 minutes

3 heaped tablespoons hulled
  tahini
10 g chopped flat-leaf parsley
2 tablespoons olive oil
75 ml white wine vinegar
1 tablespoon organic Dijon
  mustard
a squeeze of lemon juice
½ teaspoon chilli flakes (optional)
Himalayan pink rock salt and
  ground pepper
1–2 tablespoons filtered water
  (optional)

Place the tahini, parsley, olive oil, vinegar, mustard, lemon juice, chilli flakes (if using), salt and pepper in a food processor and pulse briefly. With the motor running, gradually add water if needed to achieve a smooth consistency.

Serve straight away or pour into a mason jar and store in the fridge for up to 5 days.

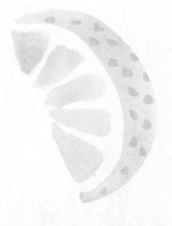

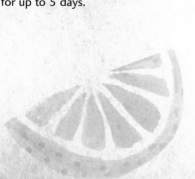

## MISO SALAD DRESSING

*This goes with just about everything so I usually make a big batch at the beginning of the week and store it in the fridge.*

MAKES about 250 ml
PREP TIME: 10 minutes

2 tablespoons white miso paste
1 tablespoon organic Dijon mustard
125 ml white balsamic vinegar
3 tablespoons sesame oil
1 teaspoon grated ginger (optional)
1 tablespoon raw honey (or stevia granules for a sugar-free version)
1 teaspoon tamari
1 teaspoon sesame seeds
1–2 tablespoons filtered water (optional)

Place the miso, mustard, vinegar, sesame oil, ginger (if using), honey, tamari and sesame seeds in a bowl and whisk until smooth and well combined. Whisk in a little water if you want to thin it down.

Serve straight away or pour into a mason jar and store in the fridge for up to 5 days.

## HEALING PEANUT SESAME DRESSING

*I love it with chicken, crisp greens and crunchy chopped peanuts.*

MAKES about 250 ml
PREP TIME: 10 minutes

75 ml white wine vinegar
2 tablespoons tamari
1 teaspoon chilli flakes (optional)
a good pinch of ground ginger
2 tablespoons sesame oil
2 tablespoons smooth or crunchy 100% peanut butter
1 tablespoon raw honey or stevia granules

Place all the ingredients in a bowl and whisk until well combined.

Serve straight away or pour into a mason jar and store in the fridge for up to 5 days.

## LEMONY TAHINI DRESSING

*This fabulous dressing is so versatile you can use it as a marinade too!*

MAKES about 125 ml
PREP TIME: 10 minutes

juice of ½ lemon
1 teaspoon finely grated lemon zest
3 tablespoons hulled tahini
1 teaspoon raw honey (optional)
a pinch of chilli flakes (optional)
½ teaspoon ground cumin
½ garlic clove, crushed
Himalayan pink rock salt and ground pepper
3 tablespoons filtered water

Place all the ingredients in a mixing bowl and whisk to combine.

Serve straight away or pour into a mason jar and store in the fridge for up to 5 days.

## JSHEALTH CLEAN LIFE DRESSING

*I couldn't forget to include my signature dressing which is an absolute household staple! Place 75 ml apple cider vinegar or white wine vinegar, 1 tablespoon organic Dijon mustard, 1 tablespoon olive oil, 1 tablespoon hulled tahini, Celtic sea salt and ground pepper, 1 teaspoon maple syrup or stevia granules (optional) in a mixing bowl and whisk to combine. Serve straight away or pour into a mason jar and store in the fridge for up to 5 days.*

## HOMEMADE HEALING DETOX TEA

*Make a big batch and drink it through the day – it will make you feel so good! If you like, store it in the fridge and drink it cool. This is a great one to drink during my 3-day liver reboot (see page 58).*

MAKES 750 ml
PREP TIME: 10 minutes

juice of 1 lemon
4 slices ginger
½ teaspoon cayenne pepper
1 teaspoon ground cinnamon
4 drops stevia
1 tablespoon virgin organic coconut oil, melted
1 tablespoon apple cider vinegar
750 ml boiling or warm filtered water

Put all the ingredients in a heatproof jug and mix well. Set aside to infuse for a few minutes, then enjoy.

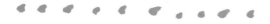

## CHOC CINNAMON MILK

*Nutritious milk that totally tastes like a treat – great for the kiddies … or you!*

SERVES 1
PREP TIME: 10 minutes

250 ml coconut or almond milk
1 heaped tablespoon raw cacao powder
½ teaspoon ground cinnamon
2 medjool dates, pitted (or 2 teaspoons stevia granules for a sugar-free version)
a handful of raw cashews
a pinch of Celtic sea salt

Put all the ingredients in a blender – and blend!

## VANILLA MILK

*Because I am a vanilla gal – my absolute favourite flavour.*

SERVES 1
PREP TIME: 10 minutes

250 ml coconut milk
2 medjool dates, pitted (or 3–4 drops vanilla stevia for a sugar-free version)
a handful of raw cashews
½ teaspoon vanilla powder
a pinch of Celtic sea salt

Put all the ingredients in a blender – and blend!

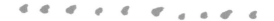

## COCONUT STRAWBERRY MILK

*Coconut and strawberry – this blissful combination tastes like summer!*

SERVES 1
PREP TIME: 10 minutes

250 ml coconut milk
4–5 fresh or frozen strawberries, hulled
2 medjool dates, pitted (or 2 teaspoons stevia granules for a sugar-free version)
a handful of raw cashews

Put all the ingredients in a blender – and blend!

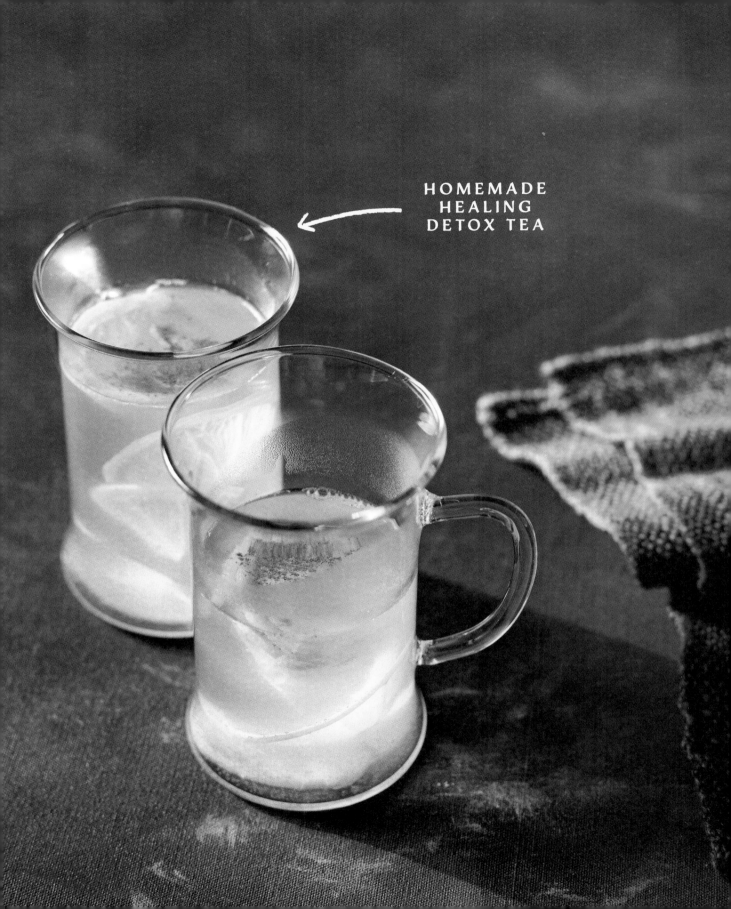

HOMEMADE
HEALING
DETOX TEA

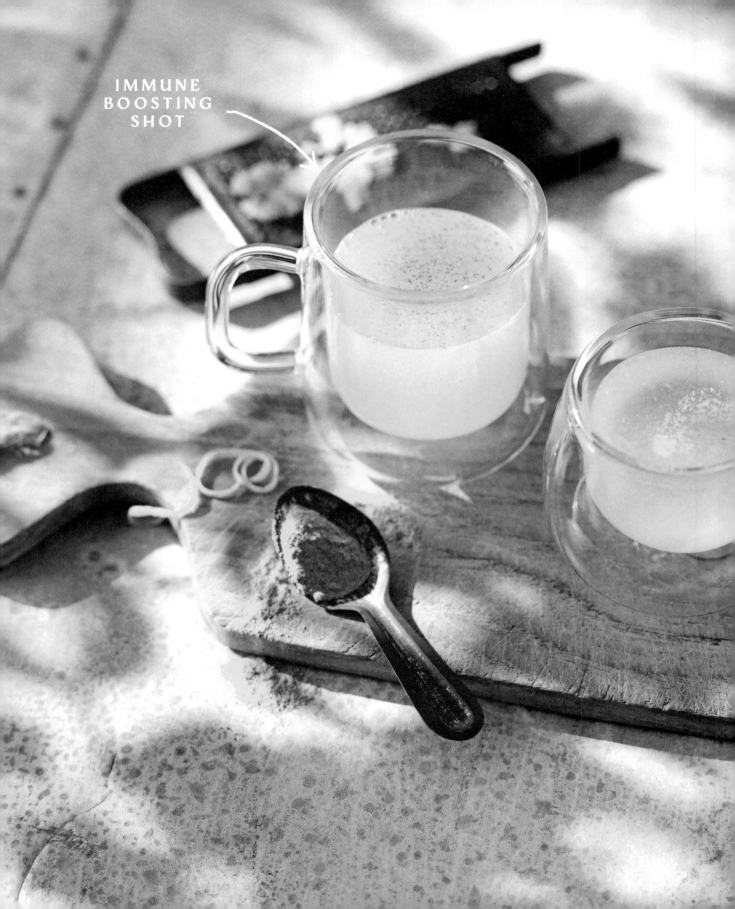

IMMUNE
BOOSTING
SHOT

## HANGOVER SHOT

*Make a big batch and drink it through the day – it will make you feel so good! If you like, store it in the fridge and drink it cool.*

SERVES 1
PREP TIME: 10 minutes

juice of ½ lemon
1 tablespoon apple cider vinegar
¼ teaspoon ground turmeric
1 teaspoon grated ginger
125 ml filtered water
finely grated lemon zest, for sprinkling (optional)

Place the lemon juice, vinegar, turmeric, ginger and water in a cup or mason jar. Mix well, sprinkle over some lemon zest (if using) and drink!

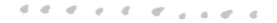

## DIGESTIVE SHOT

SERVES 1
PREP TIME: 10 minutes

juice of ½ lemon
1 teaspoon grated ginger
1 probiotic capsule or 1 teaspoon probiotic powder (be guided by your health practitioner)
1 teaspoon glutamine powder (optional)
1 tablespoon aloe vera juice
125 ml filtered water
½ teaspoon stevia granules (optional)

Place all the ingredients in a cup or mason jar. Mix well and drink!

## IMMUNE BOOSTING SHOT

SERVES 1
PREP TIME: 10 minutes

juice of ½ orange
a pinch of cayenne pepper
1 teaspoon grated ginger
¼ teaspoon ground turmeric
125 ml filtered water
1 teaspoon probiotic powder or 1 probiotic capsule (be guided by your health practitioner)
finely grated orange zest, for sprinkling (optional)

Place the orange juice, cayenne pepper, ginger, turmeric, water and probiotic powder in a cup or mason jar. Mix well, sprinkle over some orange zest (if using) and drink!

## TIP

*Glutamine powder can be found in most health-food shops.*

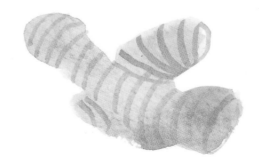

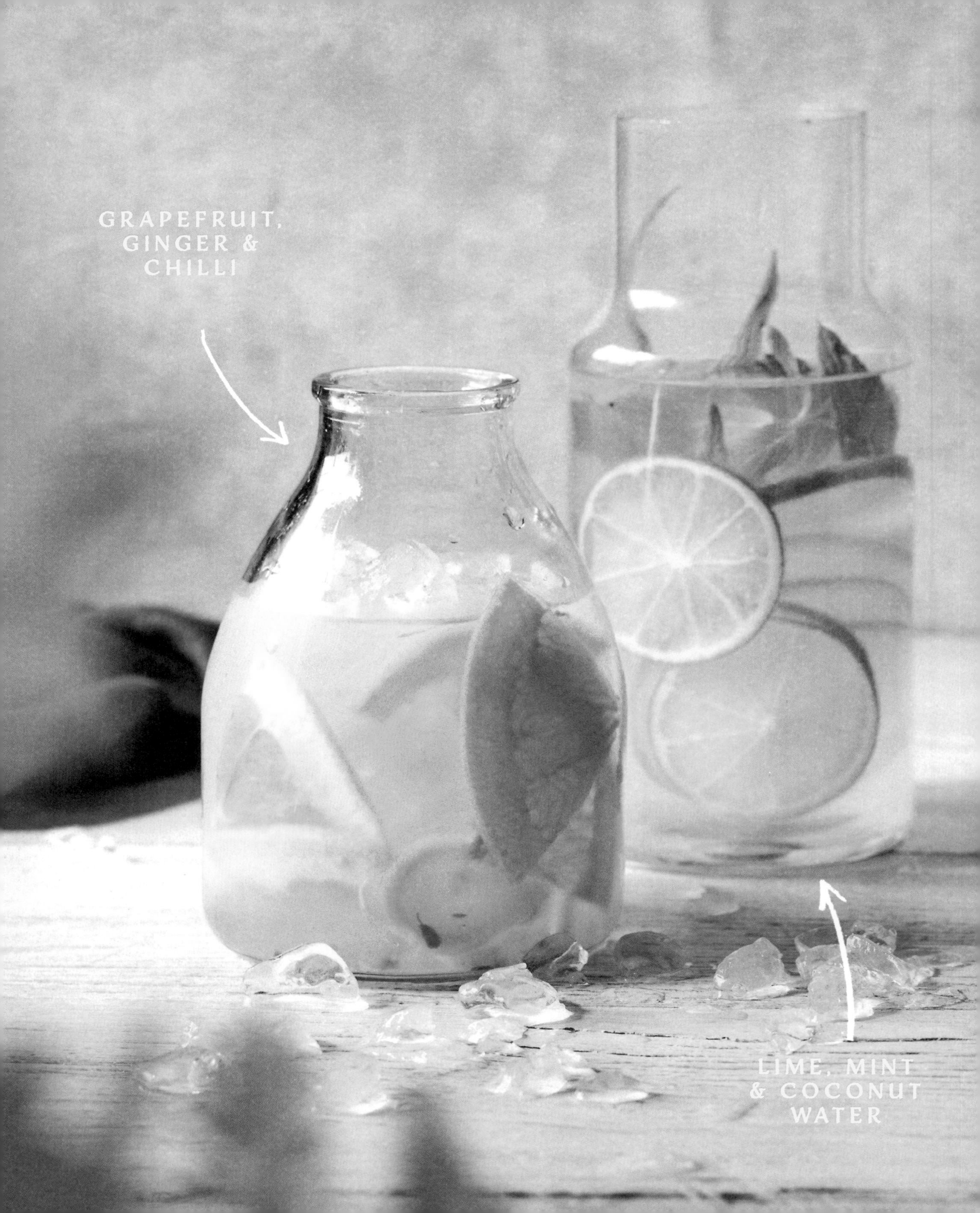

GRAPEFRUIT, GINGER & CHILLI

LIME, MINT & COCONUT WATER

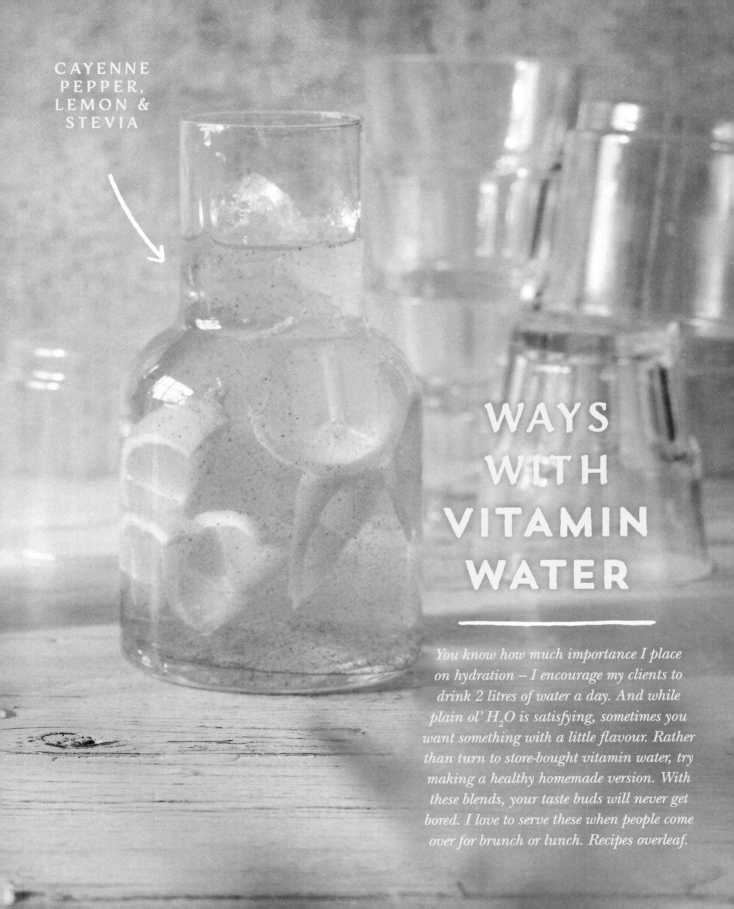

CAYENNE
PEPPER,
LEMON &
STEVIA

# WAYS WITH VITAMIN WATER

*You know how much importance I place on hydration – I encourage my clients to drink 2 litres of water a day. And while plain ol' $H_2O$ is satisfying, sometimes you want something with a little flavour. Rather than turn to store-bought vitamin water, try making a healthy homemade version. With these blends, your taste buds will never get bored. I love to serve these when people come over for brunch or lunch. Recipes overleaf.*

## GRAPEFRUIT, GINGER & CHILLI

1 large grapefruit, halved
and thinly sliced
1 teaspoon grated ginger
1 teaspoon chilli flakes,
or to taste
1 teaspoon stevia granules
750 ml filtered water or
coconut water

Place your choice of ingredients in a large serving jug, along with the filtered water or coconut water, and stir well. Don't feel like you need to add everything – just use whatever you've got. For people on the move, you can add these combos to mason jars.

## CAYENNE PEPPER, LEMON & STEVIA

1 lemon, sliced
½ teaspoon cayenne
pepper
1 teaspoon stevia
granules
750 ml filtered water

## LIME, MINT & COCONUT WATER

2 limes, sliced
a large handful of
mint leaves
750 ml coconut
water

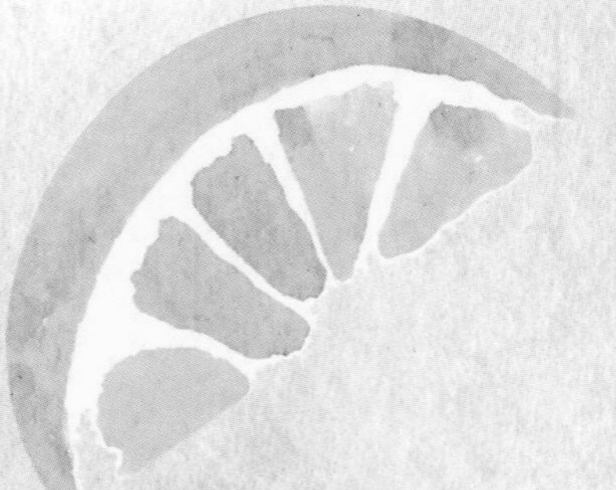

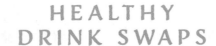

# HEALTHY
# DRINK SWAPS

**CHOCOLATE MILK:** Chocolate milk made with raw cacao powder and coconut milk or my Choc Cinnamon Milk (see page 298)

**STRAWBERRY MILK:** Coconut Strawberry Milk (see page 298)

**DIET SOFT DRINK:** Vitamin Water (see page 304) served with stevia granules to sweeten, or sparkling kombucha

**CHOC MILKSHAKE:** Bounty Smoothie (see page 146)

**SWEETENED PACKAGED JUICE:** Fresh veggie juice

**SPORTS DRINKS:** Electrolyte Elixir (see page 306)

**FRUIT JUICE:** Fresh coconut juice

## FIBRE DRINK – CONSTIPATION RELIEF!

SERVES 1
PREP TIME: 10 minutes

1 tablespoon psyllium husk
1 tablespoon chia seeds
juice of ½ lemon
1 teaspoon probiotic powder or 1 probiotic
  capsule (be guided by your health practitioner)
a few drops of stevia or 1 teaspoon stevia granules
250 ml filtered water

Place all the ingredients in a cup or mason jar.
Mix well and drink!

Make sure you drink plenty of water for the rest of
the day to avoid the fibre dehydrating your digestive
system. Try this before breakfast or after dinner.

## ELECTROLYTE ELIXIR – POST WORKOUT!

SERVES 1
PREP TIME: 10 minutes

juice of 1 lime
250 ml coconut water or the juice from 1 young
  fresh coconut
250 ml ice cubes
3–4 mint leaves
1 teaspoon stevia granules
a pinch of cayenne pepper

Put all the ingredients in your blender – and blend!

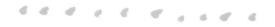

## SLIM-DOWN TONIC

SERVES 1
PREP TIME: 10 minutes

juice of ½ lemon
1 tablespoon apple cider vinegar
½ teaspoon grated ginger or a pinch or two of
  ground ginger
a pinch of ground cinnamon
a pinch of cayenne pepper
125 ml filtered water

Place all the ingredients in a cup or mason jar.
Mix well and drink!

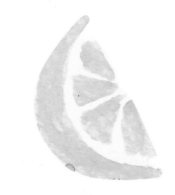

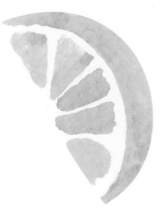

DIPS, DRESSINGS & DRINKS

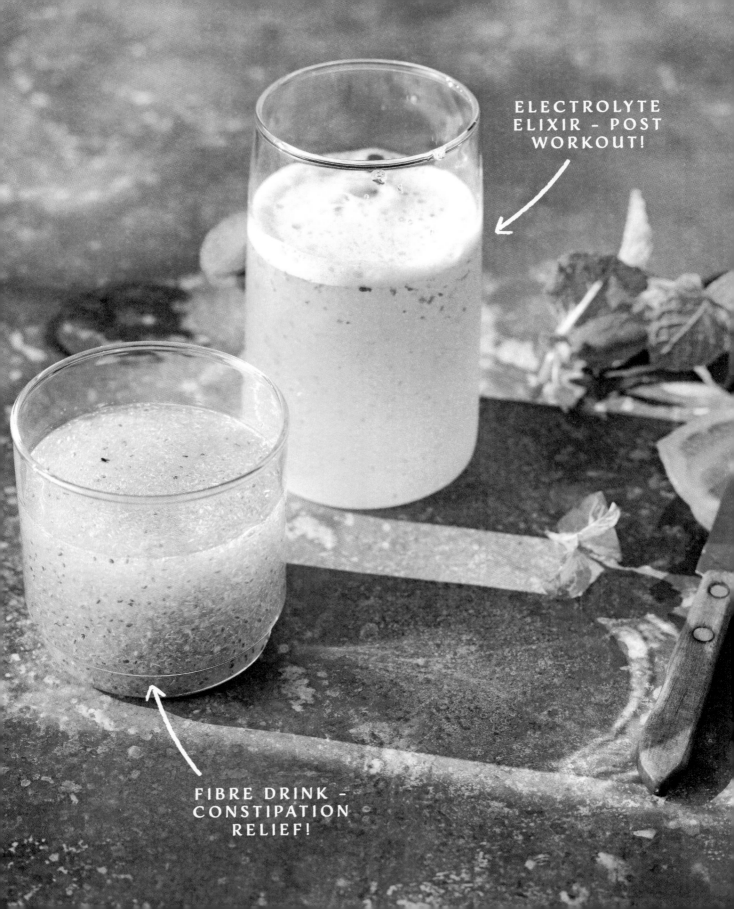

ELECTROLYTE ELIXIR - POST WORKOUT!

FIBRE DRINK - CONSTIPATION RELIEF!

# HEALTHY CHAI LATTE

*If you love a chai latte when you're at a café but you know it's full of sugar and preservatives, don't worry, I've got you! This is the cleanest and most delicious cup of chai you could ever imagine.*

SERVES 2
PREP TIME: 15 minutes

500 ml coconut milk
3 medjool dates, pitted
1 teaspoon ground cinnamon
a dash of grated nutmeg
a pinch of ground cardamom
4 cloves
2 vanilla pods, split and seeds scraped
70 g soaked raw cashews
vanilla stevia drops, to taste (optional)

Pour the coconut milk into a small saucepan.

Add the dates and spices and stir gently over medium heat until it's a little hotter than you like it. Set aside for 5 minutes to infuse.

Pour the mixture into a blender (strain out the cloves and vanilla pods if you like), add the cashews and stevia (if using) and blend until smooth and frothy.

# DANDY COFFEE

*Instead of reaching for that second or third cup of coffee, try dandy coffee. This glorious dandelion root herbal blend is like a miracle, and is readily available from grocery and health-food shops. It's a simple blend but it's full of vitamins, trace minerals and micronutrients. It also helps stimulate your digestive system, to improve the absorption of nutrients. It's a far healthier addiction than regular coffee! Remember that it's a little bitter so add sweetener to your taste.*

SERVES 1
PREP TIME: 10 minutes

1 heaped tablespoon dandelion coffee
125 ml boiling filtered water
125 ml almond milk, frothed with a milk frother
3–4 drops stevia
ground cinnamon, to taste

Infuse the dandelion coffee in the hot water for a few minutes, then strain.

Add the frothed almond milk, stevia and cinnamon to taste and you've got yourself a cosy cup.

# CINNAMON ALMOND MILK

*This nourishing drink is so easy to make, and it's a wonderful pick-me-up on a chilly day.*

SERVES 1
PREP TIME: 10 minutes

250 ml unsweetened vanilla almond milk
1 teaspoon ground cinnamon
½ teaspoon vanilla powder
a pinch of Celtic sea salt
a pinch of grated nutmeg (optional)
3–4 drops vanilla stevia or 1 teaspoon raw honey

Pour the almond milk into a small saucepan and add the remaining ingredients. Warm over medium–low heat, stirring occasionally, until it reaches the right temperature for you.

Pour the warm milk into a mug and enjoy!

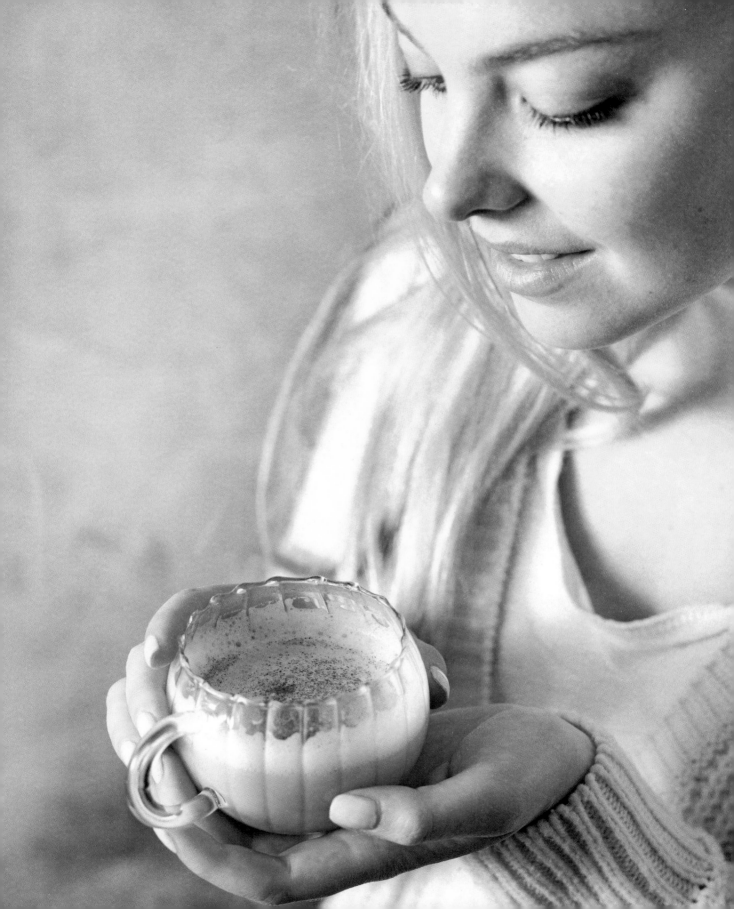

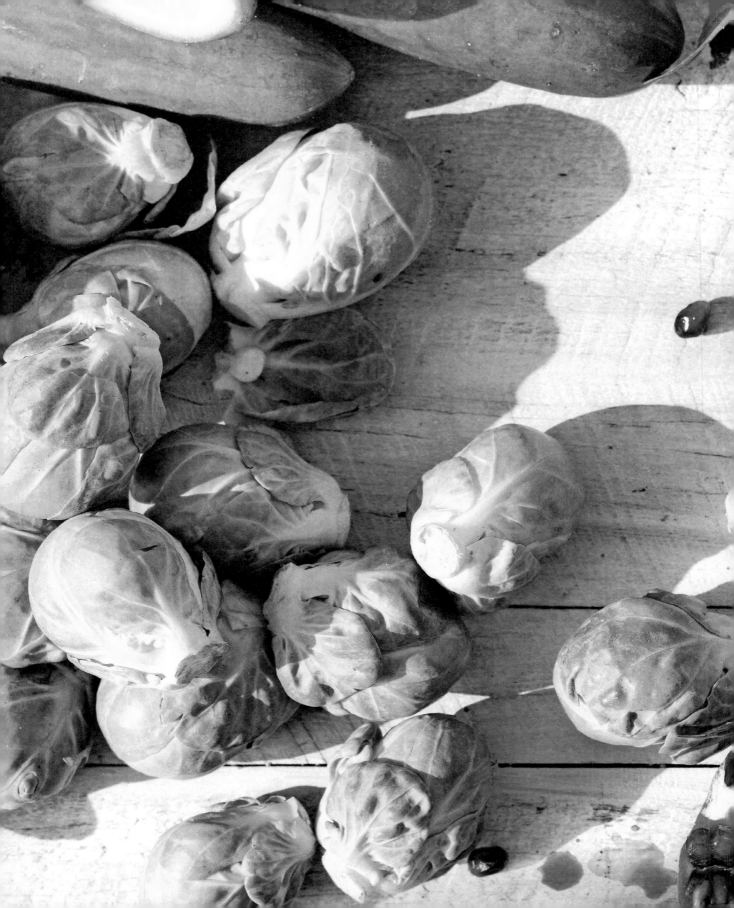

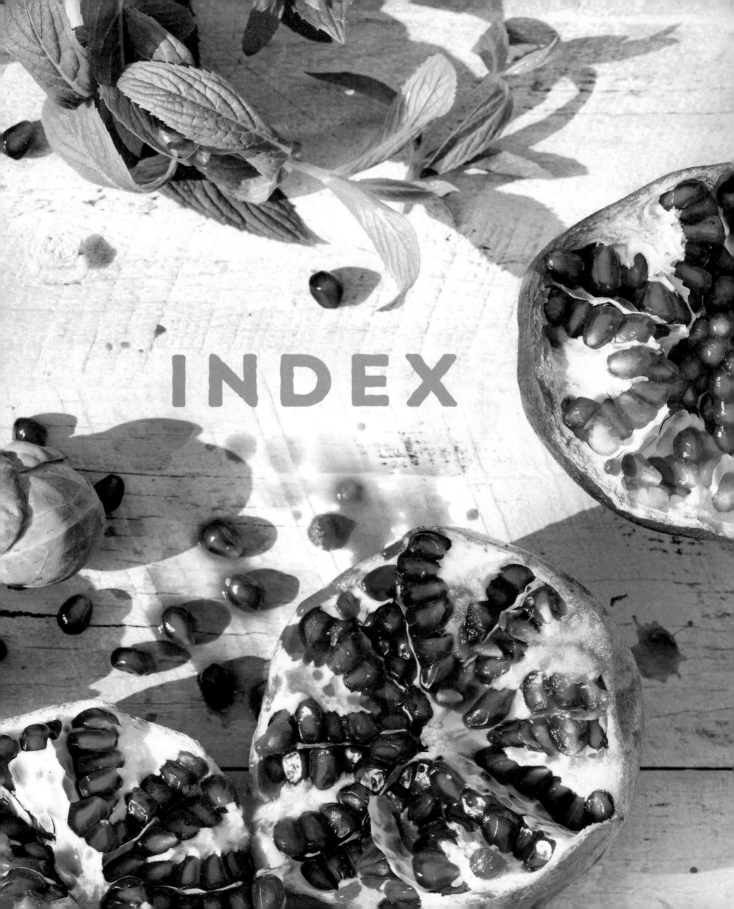

INDEX

# INDEX

## NUMBERS

3-day liver reboot 58–59
4 pm snack 17
8-week action plan 124–131
80/20 mindset 23

## A

acai bowl, peanut butter 136
adrenals
  energy and 48
  healing 44
  stress and 31–32
alcohol 114
almonds
  almond dream yoghurt 262
  almond-crusted kale chips
    257
  fried kale with 236
  maple & cardamom 251
almond milk
  choc cinnamon milk 298
  cinnamon almond milk 308
anxiety 85–89
apologising 26
apples
  apple crumble pancakes 172
  apple pie oats 152
artificial sweeteners 105
Asian greens 206
asparagus
  asparagus, avocado & almond
    salad 189
  avocado asparagus toast 160
  crispy halloumi with
    asparagus & hummus 205
  fish with baked asparagus 221
  sesame-coated 237

aubergine
  healing bruschetta 244
  miso aubergine 234
avocado asparagus toast 160

## B

bananas
  almond butter cinnamon
    halves 262
  baked with tahini caramel
    sauce 148
  banana & choc coconut
    crepes 173
  banana hazelnut chocolate
    bread 265
  chia, blueberry & banana
    breakfast muffins 143
  healing pancakes 172
  sticky banana & coconut
    granola 140
beauty seed bars 166
beef
  chilli & rosemary steak with
    sautéed greens 227
beetroot hummus, roasted
  290
berries
  berry breakfast crumble 175
  berry cocowhip 262
  berry ice-blocks 260
  chia, blueberry & banana
    breakfast muffins 143
bingeing 16–18
bircher muesli, cinnamon,
  cardamom & orange zest 148
bliss balls
  cacao sea salt truffles 268
  cookie dough balls 268

JSHealth sugar-free protein
  balls 269
Nutella 268
nut-free 269
tahini balls 269
bloating 56
body dysmorphia 19
bolognese with zoodles 212
bread
  avocado asparagus toast 160
  banana hazelnut chocolate
    265
  carrot & rosemary loaf 259
  fig & ricotta toast 160
  gluten-free green 156
  gluten-free rosemary &
    sesame focaccia 286
  mushroom, goat's cheese &
    thyme toast 160
  tahini, banana & granola
    toast 160
breakfast bars
  beauty seed 166
  choc tahini energy 166
  high-fibre 167
  for lunchboxes 167
breakfast brownies 162
breakfast cereal see also granola;
  oats
  cinnamon, cardamom &
    orange zest bircher muesli
    148
  paleo coconut, date &
    almond 136
breakfast crumble, berry 175
breakfast muffins, chia,
  blueberry & banana 143
breakfast salad, vegan 177

breathing, deep belly  34, 87
broccoli
  broccoli pizza  216
  garlic & chilli  236
  pesto chicken bowl with
    broccoli & pumpkin seeds
    184
brown rice bowl
  with sesame salmon,
    aubergine & tahini  184
  with smoked trout & avocado
    184
brownies, breakfast  162
brussels sprouts
  baked onion & tomato  247
  brussels sprout & caramelised
    onion salad  190
  crispy by Cayley  238
  lentils, cumin-spiced, with
    shaved  202
  shaved with pomegranate
    190

**C**

cacao sea salt truffles  268
candida  44, 57
caramel sauce  153
carbohydrates  100
career  81
carrots
  carrot & rosemary loaf  259
  cucumber & carrot salad with
    crunchy seeds  183
  high-protein carrot cake
    snack  252
  hummus  242
  sesame-coated chips  237
  za'atar carrot chip salad with
    cinnamon seeds  187
  za'atar carrot dip  290
cashews, rosemary chilli  270
cauliflower
  cauliflower, labneh & harissa
    salad  180
  cauliflower & Brazil nut soup
    192

cauliflower & walnut
  tabbouleh  189
cauliflower parmigiana  221
curried almond  243
harissa chicken with
  cauliflower steaks  211
sesame with crispy leeks  243
spiced on carrot hummus
  242
thai-style fried 'rice'  247
truffle purée  242
cayenne pepper, lemon & stevia
  water  304
cereal  see breakfast cereal
chai latte, healthy  308
cheese  103
cheesy chilli kale chips  257
chia, blueberry & banana
  breakfast muffins  143
chicken
  chicken & ginger stir-fry  210
  harissa with cauliflower steaks
    211
  healthy bbq  210
  moroccan skewers  210
  pesto chicken bowl with
    broccoli & pumpkin seeds
    184
  shredded san choy bau  224
chilli & lime guacamole  290
chilli & rosemary steak with
  sautéed greens  227
chilli kale chips  257
chocolate
  cacao sea salt truffles  268
  choc cinnamon milk  298
  choc cinnamon yoghurt  262
  choc date almond cookies
    272
  choc tahini energy bars  166
  chocolate almond coconut
    nice-cream  260
  chocolate bark, fig &
    pistachio  276
  chocolate skin-glow mousse
    270

salted chocolate & rosemary
  tarts  282
chop chop salad, energy  185
chop chop tuna salad  185
cinnamon scrolls  285
cleansing functions  52–59
Coco pops  162
coconut milk
  choc cinnamon milk  298
  coconut strawberry milk  298
  vanilla milk  298
coconut rough snack slice  272
coconut water  see vitamin water
coffee  61, 114–115
constipation  55–57
constipation relief fibre drink
  306
cookies
  breakfast cinnamon oat  155
  choc date almond  272
courgettes
  bolognese with zoodles  212
  courgette mushroom alfredo
    215
  tuna pasta bake  205
  za'atar courgette chips  240
crackers, rosemary chilli  251
crumble
  apple crumble pancakes  172
  berry breakfast  175
cucumber & carrot salad with
  crunchy seeds  183
cumin tahini dressing  233
curry
  curried almond cauliflower
    243
  veggie  218

**D**

daily routines  78–79
dairy foods  103
dairy substitutes  103
dandy coffee  308
dates
  choc date almond cookies  272
  paleo coconut, date &

almond cereal 136
detox soup 196
detox tea 298
dieting 20, 55, 86
digestive shot 301
digestive system 47, 53–57
dinner party ideas 201
dips
    chilli & lime guacamole 290
    roasted beetroot hummus 290
    spinach & almond 290
    za'atar carrot dip 290
dressings see also pesto; sauces; yoghurt
    cumin tahini 233
    green tahini 238, 296
    JSHealth clean life 297
    lemony tahini 297
    miso salad 297
    my aunty Jane's famous herb salad 296
    peanut sesame 297
    satay 293
    tomato 293
drink swaps 305

**E**

eating out 112
eating plans see meal plans
economy of healthy living 106
electrolyte elixir 306
emotional eating 15
energy 46–51
    adrenals and 48
    digestive system and 47
    factors affecting 48–49
    meal plans for 49, 50–51
    thyroid and 48
exercise 68, 80, 86

**F**

fats 99
fennel, sesame & leek roasted 244

fibre 104
fibre drink – constipation relief 306
figs
    caramelised with hazelnut crunch 279
    fig & pistachio chocolate bark 276
    fig & ricotta toast 160
fish see also salmon; tuna
    brown rice bowl with smoked trout & avocado 184
    fish with baked asparagus 221
    lemon herb fish in a bag 227
    tacos 225
focaccia, gluten-free rosemary & sesame 286
foods
    food philosophy 97
    healing nutrition 96–119
    to limit 107
    nourishing and grounding 161
    superfoods 107
food voice 13
fruit recommendations 102

**G**

garlic & chilli broccoli 236
garlic & mushroom san choy bau 224
gluten intolerance 100
gluten-free grains 100
gluten-free green bread 156
gluten-free rosemary & sesame focaccia 286
granola see also breakfast cereal
    chai-spiced paleo 141
    'no recipe' 140
    Nutella 141
    sticky banana & coconut 140
    tahini, banana & granola toast 160
grapefruit, ginger & chilli water 304

gratitude 28
green bread, gluten-free 156
green detox soup 196
green tahini dressing 296
guacamole, chilli & lime 290
guilt feelings 14
gut 53
    healing 44
    healing supplements 55
    inflammation and 68
    weight and 68

**H**

halloumi with asparagus & hummus 205
hangover shot 301
happiness 77
harissa chicken with cauliflower steaks 211
healing
    anxiety 84–89
    cleansing functions 52–59
    energy see energy
    lifestyle 76–83
    liver see liver
    nutrition 96–119
    relationship with food 10–23
    relationship with others 90–95
    relationship with self 24–29
    sleep 60–63
    stress see stress
    thyroid see thyroid
    weight battles see weight
herb, onion & cauliflower shakshuka 168
high-fibre bar 167
holding grudges 95
hormonal balance 69
    eating guide 70–71
    meal plan 72–73
    stress and 32
    vitamins for 69

## I

ice-blocks, berry  260
ice-cream
  healthy berry cocowhip  262
  chocolate almond coconut
    nice-cream  260
  mango chia  252
  tiramisu nice-cream  260
immune boosting shot  301
indulgence  23

## J

jetlag  81
JSHealth clean life dressing  297
JSHealth community  6–7
JSHealth eating formula  108
JSHealth smoothies  147
JSHealth sugar-free protein
 balls  269

## K

kale
  chips  256, 257
  fried with almonds  236
kiddie treats  274
kindness  95

## L

leeks
  sesame & leek roasted fennel
    244
  sesame cauliflower with crispy
    243
lemon & tahini yoghurt  228
lemon curd tart  280
lemon tahini kale chips  257
lemony tahini dressing  297
lentils, cumin-spiced, with
  shaved brussels sprouts  202
lettuce, iceberg lettuce wedge
  salad  180
lifestyle change  93
lifestyle healing  76–83
lime, mint & coconut water  304

liver  53
  3-day liver reboot  58–59
  healing  44, 58–59
  weight and  68
lunchbowls  184
lunchbox alternatives  167

## M

mango chia ice-cream  252
manifestation  82–83
maple & cardamom almonds
 251
meal plans
  8-week action plan  124–131
  daily eating guide  109
  energy  49, 50–51
  hormonal balance  72–73
  personalised  22
  thyroid  41, 42–43
  thyroid healing  44–45
  vegan/vegetarian  118–119
  week of nutritious eating
    110–111
medication  45
meditation  87
menstruating  32, 38
mercury chelation  45
milk  see almond milk; coconut
 milk
mindful eating  21
miso aubergine  234
miso salad dressing  297
mood  89
mousse, chocolate skin-glow
 270
movie-going foods  274
muffins, chia, blueberry &
 banana breakfast  143
mushrooms
  almond & herb-stuffed  234
  courgette mushroom alfredo
    215
  garlic & mushroom san choy
    bau  224
  mushroom, goat's cheese &
    thyme toast  160

  warm mushroom & ricotta
    salad  183
my aunty Jane's famous herb
  salad dressing  296

## N

natural eating  66
natural sweeteners  105
negativity  25–27
nervous system  32
Nutella bliss balls  268
Nutella granola  141
nut-free bliss balls  269
nut-free sunflower seed pesto  292
nutrients  98–100
nutrition  see foods
nuts and seeds  99

## O

oats
  apple pie  152
  breakfast cinnamon cookies
    155
  Mum's coconut & mango chia
    overnight  153
  oatmeal  152
  salted caramel  153

## P

paleo coconut, date & almond
  cereal  136
pancakes
  apple crumble  172
  banana & choc coconut
    crepes  173
  healing banana  172
parfait, vanilla, flaxseed, chia &
  banana  168
pasta, vegetable  see courgettes
peanut butter
  acai bowl  136
  vegan bars  276
peanut sesame dressing  297
pears, healing warm cinnamon
 279

peppers, tomato & red pepper soup 195
periods 32, 38
pesto
  nut-free sunflower seed 292
  pesto chicken bowl with broccoli & pumpkin seeds 184
  rocket & almond 292
pizza, broccoli 216
pomegranate, shaved brussels sprouts with 190
ponzu sesame salmon with Asian greens 206
portion sizes 108
pressure 25
probiotics 55
protein
  importance of 98
  replacements for vegans/ vegetarians 71
  types of 98
pumpkin, goat's cheese & avocado salad 177

**R**

red pepper, tomato & red pepper soup 195
reflux 56
regular bowel movements 56–57
relationship break-ups 94
relationships with others 90–95
ricotta, sweet baked rosemary 259
rocket & almond pesto 292
rosemary chilli cashews 270
rosemary chilli crackers 251
rushing 33

**S**

salads *see also* dressings
  asparagus, avocado & almond 189
  brussels sprout & caramelised onion 190
  cauliflower, labneh & harissa 180
  chop chop tuna 185
  cucumber & carrot with crunchy seeds 183
  energy chop chop 185
  iceberg lettuce wedge 180
  lunchbowls 184
  pumpkin, goat's cheese & avocado 177
  roasted vegetable & freekeh salad 233
  sweet potato with green tahini dressing 238
  vegan breakfast 177
  warm mushroom & ricotta 183
  za'atar carrot chip salad with cinnamon seeds 187
salmon
  brown rice bowl with sesame salmon, aubergine & tahini 184
  ponzu sesame salmon with Asian greens 206
  salmon & quinoa cakes with lemon & tahini yoghurt 228
  teriyaki salmon bowl 206
salted caramel oats 153
salted caramel smoothie 147
salted chocolate & rosemary tarts 282
san choy bau
  fish tacos 225
  garlic & mushroom 224
  shredded chicken 224
  tempeh 224
satay sauce 293
sauces
  caramel 153
  tahini caramel 148
scrolls, cinnamon 285
Sepel, Jessica [author] 6–7, 11–12, 39–41

sesame kale chips 257
shakshuka, herb, onion & cauliflower 168
shots 301
sleeping 61–63, 69
slim-down tonic 306
smoothies
  Bounty 146
  chai-spiced fig 147
  de-bloat green 146
  JSHealth 147
  salted caramel 147
  skin-glow 146
snack ideas 108, 274, 275
social media 88
social support 26
soups
  cauliflower & Brazil nut 192
  green detox 196
  tomato & red pepper 195
soy 103
spinach & almond dip 290
stillness 77
stress 31–35
  adrenals and 31–32
  hormones and 32
  impact 31
  rushing and 33
  stress-free eating 21
  weight and 33
stress-free zone 34
sugar 105
sugar cravings 105
sunflower seed pesto 292
supplements
  gut healing 55
  natural 87
  overuse 104
  for stress 33
  for thyroid conditions 45
sweet potato
  coconut & rosemary wedges 240
  sweet potato salad with green tahini dressing 238

# T

tabbouleh, cauliflower &
  walnut 189
tacos, fish 225
tahini
  green tahini 296
  lemony tahini dressing 297
  tahini balls 269
  tahini, banana & granola
    toast 160
  tahini caramel sauce 148
takeaway foods 113
tarts
  lemon curd 280
  salted chocolate & rosemary
    282
tea, detox 298
tempeh san choy bau 224
teriyaki salmon bowl 206
thai-style fried 'rice' 247
therapy 45, 85
thrush 57
thyroid 36–45
  energy and 48
  healing meal plan 44–45
  meal plan 41, 42–43
  protocol 44
  resources 39
  thyroid function 38
  treatment for conditions 38
  weight and 68
tiramisu nice-cream 260
tomatoes
  baked onion & tomato
    brussels sprouts 247
  sauce 293
  tomato & red pepper soup
    195
toxic friendships 92
trans fats 99
travel snack ideas 274
travelling 81–82
trout, brown rice bowl with

smoked trout & avocado 184
tuna
  chop chop tuna salad 185
  tuna pasta bake 205

# V

vanilla, flaxseed, chia &
  banana parfait 168
vanilla milk 298
vegan breakfast salad 177
vegan diets 116
vegan meal ideas 215
vegan/vegetarian meal plan
  118–119
vegan peanut butter bars 276
vegan snack ideas 275
vegetables
  recommended 101
  roasted & freekeh salad 233
  vegetable pasta see
    courgettes
  veggie curry 218
visualisation 82–83
vitamin water
  cayenne pepper, lemon &
    stevia 304
  grapefruit, ginger & chilli
    304
  lime, mint & coconut 304
vitamins
  for energy 48
  for hormonal balancing 69

# W

water 104
weight 64–74
  calorie counting 66
  eating to manage 67
  family and 16
  gain 74
  goals 65
  obsession with 14
  stress and 33

weight scales 12–13
'what ifs' 26
whey 98
working out see exercise

# Y

yoga 62–63, 86–87
yoghurt
  almond dream 262
  choc cinnamon 262
  lemon & tahini 228
  recommendations 103
  yoghurt lemon dressing 296

# Z

za'atar carrot dip 290
za'atar courgette chips 240

# ACKNOWLEDGEMENTS

*This book could only have happened with the love and support I have received from incredible people in my life. A very heartfelt thank you to:*

Dean, my darling partner. Thank you for your unconditional support during my writing of this book while we were living in Los Angeles. I will always treasure that time of our lives. Thank you for believing in me. Thank you for dreaming big with me. You are no doubt my biggest fan. I love you.

Nicky, my gorgeous mother and my biggest cooking inspiration. Thank you for teaching me what it means to eat with balance. You have taught me the essence of a healthy life. I will forever feel grateful for all those moments in the kitchen where I have watched you whip up a wholesome meal from the simple produce in the fridge. You really taught me how to cook – how can I thank you enough?

Glenn, my father. Thank you for your ongoing love and support. You are so kind with how you go around telling everyone you meet about my work. It means so much to me. You are the most incredible role model. I really value your business advice. You have such wisdom. Thank you for everything.

Gabriella and Olivia, my beautiful sisters. I am so lucky to be able to call you family. Thank you for the constant love, support and encouragement. I'm proud of you both, and that will never change. I can't wait to see what you have in store for the world.

My mother- and father-in-law, Noreen and Colin Steingold. Thank you for your unconditional love and support and of course your legal advice.

Ingrid Ohlsson, my publisher. It was the biggest compliment when you asked me to start writing a second book – because you so believe in my message. And I can't thank you enough for that. Thank you for your constant support, encouragement and dedication to making another beautiful book come to life. I have such admiration for you, both personally and professionally. Your hard work and impeccable taste is just so impressive.

Danielle Walker, my editor. I am constantly blown away by your hard work and dedication to producing such high class work. TLC comes through in everything you do. It has been such a pleasure going through another labour of love with you. Thank you for being so kind and patient during this process.

Charlotte Ree, my publicist. It is because of your faith that I could make this dream happen. You believed in me from the get-go. You are a true superstar in every sense. Thank you so much for your constant care and guidance.

Katia Lervasi, JSHealth editor. Thank you for all these years of brilliant work. You just get me and my message. I have loved working with you on all these projects. Thank you for your hard work.

Olivia Templeman, JSHealth CEO. Nothing would be possible without you. You have built JSHealth into something that I couldn't have dreamt of (and I can dream big!). Your intelligence, hard work, kindness, loyalty and business sense acumen blows Dean and me away every day. We have so much respect for you both professionally and personally. Thank you for taking care of everything while I had to sit down to write this book.

Sarah Frish, my digital content editor, and Isabelle Cleaver, my events and marketing coordinator. I am so grateful for both of you. You care so much about the brand and its message. You produce such high quality work, every time. I feel very lucky to work with you every day. Thank you for having my back during the process of putting this book together.

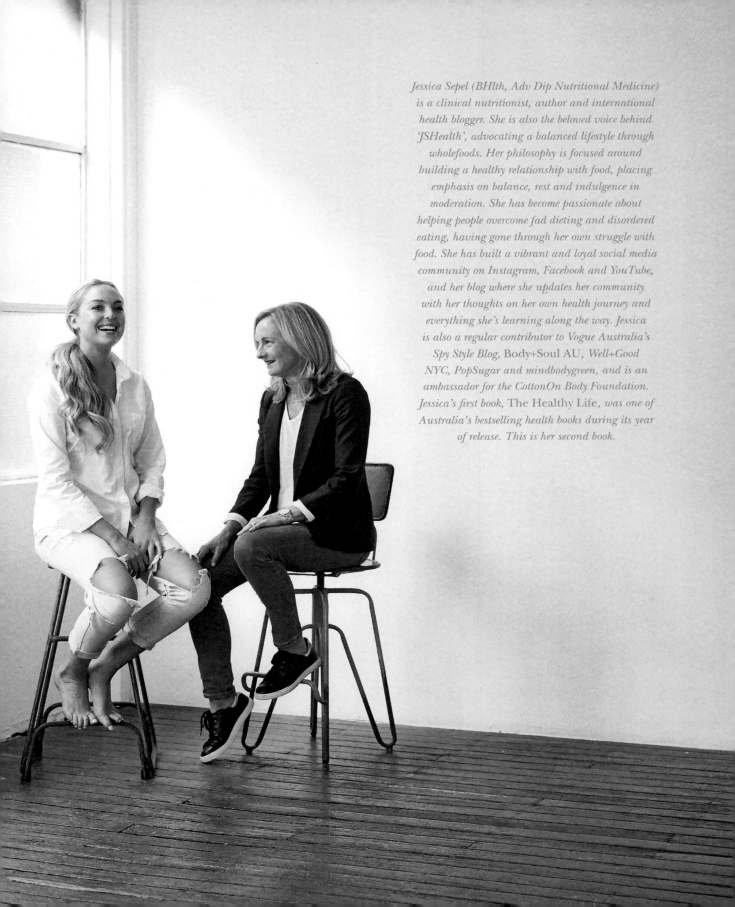

Jessica Sepel (BHlth, Adv Dip Nutritional Medicine) is a clinical nutritionist, author and international health blogger. She is also the beloved voice behind 'JSHealth', advocating a balanced lifestyle through wholefoods. Her philosophy is focused around building a healthy relationship with food, placing emphasis on balance, rest and indulgence in moderation. She has become passionate about helping people overcome fad dieting and disordered eating, having gone through her own struggle with food. She has built a vibrant and loyal social media community on Instagram, Facebook and YouTube, and her blog where she updates her community with her thoughts on her own health journey and everything she's learning along the way. Jessica is also a regular contributor to Vogue Australia's Spy Style Blog, Body+Soul AU, Well+Good NYC, PopSugar and mindbodygreen, and is an ambassador for the CottonOn Body Foundation. Jessica's first book, The Healthy Life, was one of Australia's bestselling health books during its year of release. This is her second book.

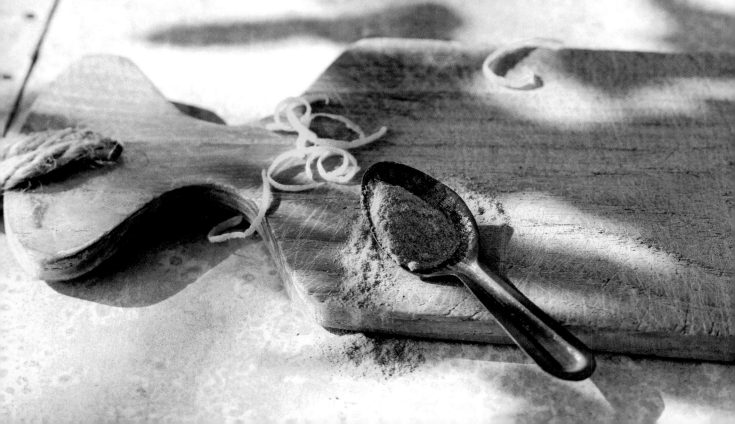

First published 2017 by Pan Macmillan Australia Pty Limited

This edition first published in the UK 2017 by Bluebird
an imprint of Pan Macmillan
20 New Wharf Road, London N1 9RR
Associated companies throughout the world
www.panmacmillan.com

ISBN 978-1-5098-2837-1

9 8 7 6 5 4 3 2 1

A CIP catalogue record for this book is available from the
British Library.

Design and illustrations by Arielle Gamble
Typeset by Kirby Jones
Editing by Samantha Sainsbury
Recipe editing by Rachel Carter

Prop and food styling by Bernadette Smithies
Styling on pages 134–35, 144–45, 178–79, 198–99,
230–31 and 288–89 by Michelle Noerianto
Jessica's styling by Gabriella Sepel
Food preparation and recipe testing by Sarah Mayoh

Colour and reproduction by Splitting Image
Colour Studio, Clayton, Victoria
Printed and bound by 1010 Printing
International Pty Ltd